Tumors
of the
Heart and Great Vessels

Atlas
of
Tumor Pathology

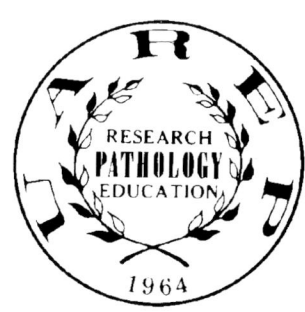

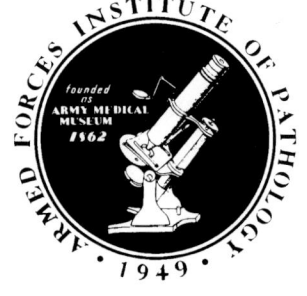

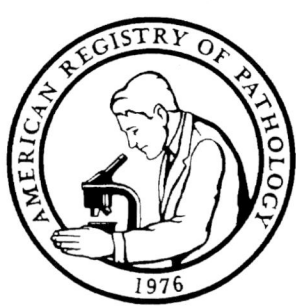

ATLAS OF TUMOR PATHOLOGY

Third Series
Fascicle 16

TUMORS OF THE HEART AND GREAT VESSELS

by

ALLEN BURKE, M.D.
Department of Cardiovascular Pathology
Armed Forces Institute of Pathology
Washington, D.C.

RENU VIRMANI, M.D.
Chair, Department of Cardiovascular Pathology
Armed Forces Institute of Pathology
Washington, D.C.

Published by the
ARMED FORCES INSTITUTE OF PATHOLOGY
Washington, D.C.

Under the Auspices of
UNIVERSITIES ASSOCIATED FOR RESEARCH AND EDUCATION IN PATHOLOGY, INC.
Bethesda, Maryland
1996

Accepted for Publication
1995

Available from the American Registry of Pathology
Armed Forces Institute of Pathology
Washington, D.C. 20306-6000
ISSN 0160-6344
ISBN 1-881041-20-4

ATLAS OF TUMOR PATHOLOGY

EDITOR
JUAN ROSAI, M.D.
Department of Pathology
Memorial Sloan-Kettering Cancer Center
New York, New York 10021-6007

ASSOCIATE EDITOR
LESLIE H. SOBIN, M.D.
Armed Forces Institute of Pathology
Washington, D.C. 20306-6000

EDITORIAL ADVISORY BOARD

EDITORS' NOTE

The Atlas of Tumor Pathology has a long and distinguished history. It was first conceived at a Cancer Research Meeting held in St. Louis in September 1947 as an attempt to standardize the nomenclature of neoplastic diseases. The first series was sponsored by the National Academy of Sciences-National Research Council. The organization of this Sisyphean effort was entrusted to the Subcommittee on Oncology of the Committee on Pathology, and Dr. Arthur Purdy Stout was the first editor-in-chief. Many of the illustrations were provided by the Medical Illustration Service of the Armed Forces Institute of Pathology, the type was set by the Government Printing Office, and the final printing was done at the Armed Forces Institute of Pathology (hence the colloquial appellation "AFIP Fascicles"). The American Registry of Pathology purchased the Fascicles from the Government Printing Office and sold them virtually at cost. Over a period of 20 years, approximately 15,000 copies each of nearly 40 Fascicles were produced. The worldwide impact that these publications have had over the years has largely surpassed the original goal. They quickly became among the most influential publications on tumor pathology ever written, primarily because of their overall high quality but also because their low cost made them easily accessible to pathologists and other students of oncology the world over.

Upon completion of the first series, the National Academy of Sciences-National Research Council handed further pursuit of the project over to the newly created Universities Associated for Research and Education in Pathology (UAREP). A second series was started, generously supported by grants from the AFIP, the National Cancer Institute, and the American Cancer Society. Dr. Harlan I. Firminger became the editor-in-chief and was succeeded by Dr. William H. Hartmann. The second series Fascicles were produced as bound volumes instead of loose leaflets. They featured a more comprehensive coverage of the subjects, to the extent that the Fascicles could no longer be regarded as "atlases" but rather as monographs describing and illustrating in detail the tumors and tumor-like conditions of the various organs and systems.

Once the second series was completed, with a success that matched that of the first, UAREP and AFIP decided to embark on a third series. A new editor-in-chief and an associate editor were selected, and a distinguished editorial board was appointed. The mandate for the third series remains the same as for the previous ones, i.e., to oversee the production of an eminently practical publication with surgical pathologists as its primary audience, but also aimed at other workers in oncology. The main purposes of this series are to promote a consistent, unified, and biologically sound nomenclature; to guide the surgical pathologist in the diagnosis of the various tumors and tumor-like lesions; and to provide relevant histogenetic, pathogenetic, and clinicopathologic information on these entities. Just as the second series included data obtained from ultrastructural (and, in the more recent Fascicles, immunohistochemical) examination, the third series will, in addition, incorporate pertinent information obtained with the newer molecular biology techniques. As in the past, a continuous attempt will be made to correlate, whenever possible, the nomenclature used in the Fascicles with that proposed by the World Health Organization's International Histological Classification of Tumors. The format of the third series has been changed in order to incorporate additional items and to ensure a consistency of style throughout. Close cooperation between the various authors and their respective liaisons from the editorial board will be emphasized to minimize unnecessary repetition and discrepancies in the text and illustrations.

To its everlasting credit, the participation and commitment of the AFIP to this venture is even more substantial and encompassing than in previous series. It now extends to virtually all scientific, technical, and financial aspects of the production.

The task confronting the organizations and individuals involved in the third series is even more daunting than in the preceding efforts because of the ever-increasing complexity of the matter at hand. It is hoped that this combined effort—of which, needless to say, that represented by the authors is first and foremost—will result in a series worthy of its two illustrious predecessors and will be a suitable introduction to the tumor pathology of the twenty-first century.

Juan Rosai, M.D.
Leslie H. Sobin, M.D.

ACKNOWLEDGMENTS

The illustrations in this Fascicle are possible only because of the many practicing pathologists who have sent cases to the Armed Forces Institute of Pathology (AFIP) over the years. By publishing this Fascicle, we hope to share the case repository of the AFIP with pathologists throughout the world. We are especially grateful for the submitted gross illustrations of cardiac tumors which we have taken the liberty to use in this publication.

The microscopic illustrations, and most of the gross illustrations, were photographed here at the AFIP. We acknowledge the support of Mr. George Jones and his colleagues for the high quality representations of histologic sections, the Institute as a whole for its photographic support, and Kenneth Stringfellow, who performed the color separations and image scanning.

We would like to acknowledge the many pathologists who have shaped our understanding of cardiac tumor pathology and have provided the foundation for the knowledge we have today. This Fascicle would not be possible without the work of Hugh McAllister, former chairman of cardiovascular pathology at the AFIP, and the late John J. Fenoglio Jr., co-authors of the previous Fascicle on tumors of the cardiovascular system. We would like to thank Dr. McAllister and Dr. William C. Roberts for their monumental contributions to the development of cardiac pathology as a subspecialty. Drs. Leslie Sobin and Franz Enzinger contributed greatly to our understanding of the classification and diagnosis of benign and malignant neoplasms.

Finally, we would like to thank several people who have spent long hours reading and editing the manuscript. These include Dr. Mark Brown; the editors provided by the advisory board; and Dian Thomas, Audrey Kahn, and Andrew Male of the editorial office.

Allen Burke, M.D.
Renu Virmani, M.D.

Permission to use copyrighted illustrations has been granted by:

American Medical Association:
  Arch Pathol Lab Med 1990;114:1057–62. For figures 11-13, 11-14, and 11-15.

Elsevier Science Publishing:
  Ann Thorac Surg 1991;52:1127-31. For figures 4-1 and 4-2.
  J Am Coll Cardiol 1993;22:226–38. For figure 8-1.

Excerpta Medica:
  Am J Cardiol 1976;38:241–51. For figure 5-2.

Field & Wood:
  Am J Cardiovasc Pathol 1990;3:283–90. For figures 7-9 and 7-10.

JB Lippincott:
  Am J Clin Pathol 1993;100:671–80. For figures 3-14, 3-15, 3-21, 3-26, 3-31, 3-32.
  Cancer 1992;69:387–95. For figure 12-7.
  Cancer 1993;71:1761–73. For figure 16-7.

Mosby-Year Book, Inc.:
  Am Heart J 1988;116:1105–7. For figures 12-59 and 12-60.
  J Thorac Cardiovasc Surg 1994;108:862–70. For figure 2-6.
  Current Problems in Cardiology 1992:80–137. For Table 2-1.

Raven Press:
  Am J Surg Pathol 1985;9:890–7. For figures 16-2 and 16-3.

Williams & Wilkins:
  Mod Pathol 1991;4:70–4. For figures 5-5 and 5-7.
  Moss' Heart Disease in Infants, Children, and Adolescents. 4th ed. 1983:5. For figure 1-1.

TUMORS OF THE HEART AND GREAT VESSELS

Contents

TUMORS OF THE HEART AND GREAT VESSELS

1
CLASSIFICATION AND INCIDENCE OF CARDIAC TUMORS

Historical Background

It has been at least 150 years since a primary tumor of the heart was first described. Although the date of initial postmortem documentation is debated, several early milestones are historically important: in 1835, Albers described a cardiac tumor that was most likely a primary cardiac fibroma; one decade later, King illustrated the first left atrial myxoma; von Recklinghausen described a cardiac rhabdomyoma in 1862; and Bodenheimer reported a primary cardiac sarcoma in 1865, by which time four major primary cardiac tumors, both benign and malignant, were recognized (30).

Although primary cardiac tumors were described over a century ago, their clinical diagnosis is a relatively recent phenomenon. One of the first major English language reviews of cardiac tumors was that of Prichard in 1951 (22), who wrote, "surgical treatment of these neoplasms is virtually unheard of...and the [antemortem] diagnosis of cardiac tumors is either impossible or a matter of chance." Within a year of this pronouncement, Goldberg et al. (9) diagnosed the first cardiac myxoma premortem; Crafoord (7) successfully resected a cardiac myxoma in 1954. In the ensuing decades, increasing surgical resections of benign and malignant primary cardiac tumors, including metastatic lesions, have mirrored the advances in cardiac catheterization, echocardiography, and surgery.

In barely 40 years, cardiac tumors of the heart evolved from a medical curiosity to a small but diverse field of medicine. Clinicians now recognize dozens of cardiac tumor types, and virtually all major technologic advances in imaging, surgery, and pathology are now employed in their diagnosis and treatment.

Embryology of the Heart and Cardiac Tumor Classification

The cardiac embryology that affects the histogenesis and classification of some cardiac neoplasms is discussed briefly. For a more detailed review of cardiac embryology, the reader is referred to a succinct review by Clark and von Mierop (6).

At about 15 days after fertilization, a crescentic zone of thickened mesoderm, the precursor of the heart and pericardium, appears adjacent to the margin of the embryonic disk. A day or two later, this thickened zone of mesoderm splits into somatic and splanchnic layers, which surround the pericardial portion of the coelomic cavity forming the pericardial coelom. Cardiac primordia form as paired lateral structures from the splanchnic mesodermal layer of the primitive pericardial cavity where it lies against the developing foregut (fig. 1-1). The mesodermal cardiogenic plate originally lies between the ectoderm of the neural plate and the endoderm of the foregut. With formation of the head and closure of the foregut from the yolk sac, the foregut swings into position between the primitive heart and neural groove.

By 2 1/2 weeks, the bilateral cardiac primordia fuse in the midline, and the heart is suspended as a double-walled tube supported dorsally by mesocardium. By 22 days, in an 8-somite embryo, the lateral endocardial tubes have fused in the midline, and the cardiac primordium is in proximity to the foregut only in a narrow dorsal portion adjacent to the dorsal mesocardium.

The early heart tube is formed by three layers: the endocardial layer, intervening cardiac "jelly," and a mesothelial layer lining the pericardial coelom. These three layers are formed very early in development, in the presomite stage, at approximately 18 days. Eventually, cardiac muscle cells arise adjacent to the mesothelial layer,

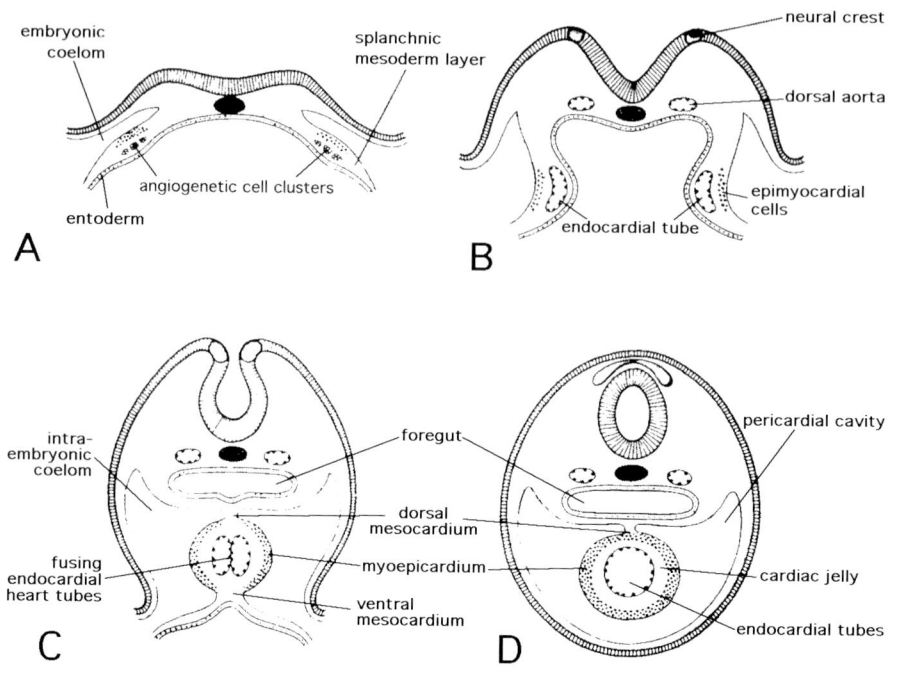

Figure 1-1
EARLY CARDIAC DEVELOPMENT

A: The heart develops from angiogenetic cell clusters situated laterally between the entoderm and ectoderm (17 days).

B: At approximately 18 days, these cell clusters differentiate into epimyocardial cells adjacent to the mesothelial-lined coelom (which later becomes the pericardial sac) and endocardial cells adjacent to the entoderm (later forming the foregut).

C: At about 21 days, the endocardial tubes fuse in the midline, and the proximity between the foregut and heart is restricted dorsally to the area of the dorsal mesocardium.

D: After fusion of the heart tubes (22 days), the three layers of the heart are now circumferentially developed. These are, from outward to center, the myoepicardium (lined externally by mesothelial cells), the cardiac jelly, and the endocardial layer. (Fig. 1.8 from Clark EB, Mierop LH. Development of the cardiovascular system. In: Adams FH, Emmanouilides GC, Riemenschneider TA, eds., Moss' heart disease in infants, children and adolescents, 4th ed., Baltimore: Williams & Wilkins, 1983.)

forming the epimyocardium. Primitive cardiac myocytes acquire myofibrils and a longitudinal orientation in embryos that are 5 to 9 mm in length. Cross striations are present when the embryo reaches 4.5 cm. During this time, endocardial cushion tissue or primitive plastic connective tissue begins to invade the cardiac jelly lying between the endodermal and mesothelial layers. In the second month of development, the atrial and ventricular septa begin to form. Cushion tissue begins to project into the primitive cardiac ventricles in the 8- to 9-mm embryo, with completed valve development by 12 to 14 weeks.

It follows from this brief overview that the heart and pericardium are derived entirely from mesodermal structures. All primary tumors of the heart and pericardium are of mesodermal origin, with two general exceptions: tumors of

misplaced endodermal rests and neural tumors, which are of ectodermal origin. Neural tumors of the heart are rare and are virtually limited to paragangliomas and granular cell tumors of the epicardial surfaces and atria.

Cardiac proliferation with endodermal elements, such as glandular structures present in bronchogenic cysts and tumors of the atrioventricular (AV) node, are presumed to arise from embryologically misplaced tissues. Theoretically, endodermal structures could be incorporated into cardiac tissue early in embryogenesis, when the foregut is adjacent to the laterally placed cardiogenic plates. With elongation and bending of the cardiac tube, which begins at 2 1/2 weeks, the endocardium and foregut are no longer in proximity, suggesting that incorporation of misplaced endodermal tissues occurs prior to this time.

The histogenesis of cardiac myxoma is particularly controversial (see chapter 3). The cardiac jelly, which supports the epimyocardial and endothelial layers, is present before 2 weeks (4-somite embryo), and becomes infiltrated from the endothelial surface by endocardial cushion cells. These cells are the putative cells of origin of cardiac myxoma, and are believed to persist in some adults near the fossa ovalis. Because of its origin in the primitive endocardium, myxoma may loosely be considered a neoplasm of vascular origin. The rare occurrence of glandular structures within cardiac myxoma should not be mistaken for adenocarcinoma. It is difficult to satisfactorily explain their presence from an embryologic point of view. Because glandular structures in cardiac myxomas appear to arise within cardiac myxoma cells, it is unlikely that they are endodermal rests accidentally caught within the cardiac myxoma. It is hypothesized that cardiac myxoma is a true neoplasm of pluripotential mesodermal cells (endocardial cushion cells). This neoplastic alteration is apparently capable of inciting these cells, which are of mesodermal origin, to form mucin-producing glands.

These embryologic principles help explain the histogenesis of cardiac myxoma and heterotopic cardiac tissues, such as AV nodal tumors. The histogenesis of individual cardiac tumors is further discussed with the pathologic features of each tumor in ensuing chapters.

Methods of Classification

There is no standard classification of cardiac tumors. Mahaim (12), in his monumental treatise on the subject, divided cardiac tumors into "polyps" (largely myxomas) and "tumors." Such a simplified division is clearly not useful today. In a classification by Heath in 1968 (10), the major entities were simply listed, largely in order of incidence. In the second series Fascicle on cardiac tumors (13), and in a recent review from the University of Minnesota (17), the tumors were separated into benign and malignant, but no systematic attempt was made to further categorize them.

Tumors may be classified either on the basis of cellular organization (reactive proliferations, hamartomas, cysts, benign neoplasms, malignant neoplasms) or tissue type (mesenchymal, epithelial, serosal). Classification of cardiac tumors by cellular organization is problematic,

especially for benign conditions. The nature of the more common primary cardiac tumors is unclear. Although most authorities believe that myxoma is a benign neoplasm, the theory that it is organized thrombi refuses to die. Whether papillary fibroelastomas are exaggerated Lambl excrescences or a form of hamartoma is not resolved. Lipomatous hypertrophy of the interatrial septum may be a metabolic disturbance related to obesity, or a true hamartoma. Although rhabdomyoma is universally considered hamartoma, such is not the case for fibroma, even though both are benign congenital lesions of single cell type associated with inherited syndromes.

The cell of origin of several primary cardiac tumors is unknown; classification of cardiac tumors by tissue type is, therefore, difficult. There is ongoing debate as to the nature of the "myxoma cell," with suggested derivations including endothelial, epithelial, neural, or primitive mesenchymal. A large number of primary cardiac sarcomas are likewise "undifferentiated": that is, the malignant mesenchymal cells do not show ultrastructural or immunohistochemical evidence of a particular connective tissue cell.

Classification of cardiac tumors is difficult partly because they are not analogous to extracardiac soft tissue tumors, which have been relatively well characterized. Several of the entities already mentioned, such as myxoma, papillary fibroelastoma, lipomatous hypertrophy, and rhabdomyoma, either have no identical extracardiac counterparts or are histologically distinct from noncardiac lesions of similar name.

In this Fascicle, cardiac tumors are classified as benign or malignant because of historic precedent in virtually all reported pathologic and clinical series (Table 1-1). Benign lesions are classified by cellular differentiation, and include tumors of fibrous, muscle, nerve, fat, mesothelial, and ectopic cells. Malignant tumors are classified by tissue type, namely, mesenchymal (sarcomas), metastatic, lymphoid, and mesothelial tissues. Myxoma and papillary fibroelastoma, which do not fit in any of these categories, are discussed separately.

Tumors of the pericardium are discussed by tissue type, together with cardiac tumors of similar cellular differentiation. Pericardial tumors and cysts of mesothelial derivation are discussed with benign and malignant mesothelial tumors

Table 1-1

CLASSIFICATION OF TUMORS OF THE HEART, PERICARDIUM, AND GREAT VESSELS

Benign Cardiac Tumors

Tumors of unknown histogenesis
  Myxoma
  Papillary fibroelastoma

Tumors of cardiac muscle
  Rhabdomyoma
  Histiocytoid cardiomyopathy (Purkinje cell
    hamartoma)
  Miscellaneous hamartomas

Tumors of fibrous tissue
  Fibroma
  Solitary fibrous tumor of pericardium
  Benign fibrous histiocytoma
  Inflammatory pseudotumor

Vascular tumors and tumor-like lesions
  Varix
  Hemangioma
  Hemangioendothelioma
  Hemangiopericytoma
  Lymphangioma

Tumors and proliferations of fat
  Lipomatous hypertrophy, interatrial septum
  Lipomatous hamartomas of cardiac valves
  Lipoma
  The fatty heart

Tumors and tumor-like lesions of mesothelial cells
  Mesothelial cysts
  Mesothelial/monocytic incidental cardiac
    excrescences
  Mesothelial papilloma

Tumors of neural tissue
  Granular cell tumor
  Schwannoma/neurofibroma
  Paraganglioma

Tumors of smooth muscle
  Leiomyoma
  Intravascular leiomyomatosis

Heterotopias and tumors of ectopic tissue
  Bronchogenic/foregut cysts
  Tumors of the atrioventricular nodal region
  Teratoma
  Ectopic thyroid
  Intrapericardial thymoma

Malignant Cardiac Tumors

Sarcomas
  Angiosarcoma
  Malignant fibrous histiocytoma
  Unclassified sarcoma
  Myxosarcoma
  Fibrosarcoma
  Leiomyosarcoma
  Rhabdomyosarcoma
  Osteosarcoma
  Synovial sarcoma
  Malignant schwannoma (malignant peripheral
    nerve sheath tumor)
  Malignant mesenchymoma
  Malignant hemangiopericytoma
  Kaposi's sarcoma

Malignant germ cell tumors

Hematologic tumors
  Lymphoma
  Granulocytic sarcoma

Mesothelial malignancies
  Malignant mesothelioma

Metastatic tumors to the heart

Sarcomas of the Aorta and Pulmonary Artery

Luminal (intimal) sarcoma
  Unclassified sarcomas
  Malignant fibrous histiocytoma
  Angiosarcoma
  Osteosarcoma
  Chondrosarcoma
  Leiomyosarcoma
  Malignant mesenchymoma

Mural sarcomas
  Leiomyosarcoma
  Angiosarcoma
  Malignant fibrous histiocytoma (MFH)
  Unclassified sarcomas

Sarcomas of the Inferior Vena Cava

Mural leiomyosarcoma

Luminal (intimal) sarcoma

Leiomyomas of Veins

(chapters 9 and 14). Other primary tumors of the pericardium are rare. Sarcomas of the pericardium are discussed with cardiac sarcomas, because they are histologically similar to their cardiac counterparts and often involve both the pericardium and myocardium. Germ cell tumors and bronchogenic cysts may occur in the pericardium or myocardium, and are discussed together in chapter 11; benign fibrous tumor of the peri-

cardium is discussed with other fibrous tumors of the heart in chapter 6.

A brief discussion of histogenesis accompanies each chapter; however, some difficulties in classification occur. There is some confusion regarding tumors that have at one time or other been classified as fibromas. In this Fascicle, papillary endocardial tumors that lack the histologic features of myxoma are classified as papillary fibroelastoma.

This is the most commonly used term, and we adopt it despite the fact that elastic fibers are not always prominent and smooth muscle cells may be present. Fibrous tumors located within the myocardium are termed fibromas, whether or not elastic fibers are prominent, and are considered separate from pericardial fibromas or solitary fibrous tumors (mesotheliomas).

Purkinje cell hamartoma and histiocytoid cardiomyopathy are terms used for rare congenital tumors of cardiac myocytes. Neither term is completely accurate, but we use histiocytoid cardiomyopathy, which is more widely used, in this Fascicle.

Several rare lesions, which are discussed in chapter 11, are derived from noncardiac tissues that have migrated to cardiac sites during embryogenesis. Although cystic tumors of the AV node were considered mesotheliomas in the previous cardiac Fascicle (13), they are currently believed to originate from endodermal rests, and are also discussed in chapter 11.

Tumors of multiple cell types are classified by the predominant cell type. Cardiac hemangiomas, similar to intramuscular hemangiomas of soft tissue, may contain fatty elements; conversely, hamartomas of cardiac valves are composed predominantly of fatty tissue, but may have a minor fibrous component.

Most of the other terms used are standard, with the possible exception of MICE (mesothelial/monocytic incidental cardiac excrescences). This recently described entity is most likely not a tumor at all, but an artifact of open heart surgery. Because it may simulate a tumor, it is discussed with other lesions that contain mesothelial cells.

Incidence of Cardiac Tumors

Primary Cardiac Tumors. McAllister and Fenoglio (13) estimated that 800 to 1,000 primary cardiac tumors were described before 1977. Since then, at least 1,000 cases have been reported.

Because the premortem diagnosis of cardiac tumor has only recently been possible, the incidence of cardiac tumors is generally based on autopsy studies. The estimated incidence of cardiac tumors in the United States ranges from 0.001 to 0.03 percent (8,19). However, incidence figures from autopsy series vary by a factor of greater than 100 (30). The reason for this great variation is unknown, but is likely related to selection of au-

topsies, inaccuracies due to the retrospective nature of the series, and populations studied.

The highest incidence of cardiac tumors at autopsy was cited as 0.33 percent by Pollia and Gogol (21): 154 primary cardiac tumors were found in a series of 46,072 autopsies from a selected population composed largely of cancer patients. From 1915 to 1931 the incidence of primary cardiac tumors at the Mayo Clinic was 0.05 percent of all autopsies performed (11); this rate more than tripled (0.17 percent) between 1954 and 1979 (30). It is likely that this latter figure is an overrepresentation of primary cardiac tumors because of referral bias at the Mayo Clinic. In a compilation of six autopsy series reported from the American Medical Association Internship Hospitals, the incidence of primary cardiac tumors was a mere 0.0017 percent (27). This reflects the general population more closely than a single institution study, but may be limited by a lack of uniformity of data collection and diagnostic criteria. In a recent series of 7,200 autopsies in a university hospital in Paris, the incidence was over 0.1 percent (5), which is significantly higher than a recent Japanese study, in which the rate was 0.038 percent (18). Nadas and Ellison (20) reported a 0.01 percent incidence of primary cardiac tumors in an autopsy series of infants, which falls in the estimated range of 0.001 to 0.03 percent, based on autopsies performed on patients of all ages.

The relative incidence of individual cardiac tumors has changed over the years (fig. 1-2). Of the cardiac tumors diagnosed at autopsy before the advent of cardiopulmonary bypass, the incidence of cardiac myxoma, the most common primary tumor of the heart, was only slightly greater than that of cardiac sarcoma, the second most common primary tumor of the heart. Approximately 125 cases of cardiac myxoma had been reported before 1951 in comparison to 113 primary cardiac sarcomas (22). Of 329 primary cardiac tumors seen by Mahaim, who wrote an extensive monograph on cardiac tumors in 1945 (12), 105 cases (32 percent) were cardiac myxoma, and 87 cases (26 percent) were cardiac sarcoma; the remaining 42 percent were rhabdomyoma (18 percent), fibroma (12 percent), angioma (4 percent), lipoma (4 percent), and miscellaneous benign tumors (4 percent). In the second series Fascicle on tumors of the heart (13),

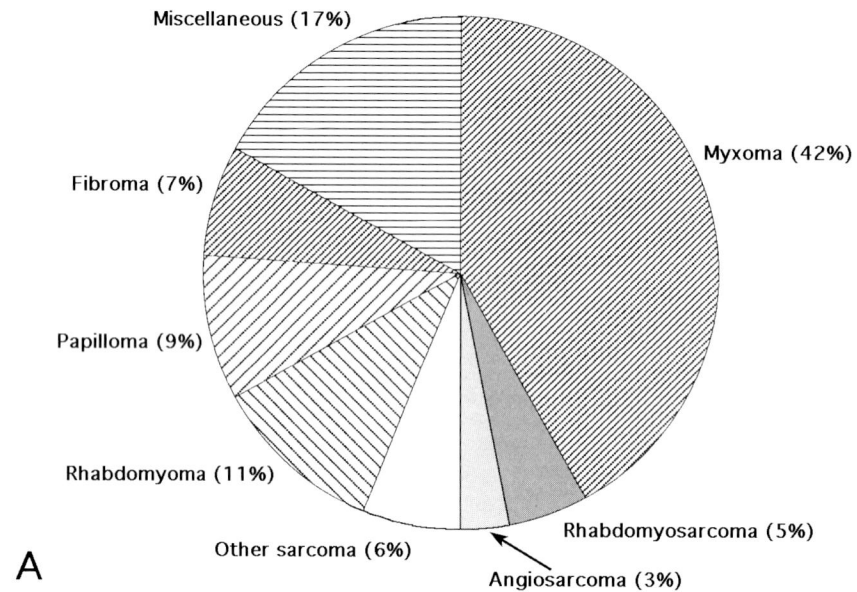

Primary Cardiac Tumors
University of Minnesota

Miscellaneous (17%)

Myxoma (42%)

Fibroma (7%)

Papilloma (9%)

Rhabdomyoma (11%)

Other sarcoma (6%)

Rhabdomyosarcoma (5%)

Angiosarcoma (3%)

A

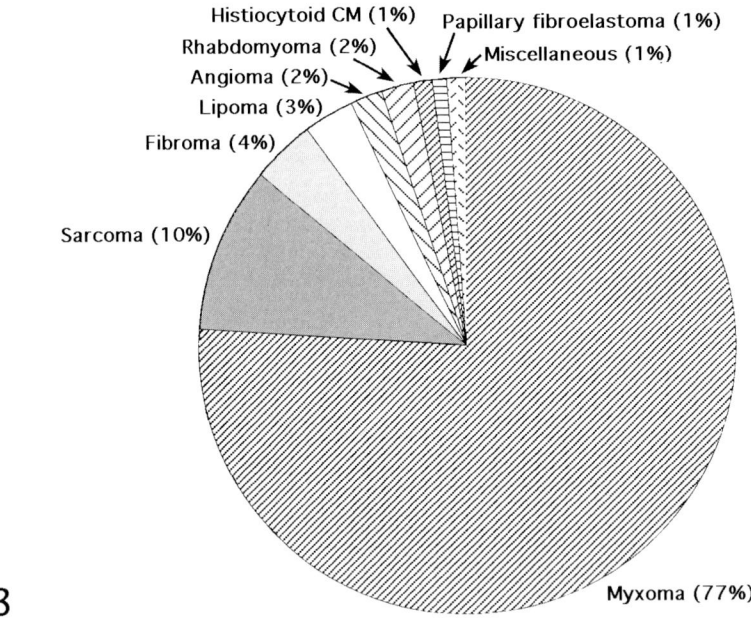

Cardiac Tumors, Surgical Series

Histiocytoid CM (1%)   Papillary fibroelastoma (1%)

Rhabdomyoma (2%)   Miscellaneous (1%)

Angioma (2%)

Lipoma (3%)

Fibroma (4%)

Sarcoma (10%)

Myxoma (77%)

B

Figure 1-2
RELATIVE INCIDENCE OF CARDIAC TUMORS

The proportion of surgical cases greatly influences the relative incidence of primary cardiac tumors.

A: If both surgical and autopsy cases are considered, there is a wide variety of tumors encountered (data obtained from reference 15).

B: In exclusively surgical series, myxomas account for over 75 percent of cases, compared to about 40 percent of autopsy and surgical cases combined (see Table 1-2 for references). CM = cardiomyopathy.

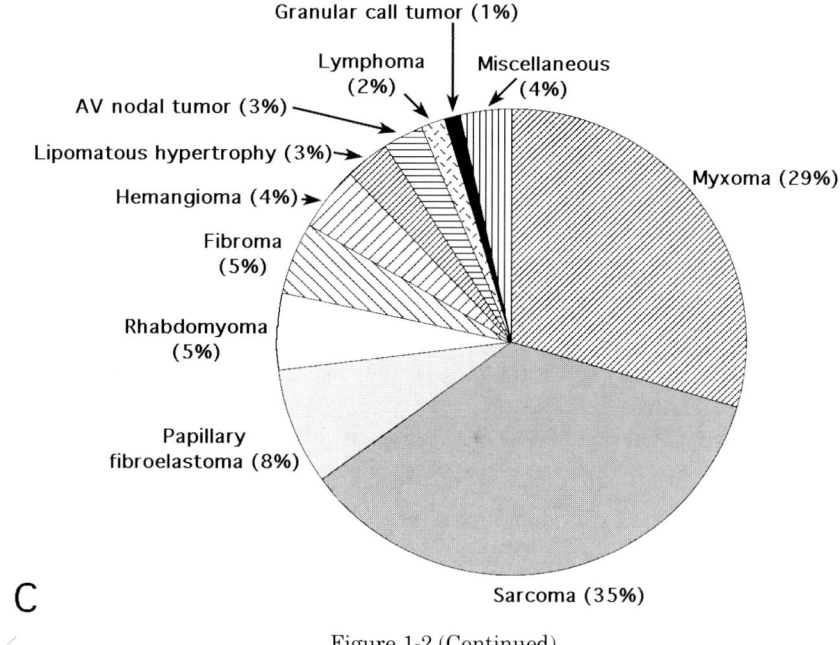

Primary Cardiac Tumors, AFIP, 1976-1993

Granular call tumor (1%)

Lymphoma (2%)

Miscellaneous (4%)

AV nodal tumor (3%)

Lipomatous hypertrophy (3%)

Hemangioma (4%)

Fibroma (5%)

Rhabdomyoma (5%)

Papillary fibroelastoma (8%)

Myxoma (29%)

Sarcoma (35%)

C

Figure 1-2 (Continued)
RELATIVE INCIDENCE OF CARDIAC TUMORS
C: There is a greater diversity of tumors seen at a referral institution, such as the AFIP, than at a single institution, especially for malignant lesions. Myxomas account for only 29 percent and sarcoma 35 percent of tumors. These tumors largely represent surgical specimens.

91 of 444 primary tumors were cardiac sarcomas, 20 percent of all tumors excluding cysts. Although still the second most common primary tumor after myxoma (30 percent of cases in the second series Fascicle), the relative number of sarcomas is lower than in Mahaim's series. In the largest single-institution series of primary cardiac tumors (other than at the Armed Forces Institute of Pathology [AFIP]), of 124 cases diagnosed both at autopsy and surgery over 40 years (fig. 1-2) (17), 42 percent were cardiac myxomas and 16 percent were cardiac sarcomas.

The gradual increase in the proportion of cases of cardiac myxoma as compared to cardiac sarcoma is a reflection of the increase in surgically excised cardiac tumors. Myxomas are detected more frequently and in younger individuals than previously because of the increased use of noninvasive cardiac imaging techniques; they are also more easily excised than sarcomas, fibromas, and rhabdomyomas. In almost 1,000 surgically resected cardiac tumors from several series of the last 10 years, the proportion of

cardiac sarcomas was only 10 percent, while the proportion of cardiac myxomas was 77 percent (Table 1-2) (3,8,14–16,19,23,26,28,29).

Unusual cardiac and pericardial tumors are present in relatively large proportions in the AFIP files because of referral bias (Tables 1-3, 1-4).

Primary cardiac tumors in children are uncommon, and are usually rhabdomyomas, fibromas, or teratomas (fig. 1-3, Table 1-5). Pediatric cardiac malignancies are extremely rare and only a few cases have been reported (2,5,9,20): in a literature review of the subject in 1980, only three cases were found (2).

Metastatic Tumors to the Heart. Primary cardiac tumors are far less frequent than metastatic tumors to the heart: a ratio of 1:20 to 1:40 is estimated (11), but may be as low as 1:500 (see below). As with primary cardiac tumors, the autopsy incidence of metastatic tumors to the heart varies greatly by study. In a series of 4,375 autopsies performed on cancer patients in 1940 (22), Prichard found 3.4 percent to have metastases to heart. In a literature review of cancer autopsies

Table 1-2

CARDIAC TUMORS, SURGICAL SERIES

	Total (%)	Blondeau	Tazelaar et al.	Miralles et al.	Murphy et al.	Reece et al.	Dein et al.	Melo et al.	Verkkala et al.
Myxoma	758 (77%)	444	80	63	58	51	27	19	16
Sarcoma	95 (10%)	52*	8	12	7	5	8	1	2
Fibroma	35 (4%)	9	9	7	3	5	1	1	0
Lipoma	26 (3%)	9	5	4	2	3	1	0	2
Angioma	22 (2%)	7	0	3	3	2	7	0	0
Rhabdomyoma	19 (2%)	5	0	9	0	5	0	0	0
Histiocytoid cardiomyopathy**	14 (1%)	0	1	0	13	0	0	0	0
Papilloma	9 (1%)	0	7	0	0	0	2	0	0
Hamartoma	5	4	0	0	0	0	1	0	0
Ectopic thyroid	2	2	0	0	0	0	0	0	0
Lymphoma	1	1	0	0	0	0	0	0	0
Total	**986**	**533**	**110**	**98**	**86**	**71**	**47**	**21**	**20**

* Includes two malignant neoplasms that were considered unclassifiable.
** Histiocytoid cardiomyopathy is synonymous with Purkinje cell hamartoma.

Primary Tumors and Cysts of the Heart and Pericardium AFIP, 1976-1993, Patients 0-16 Years of Age

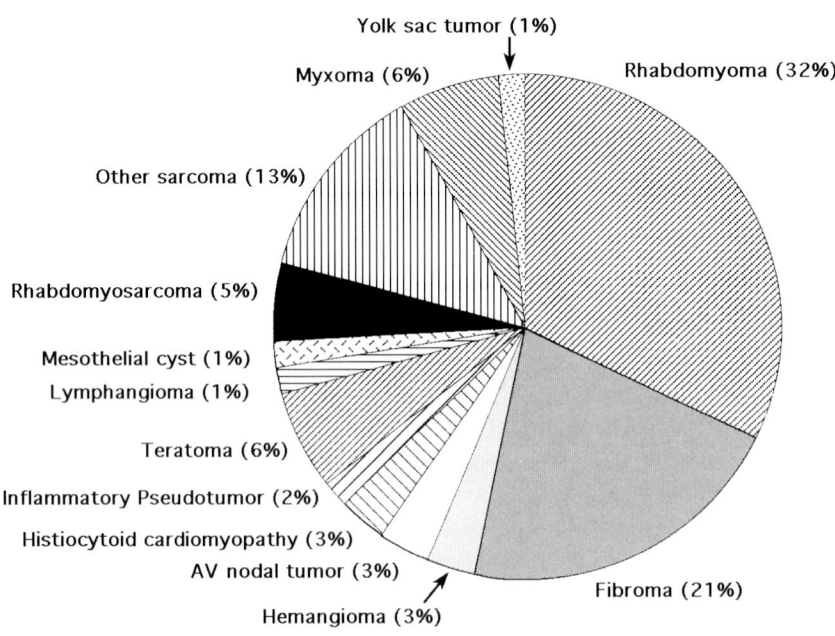

Yolk sac tumor (1%)
Myxoma (6%)
Rhabdomyoma (32%)
Other sarcoma (13%)
Rhabdomyosarcoma (5%)
Mesothelial cyst (1%)
Lymphangioma (1%)
Teratoma (6%)
Inflammatory Pseudotumor (2%)
Histiocytoid cardiomyopathy (3%)
AV nodal tumor (3%)
Hemangioma (3%)
Fibroma (21%)

Figure 1-3
CARDIAC TUMORS IN CHILDREN
Primary cardiac tumors of children differ greatly from those of adults. Rhabdomyomas, fibromas, and sarcomas are the most common tumors in the AFIP files. Myxomas are relatively rare. All three in this figure were removed from 16-year-old patients.

Table 1-3
386 PRIMARY TUMORS OF THE HEART: AFIP 1976–1993

Benign Tumors	Total (%)	Surgical Cases	<16 Years*	<1 Year*
Myxoma	114 (29%)	102	4	0
Papillary fibroelastoma	31 (8%)	8	0	0
Rhabdomyoma	20 (5%)	6	20	19
Fibroma	20 (5%)	18	13	8
Hemangioma	17 (4%)	10	2	1
Lipomatous hypertrophy, atrial septum	12 (3%)	7	0	0
AV nodal tumor	10 (3%)	0	2	1
Granular cell tumor	4 (1%)	0	0	0
Lipoma	2	2	0	0
Paraganglioma	2	2	0	0
Myocytic hamartoma, not further classified	2	2	0	0
Histiocytoid cardiomyopathy	2	0	2	2
Inflammatory pseudotumor	2	2	1	0
Benign fibrous histiocytoma	1	0	0	0
Epithelioid hemangioendothelioma	1	1	0	0
Bronchogenic cyst	1	1	0	0
Teratoma	1	0	1	1
Total Benign Tumors	**242**	**161**	**45**	**32**

Malignant Tumors	Total (%)	Surgical Cases	<16 Years*	<1 Year*
Sarcoma	137 (35%)	124	11	3
Angiosarcoma	33	22	1	0
Unclassified	33	30	3	1
Malignant fibrous histiocytoma (MFH)	16	16	1	0
Osteosarcoma	13	13	0	0
Leiomyosarcoma	12	11	1	1
Fibrosarcoma	9	9	1	0
Myxosarcoma	8	8	1	0
Rhabdomyosarcoma	6	2	3	1
Synovial sarcoma	4	4	0	0
Liposarcoma	2	0	0	0
Malignant schwannoma	1	1	0	0
Lymphoma	7 (2%)	1	0	0
Total Malignant Tumors	**144**	**125**	**11**	**3**
TOTAL TUMORS	**386**	**286**	**56**	**35**

* Age of patient at time of diagnosis.

Table 1-4

64 PRIMARY CYSTS AND TUMORS OF THE PERICARDIUM: AFIP 1976–1993

Benign Tumors	Total (%)	Surgical Cases	<16 Years*	<1 Year*
Mesothelial cyst	37 (58%)	35	1	0
Teratoma	3 (5%)	3	3	2
Bronchogenic cyst	2 (3%)	2	0	0
Benign fibrous tumor	2 (3%)	2	0	0
Lymphangioma	2 (3%)	1	1	0
Giant lymph node hyperplasia	1 (2%)	1	0	0
Malignant Tumors				
Malignant mesothelioma	8 (13%)	4	0	0
Sarcoma	8 (13%)	8	0	0
Angiosarcoma	4 (6%)			
Unclassifiable	2 (3%)			
Synovial sarcoma	1 (2%)			
Malignant schwannoma	1 (2%)			
Yolk sac (endodermal sinus) tumor	1 (2%)	1	1	1
TOTALS	**64**	**61**	**6**	**3**

* Age of patient at time of diagnosis.

Table 1-5

SELECTED PRIMARY CARDIAC TUMORS LISTED BY MEAN AGE AT PRESENTATION: AFIP EXPERIENCE

Tumor Type	Mean Patient Age at Diagnosis
Teratoma	16 weeks
Rhabdomyoma	33 weeks
Fibroma	13 years
Rhabdomyosarcoma	15 years
Hemangioma	31 years
AV nodal tumor	33 years
Sarcoma (all)	41 years
Myxoma	50 years
Mesothelioma	57 years
Papillary fibroelastoma	59 years
Lipomatous hypertrophy	64 years

(21,22,24,25) Prichard calculated a similar incidence (326 of 8,414 autopsies, 3.9 percent). Extrapolating from these data, one would expect an incidence of no more than 1.3 percent cardiac metastases in the total autopsy population, assuming generously that one third of autopsies are performed on cancer patients. However, in a recent review of 3,314 consecutive autopsies, Abraham et al. (1) found a 2.9 percent incidence of metastatic tumors of the heart; of 806 autopsies of cancer patients, the incidence of metastatic cardiac deposits was 12 percent. This figure is nearly identical to that of a recent study from France (5). There are several possible explanations for the increase in incidence between earlier series in the 1940s and more recent studies. The definitions of cardiac involvement by metastatic tumor were not clearly defined in many earlier reports, and the recent data include cases of pericardial, as well as myocardial, involvement. It is possible that earlier studies included only cases of bulky myocardial metastases, and did not rely on histologic examination to verify the presence of microscopic metastases. Additionally, more intensive treatment modalities that have been introduced in the last 30 years have resulted in prolonged life of cancer patients, and increased probability of spread to the myocardium.

If one accepts a rate of 1 to 3 percent for cardiac metastases seen at autopsy, and a rate of 0.001 to 0.03 percent for primary cardiac tumors seen at autopsy (see above), then the ratio of cardiac metastases to primary cardiac tumor is 100:1 to 1,000:1. This estimate is far higher than previous estimates of 1:20 to 1:40 (11). The ratio of metastatic to primary cardiac tumors was 400:1 in one large autopsy series (18), a ratio that falls within the calculated range of 100 to 1000:1, and is likely an accurate estimate of the true ratio of metastatic to primary tumors of the heart.

REFERENCES

1. Abraham DP, Reddy V, Gattusa P. Neoplasms metastatic to the heart: review of 3314 consecutive autopsies. Am J Cardiovasc Pathol 1990;3:195–8.
2. Arciniegas E, Hakimi M, Farooki ZQ, Truccone NJ, Green EW. Primary cardiac tumors in children. J Thorac Cardiovasc Surg 1980;79:582–91.
3. Blondeau P. Primary cardiac tumors—French studies of 533 cases. Thorac Cardiovasc Surg 1990;38:192–5.
4. Chan HS, Sonley MJ, Moes CA, Daneman A, Smith CR, Martin DJ. Primary and secondary tumors of childhood involving the heart, pericardium, and great vessels. A report of 75 cases and review of the literature. Cancer 1985;56:825–36.
5. Chomette G, Auriol M, Cabrol C, Tranbaloc P. Primary malignant tumors of the heart. Anatomo-clinical study of 12 cases. Ann Med Interne (Paris) 1985;136:301–5.
6. Clark EB, Van Mierop LH. Development of the cardiovascular system. In: Adams FH, Emmanouilides GC, Riemenschneider TA, eds. Moss' heart disease in infants, children, and adolescents. Baltimore: Williams & Wilkins, 1983:2–15.
7. Crafoord C. Panel discussion on late results of mitral commissurotomy. In: Lam CR, ed. International symposium on cardiovascular surgery. Philadelphia: WB Saunders, 1955:161–78.
8. Dein JR, Frist WH, Stinson EB, et al. Primary cardiac neoplasms. Early and late results of surgical treatment in 42 patients. J Thorac Cardiovasc Surg 1987;93:502–11.
9. Goldberg HP, Glenn F, Dotter CT, Steinberg I. Myxoma of the left atrium: diagnosis made during life with operative and post-mortem findings. Circulation 1952;6:762–7.
10. Heath D. Pathology of cardiac tumors. Amer J Cardiol 1968;21:315–27.
11. Lymburner RM. Tumours of the heart: histopathologic and clinical study. Can Med Assoc J 1934;30:368–73.
12. Mahaim K. Les tumeurs et les polypes de coeur: etude anatomo-clinique. Paris: Masson, 1945.
13. McAllister HA, Fenoglio JJ Jr. Tumors of the cardiovascular system. Atlas of Tumor Pathology, 2nd Series, Fascicle 15. Washington, D.C.: Armed Forces Institute of Pathology, 1978.
14. Melo J, Ahmad A, Chapman R, Wood J, Starr A. Primary tumors of the heart: a rewarding challenge. Am Surg 1979;45:681–3.
15. Miralles A, Bracamonte L, Oncul H, Diaz del Castillo R, et al. Cardiac tumors: clinical experience and surgical results in 74 patients. Ann Thorac Surg 1991;52:886–95.
16. Moggio RA, Pucillo AL, Schechter AG, Pooley RW, Sarabu MR, Reed GE. Primary cardiac tumors. Diagnosis and management in 14 cases. N Y State J Med 1992;92:49–52.
17. Molina JE, Edwards JE, Ward HB. Primary cardiac tumors: experience at the University of Minnesota. Thorac Cardiovasc Surg 1990;38[Supp 2]:183–91.
18. Mukai K, Shinkai T, Tominaga K, Shimosato Y. The incidence of secondary tumors of the heart and pericardium: a 10-year study. Jpn J Clin Oncol 1988;18:195–201.
19. Murphy MC, Sweeney MS, Putnam JB Jr, et al. Surgical treatment of cardiac tumors: a 25-year experience. Ann Thorac Surg 1990;49:612–7.
20. Nadas AS, Ellison RC. Cardiac tumors in infancy. Am J Cardiol 1968;21:363–6.
21. Pollia JA, Gogol LJ. Some notes on malignancies of the heart. Am J Cancer 1936;27:329–33.
22. Prichard RW. Tumors of the heart: review of the subject and report of one hundred and fifty cases. Arch Pathol 1951;51:98–128.
23. Reece IJ, Cooley DA, Frazier OH, Hallman GL, Powers PL, Montero CG. Cardiac tumors. Clinical spectrum and prognosis of lesions other than classical benign myxoma in 20 patients. J Thorac Cardiovasc Surg 1984;88:439–46.
24. Ritchie G. Metastatic tumors of the myocardium: a review of 16 cases. Am J Pathol 1941;17:483–91.
25. Scott RW, Garvin CF. Tumors of the heart and pericardium. Am Heart J 1939;17:431–6.
26. Silverman NA. Primary cardiac tumors. Ann Surg 1980;191:127–38.
27. Straus R, Merliss R. Primary tumor of the heart. Arch Pathol 1945;39:74–8.
28. Tazelaar HD, Locke TJ, McGregor CG. Pathology of surgically excised primary cardiac tumors. Mayo Clin Proc 1992;67:957–65.
29. Verkkala K, Kupari M, Maamies T, et al. Primary cardiac tumours—operative treatment of 20 patients. Thorac Cardiovasc Surg 1989;37:361–4.
30. Wold LE, Lie JT. Cardiac myxomas: a clinicopathologic profile. Am J Pathol 1980;101:219–40.

2
CLINICAL AND DIAGNOSTIC CONSIDERATIONS

A primary tumor of the heart was first diagnosed clinically by Goldberg in 1952 (8), who described the angiographic findings of a cardiac myxoma. The advent of cardiopulmonary bypass surgery in the early 1960s allowed successful excision of cardiac myxomas routinely. Prior to the establishment of two-dimensional echocardiography in the late 1970s, antemortem diagnosis of cardiac tumor was possible only when the lesion was large, the cardiac silhouette was distorted, or hemodynamic effects from valve encroachment were produced (18). Current noninvasive technologies, including transesophageal echocardiography, computed tomography (CT), and magnetic resonance imaging (MRI), provide precise anatomic location, and in some cases, tissue assessment for diagnosing and characterizing cardiac tumors (3,4,7,13).

Clinical Manifestations of Cardiac Tumors

Tumors of the heart result in a wide range of clinical signs and symptoms. The presenting symptoms are usually related to congestive heart failure, thromboembolism, or arrhythmias, and may initially manifest in the central nervous system, lungs, extremities, and other extracardiac sites. Because cardiac tumors are rare, clinicians often consider the correct diagnosis relatively late in the disease course. The protean manifestations of cardiac myxoma, for example, are well known; so is its propensity to present as a systemic illness rather than as a primary cardiac disease (3,18).

The anatomic location of the tumor, rather than its size, often determines the clinical findings. Large infiltrative tumors of the myocardium may be clinically silent; yet small, strategically located tumors may cause obstruction to blood flow across a valve and result in dramatic symptoms (3,9,18).

Endocardial tumors, such as myxomas, papillary fibroelastomas, and sarcomas, can embolize to the coronary, renal, cerebral, or peripheral circulation resulting in ischemia of the particular arterial bed affected. Left atrial tumors that are mobile and pedunculated, especially myxo-mas, may prolapse into the mitral valve orifice causing obstruction to the blood flow with resultant signs and symptoms of mitral valve disease (3). Mitral stenosis or regurgitation may result in dyspnea, orthopnea, paroxysmal nocturnal dyspnea, pulmonary edema, fatigue, cough, hemoptysis, and chest pain. Right atrial tumors often produce signs and symptoms of right heart failure, including peripheral edema, ascites, hepatomegaly, and prominent "a" waves in the jugular venous pulse (8,17). If large, right atrial tumors can obstruct the tricuspid valve or cause tricuspid regurgitation. Intracavitary tumors of the right atrium, and less commonly the right ventricle, may cause pulmonary hypertension and thromboembolic disease (19).

Left ventricular tumors may be intramural or intracavitary. Intramural tumors are often asymptomatic or may present with arrhythmias. Infiltrative tumors may cause hemodynamic compromise or, if there is infiltration of the conduction system, conduction defects and sudden death. Intracavitary tumors, if large, may cause left ventricular failure (3). Chest pain can be caused by an embolus into the coronary artery or from compression of the coronary artery by a left ventricular tumor (20).

Right ventricular tumors may obstruct the right ventricular outflow, resulting in right heart failure and signs and symptoms similar to those caused by right atrial tumors: peripheral edema, hepatomegaly, ascites, shortness of breath, syncope, and sudden death (3). Right axis deviation, right ventricular hypertrophy, and right bundle branch block electrocardiographically should suggest an intracavitary right ventricular tumor (3).

Pericardial involvement by tumor may cause pericardial pain, constrictive pericarditis, and pericardial tamponade.

Constitutional symptoms such as anorexia, weight loss, lethargy, or malaise may be the initial presentation of cardiac tumors, especially myxoma (3,18). These symptoms may or may not be accompanied by anemia, polycythemia, thrombocytosis, leukocytosis, elevated sedimentation rate, and hypergammaglobulinemia. The

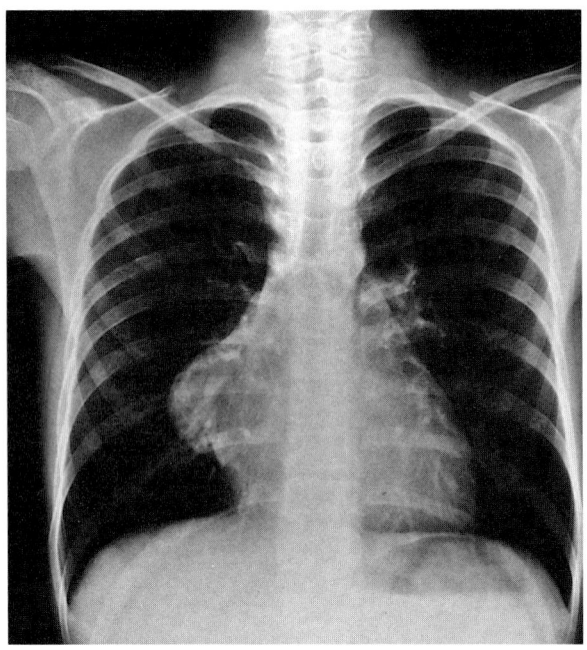

Figure 2-1
CARDIAC SARCOMA
Posterior-anterior (PA) chest radiograph from a 12-year-old boy with chest pain and arrhythmias. There is a sharply marginated mass silhouetting the right cardiac border; histologic examination demonstrated rhabdomyosarcoma.

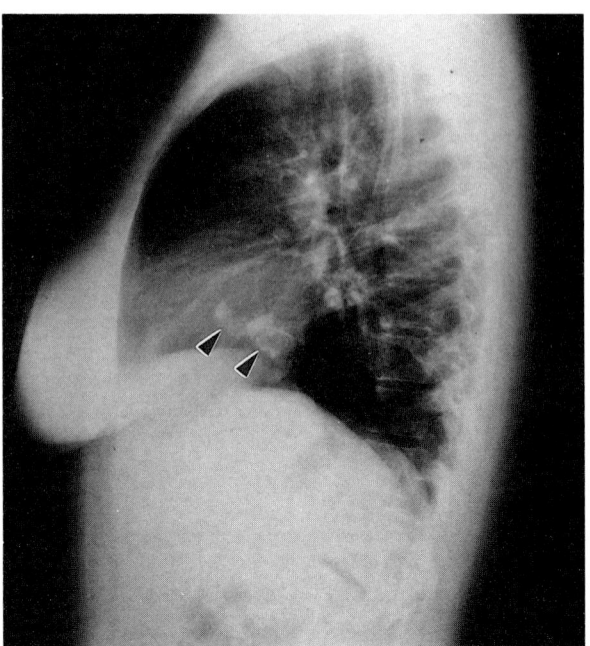

Figure 2-2
CARDIAC MYXOMA
Lateral chest radiograph from a 16-year-old girl with syncope and bacterial endocarditis. The radiograph demonstrates two areas of dense calcification (arrowheads) overlying the posterior aspect of heart. The posterior-anterior (PA) view confirmed location in the heart (not shown). At surgery a calcified myxoma of the right atrium was removed.

mechanism underlying these symptoms remains obscure but has been attributed to tumor necrosis, tumor secretion products (14), and secretion of interleukin-6 in the case of myxoma (10).

Clinical Diagnosis of Cardiac Tumors

Auscultation and Electrocardiography. Although there are few auscultatory signs specific for cardiac tumors, left atrial myxomas may cause a classic "tumor plop," as well as a variety of murmurs (see chapter 3). Pericardial friction rubs indicate pericardial invasion by tumor. Electrocardiographic (ECG) changes are usually nonspecific and include tachyarrhythmias, conduction deficits, low voltage, and ST-T wave changes (3). In clinically stable patients with malignancy and no cardiac symptoms suggestive of ischemia, any new ECG changes should raise the suspicion of cardiac metastasis. ECG findings of myocardial ischemia or injury is a highly specific (96 percent), but not sensitive (40 percent), indicator of cardiac metastases (2). Myocardial tumor invasion can produce a wide vari-

ety of electrical disturbances such as atrial fibrillation, atrial flutter, paroxysmal atrial tachycardia with or without blocks, nodal rhythm, premature ventricular contraction, ventricular tachycardia, and ventricular fibrillation (3,8).

Chest Roentgenograms. These are often normal or show nonspecific findings. Abnormal cardiac contours (fig. 2-1) are indicative of massive tumor infiltration of the myocardium, pericardium, and contiguous mediastinum. Increased pulmonary vascular markings are indicative of pulmonary hypertension or mitral valve obstruction from left atrial myxoma or emboli. Tumor calcification has been described in teratomas, rhabdomyosarcomas, myxomas (fig. 2-2), fibromas, and primary osteogenic sarcomas of the heart (3,18).

Angiography. Cardiac angiography was at one time the standard for cardiac tumor diagnosis. Compression or deformity of cardiac chambers, filling defects, variation in the thickness of the myocardium, and wall motion abnormalities

Table 2-1

IMAGING TECHNIQUES FOR THE DIAGNOSIS OF CARDIAC TUMORS*

	Radiography	CT	Angiography	MRI	Echocardiography
Primary Benign Tumors					
Myxoma	+**	++	+++	++++	+++++
Pericardial cyst	++	+++	0	+++++	+
Lipoma	+	+++	+	+++++	+++
Fibroelastoma	0	0	0	+++	+++++
Rhabdomyoma	0	+	+	++++	+++++
Fibroma	0	+		++++	++++
Primary Malignant Tumors					
Sarcoma	+	++	++	+++++	+++
Mesothelioma	+	+++	+	+++++	++
Lymphoma	++	+++	+	+++++	++
Secondary Tumors					
Direct extension	+	+++	++	+++++	+++
Venous extension	0	+	+++	++++	++++
Metastatic spread	+	++	+	++++	++

*From reference 18.
**0 = of no use; + = of limited use; ++ = may be of use; +++ = useful; ++++ = very useful; +++++ = preferred diagnostic tool.

allowed for localization of the tumor. In addition, valvular function, coronary artery obstruction, and encroachment of the great vessels could also be assessed and were critical in preoperative evaluation. Two-dimensional echocardiography, CT, and MRI have largely replaced angiography in cardiac tumor diagnosis (Table 2-1). However, there are some situations that justify the risk and expense of cardiac catheterization for evaluation of cardiac tumors (3): if noninvasive evaluation does not adequately define the location of the tumor or its attachment, when all cardiac chambers are not fully visualized, when there is a presumed malignant cardiac tumor, and when there is a suspicion of other cardiac diseases, especially coronary artery disease.

Echocardiography. M-mode echocardiography was the first imaging modality used to detect the exact location of cardiac tumors, but its usefulness was limited to the recognition of pedunculated tumors, especially left atrial myxomas. Two-dimensional echocardiography provides in-

formation regarding tumor size, location, attachment (fig. 2-3), and mobility, and its use has resulted in an increase in the rate of detection of many types of cardiac tumors (3,7). It is sensitive enough to detect small tumors and can diagnose cardiac tumors in neonates and in utero (4). It can differentiate a thrombus which produces a layered appearance and a myxoma which is mottled (3). Hemorrhage into a tumor can be detected as an area of echolucency. By utilizing Doppler ultrasound, hemodynamic consequences of the cardiac tumor can be assessed. Although the overall sensitivity of two-dimensional echocardiography in the diagnosis of cardiac tumors is high, pericardial tumors may be difficult to detect by this method (18).

Transesophageal echocardiography provides high quality images of left and right atria, interatrial septum, pulmonary veins, and superior and inferior venae cavae. The accuracy of transthoracic and transesophageal echocardiography was compared recently in 47 patients with cardiac

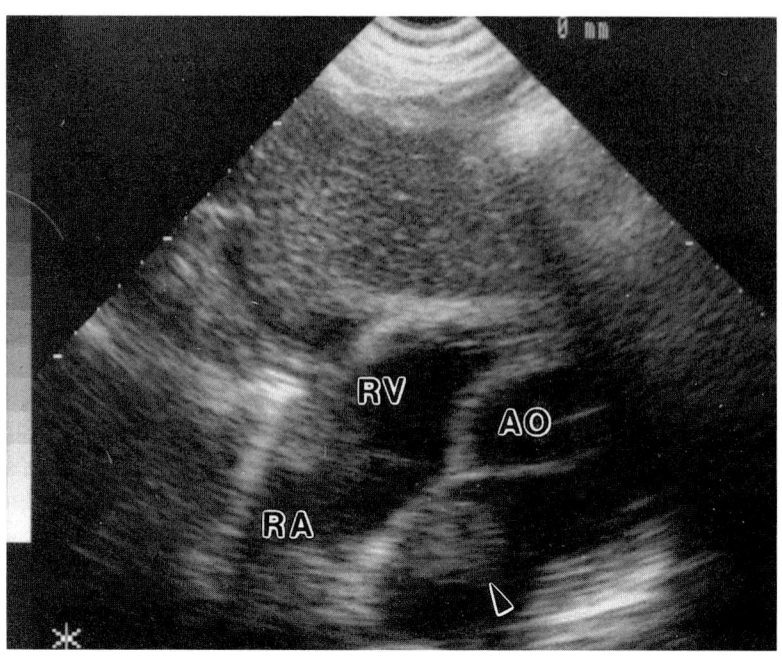

Figure 2-3
CARDIAC MYXOMA
Transthoracic echocardiogram (short axis, parasternal view) through the level of the atria shows a round, echogenic mass (arrowhead) within the left atrium attached to the atrial septum. The patient was a 44-year-old woman with chest pain and left atrial myxoma. AO = aorta; RA = right atrium; RV = right ventricle.

masses (15). Transesophageal echocardiography was superior to transthoracic echocardiography in visualizing left atrial appendage thrombi, small and flat thrombi in left atrial cavity, thrombi and tumors of the superior vena cava, and masses attached to the right heart and the descending thoracic aorta. However, apical thrombi were better detected by precordial echocardiography. Atrial myxomas and left sided cardiac tumors were detected with equal accuracy by both.

Computed Tomography. Conventional, nongated CT has been shown to be of value in assessing the presence of lung and mediastinal pathology, and of lesser value in assessing the heart because of cardiac motion artifacts. CT is the most useful method for finding paracardiac masses in the region of the pericardium and for assessing the extent of tumor spread in the lung, mediastinum, pericardium, and cardiac chambers (18). Fat, which has low radiodensity, can be distinguished from myxoma and thrombus (12). Contrast-enhanced CT may be useful in diagnosing heterogeneous tumors like teratomas (18). With ECG-gated CT, the resolution is improved, especially for the evaluation of shape, motion, and attachment of tumors (3,18). Ultrafast CT (cine-CT) facilitates the evaluation of paracardiac and intracardiac tumors (18) and lessens the artifact due to cardiac motion.

Magnetic Resonance Imaging. This modality enables high-resolution tomography in three dimensions and generates intravascular and soft tissue contrast without a contrasting agent (figs. 2-4–2-6). With the addition of ECG-gating of MRI it is possible to get high resolution of cardiac morphology (6). Two-dimensional echocardiography is the technique of choice in the evaluation of intracardiac tumors but MRI yields additional information of the entire thorax including mediastinum, lungs, and great vessels. MRI delineates not only the presence and extent of the cardiac tumor mass, but also distinguishes the tumor as pericardial, intramural, or intracavitary (18). MRI also can determine tissue composition, especially for the separation of lipomatous lesions from myxoma or thrombi (12,13). Use of MRI is limited by high cost and lack of availability in all institutions. Like other radiologic modalities, MRI does not separate benign and malignant tumors (18).

Tissue Sampling

Open Biopsy. The majority of cardiac tumors are biopsied or resected by open techniques. Most cardiac tumors are intracavitary and require cardiac bypass for excision. Epicardial tumors and those restricted to the atrial appendages are occasionally resected without entry into

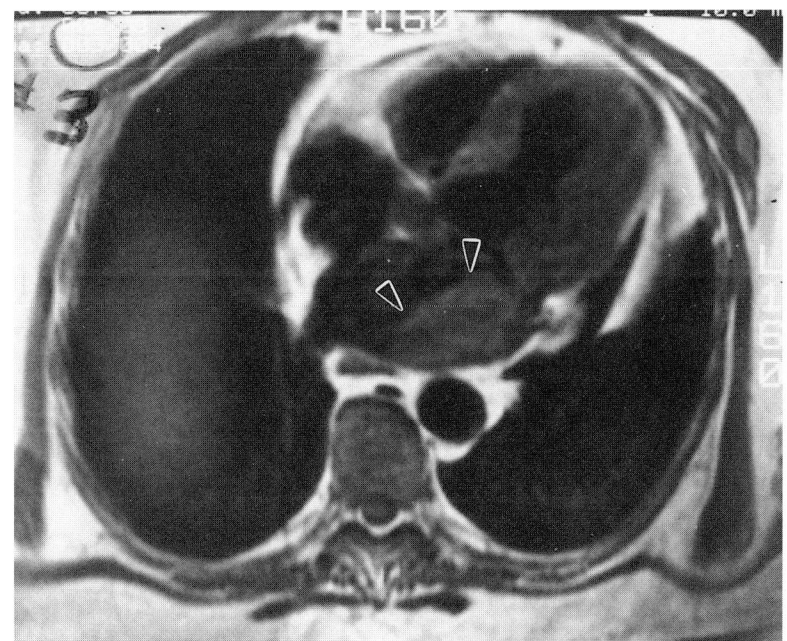

Figure 2-4
CARDIAC MYXOMA
Axial T1-weighted MRI shows a soft tissue mass within the left atrium isointense to skeletal muscle (arrowheads). A friable myxoma was removed from the left atrium of a 53-year-old man with cerebrovascular accidents.

the cardiac chambers, obviating the need for extracorporeal circulation. In some instances, a tumor is found to be inoperable after the chest is opened, and a needle biopsy is done purely for diagnostic purposes.

In cases of surgical excision, it is recommended that the pathologist ink the specimen to evaluate surgical margins. If possible, it is best to preserve a viable portion of tumor in fixative that optimally preserves ultrastructural detail, in the event that electron microscopic studies are necessary. Tissue cultures for chromosomal studies are helpful in diagnosing cardiac sarcomas, especially synovial sarcoma (see chapter 12).

Endomyocardial Biopsy. Endomyocardial biopsy is an established technique in the diagnosis of primary or metastatic cardiac tumors (5). Right ventricular biopsy via a transvenous approach is the standard for cardiac biopsy. However, a transarterial approach may be necessary for left-sided tumors. At the Armed Forces Institute of Pathology (AFIP), three cases of cardiac malignancy have been diagnosed by endocardial biopsy. Most cardiac tumors so diagnosed have been metastatic hematologic malignancies, metastatic melanoma, primary undifferentiated sarcomas, and primary angiosarcoma. The diagnostic yield depends upon obtaining adequate tissue: three tissue pieces from a 9-French

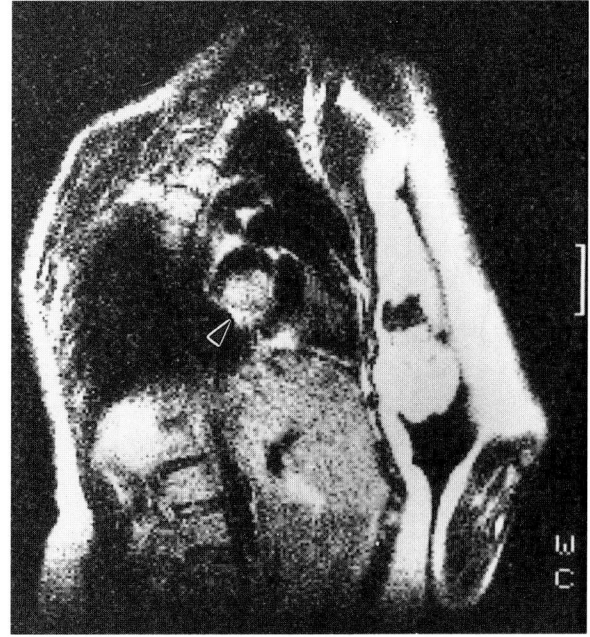

Figure 2-5
CARDIAC MYXOMA
Oblique sagittal T1-weighted MRI showing a soft tissue mass in the left atrium (arrowhead). The resected tumor was a heavily calcified myxoma with gamna bodies; the calcification accounts for the bright signal on T1-weighted imaging. The patient was a 61-year-old woman with a 2-year history of unexplained syncope.

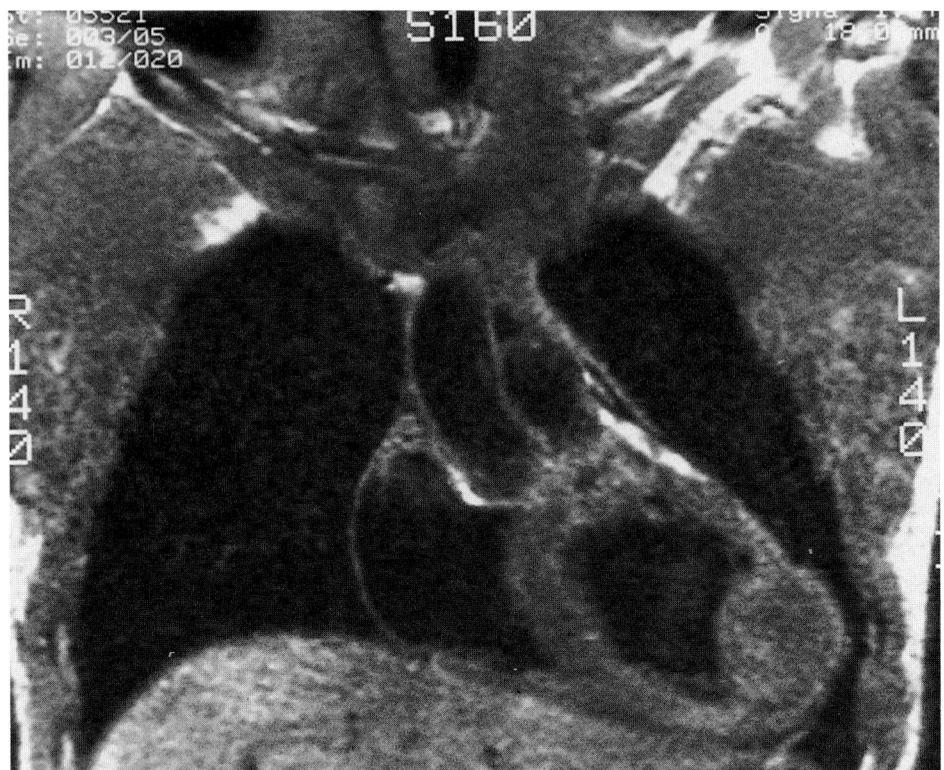

Figure 2-6
CARDIAC FIBROMA

A 19-year-old previously healthy male developed arrhythmias during nasal septal surgery. Coronal cardiac-gated T1-weighted MRI (TR 1090/TE 11) shows a round homogeneous mass at the left ventricular apex which is isointense to skeletal muscle. The resected tumor was a benign fibroma that was completely excised. (Fig. 3 from Burke AP, Rosado-de-Christenson M, Templeton PA, Virmani R. Cardiac fibroma: clinicopathologic correlates and surgical treatment. J Thorac Cardiovasc Surg 1994;108:862–70.)

biotome is the minimum (5). To further increase the yield, more specimens are removed and the biopsy is taken from the chamber with the greatest clinical involvement (5). Embolization of tumor is a theoretical complication that as yet has not been reported. Endomyocardial biopsy has the advantage of being an outpatient procedure with low morbidity and mortality.

Transcutaneous Needle Biopsy. For bulky neoplasms, especially pericardial tumors such as mesothelioma, CT-guided transcutaneous core needle biopsies may be utilized for diagnosis.

Cytologic Diagnosis. Cytologic aspirates, especially of pericardial fluid, are used for the diagnosis of cardiac tumors with pericardial involvement, such as mesothelioma or rhabdomyosarcoma. Fine-needle aspirates are also used. Special techniques, such as electron microscopy or immunohistochemistry, may be performed on exfoliated cells to facilitate a specific diagnosis.

Treatment

Surgical removal is the treatment of choice for benign cardiac tumors because a complete cure is often possible. Surgery should be performed as soon as possible after diagnosis, because patients may experience complications, especially embolization, while awaiting surgery. Except for some epicardial tumors, cardiac tumors are removed under extracorporeal circulation using standard cardiopulmonary bypass (3). All cardiac tumors are removed under direct visualization because of the danger of embolization or micrometastasis. The site of tumor attachment is determined after removal of blood in order to ensure complete excision (3). For myxomas, some surgeons advocate removal of 5 mm of tissue beyond the site of attachment, and others advocate excision of the entire fossa ovalis region. To avoid creating an atrial septal defect, laser photocoagulation around the stalk is recommended for pedunculated tumors and those that do not required excision of atrial septal tissue (3). Care must be taken to prevent damage to the atrioventricular valves, to preserve the conduction tissue, and to leave sufficient ventricular muscle for adequate function. Rhabdomyomas are excised conservatively, with dissection limited to the area of the tumor. Fibromas are removed by a blunt and sharp dissection and the ventricle is reconstructed (11).

Surgery is not a definitive treatment for primary cardiac sarcomas because recurrence and eventual death from tumor is the rule. The major role of surgery is to establish histologic diagnosis and palliate obstructive lesions for the restoration of hemodynamic function. However, surgery with or without combination chemotherapy has been shown to prolong life in patients with primary sarcomas of the heart (1) and is currently routinely performed.

In a recent report of surgical treatment for a large series of cardiac tumors (102 benign and 12 malignant), the operative survival was 91 percent: operative survival for primary cardiac malignancy was 83 percent and for metastatic malignancy, 68 percent (16). Of the 10 patients with primary malignant disease who survived surgery, mean survival for 7 was 9 months and 6, 17, and 54 months for the other 3 (16).

REFERENCES

1. Burke AP, Cowan D, Virmani R. Primary sarcomas of the heart. Cancer 1992;69:387–95.
2. Cates CU, Virmani R, Vaughn WK, Robertson RM. Electrocardiographic markers of cardiac metastasis. Am Heart J 1986;112:1297–303.
3. Colucci WS, Braunwald E. Primary tumors of the heart. In: Braunwald E, ed. Heart disease. A textbook of cardiovascular medicine. Philadelphia: WB Saunders, 1992:1451–64.
4. Dennis MA, Appareti K, Manco-Johnson ML, Clewell W, Wiggins J. The echocardiographic diagnosis of multiple fetal cardiac tumors. J Ultrasound Med 1985;4:327–93.
5. Flipse TR, Tazelaar HD, Holmes DR. Diagnosis of malignant cardiac disease by endomyocardial biopsy. Mayo Clin Proc 1990; 65:1415–22.
6. Freedberg RS, Kronzon I, Rumancik WM, Liebeskind D. The contribution of magnetic resonance imaging to the evaluation of intracardiac tumors diagnosed by echocardiography. Circulation 1988;77:96–103.
7. Fyke FE III, Seqard JB, Edwards WD, et al. Primary cardiac tumors: experience with 30 consecutive patients since the introduction of two-dimensional echocardiography. J Am Coll Cardiol 1985;5:1465–73.
8. Harvey WP. Clinical aspects of cardiac tumors. Am J Cardiol 1968;21:328–43.
9. Jack CM, Cleland J, Geddes JS. Left atrial rhabdomyosarcoma and the use of digital gated computed tomography in its diagnosis. Br Heart J 1986;55:305–7.
10. Jourdan M, Bataille R, Seguin J, Zhang XG, Chaptal PA, Klein B. Constitutive production of interleukin-6 and immunologic features in cardiac myxomas. Arthritis Rheum 1990;33:398–402.
11. Kirklin JW, Barratt-Boyes BG. Cardiac tumors. Morphology, diagnostic criteria, natural history, techniques, results, and indications. In: Cardiac surgery. JW Kirklin, BG Barratt-Boyes, eds. New York: John Wiley & Sons, 1986;1393–407.
12. Levine RA, Weyman AE, Dinsmore RE, et al. Noninvasive tissue characterization: diagnosis of lipomatous hypertrophy of the atrial septum by nuclear magnetic resonance imaging. J Am Coll Cardiol 1986;7:688–92.
13. Lund JT, Ehman RL, Julsrud PR, Sinak LJ, Tajik AJ. Cardiac masses: assessment by MR imaging. Am J Roentgenol 1989;152:469–73.
14. MacGregor GA, Cullen RA. The syndrome of fever, anemia and high sedimentation rate with an atrial myxoma. Br Med J 1959;2:991–6.
15. Mugge A, Daniel WG, Haverich A, Lichtlen PR. Diagnosis of noninfective cardiac mass lesions by two-dimensional echocardiography. Comparison of the transthoracic and transesophageal approaches. Circulation 1991;83:70–8.
16. Murphy MC, Sweeney MS, Putman JB Jr, et al. Surgical treatment of cardiac tumors: a 25-year experience. Ann Thorac Surg 1990;49:612–8.
17. Panidis IP, Kotler MN, Mintz GS, Ross J. Clinical and echocardiographic features of right atrial masses. Am Heart J 1984;107:745–58.
18. Salcedo EE, Cohen GI, White RD, Davison MB. Cardiac tumors: diagnosis and management. In: Current problems in cardiology. O'Rourke RA, McCall D, eds. St Louis:Mosby-Year Book, 1992;80–137.
19. Virmani R, Clark MA, Posey DM, McAllister HA. Right atrial myxoma causing pulmonary emboli and pulmonary hypertension. Am J Forensic Med Pathol 1982;3:249–52.
20. _____, Khedekar RR, Robinowitz M, McAllister HA. Tumor embolization in coronary artery causing myocardial infarction. Arch Path Lab Med 1983;107:243–5.

3
CARDIAC MYXOMA

Definition. Cardiac myxoma is a benign neoplasm of uncertain histogenesis that occurs exclusively on the endocardial surface, usually in the atrium near the fossa ovalis. The histologic diagnosis depends on finding typical cardiac myxoma cells in a myxoid background. Cardiac myxoma shares its name and the presence of a mucopolysaccharide matrix with myxomas of soft tissue. However, the cardiac myxoma cell is histologically and histogenetically distinct from spindle cells of soft tissue myxomas.

Incidence. Cardiac myxomas account for approximately 50 percent of all primary cardiac tumors, and in surgical series for 75 to 80 percent of cardiac tumors. They are nevertheless rare, because primary cardiac tumors of all types occur in about 0.001 to 0.03 percent of autopsy cases (see chapter 1).

Histogenesis. There is a long history of debate concerning the histogenesis of cardiac myxomas. The theory that they are peculiar organizing thrombi or reactive lesions was first put forth over 100 years ago, and even today this theory receives some support (41,48). The current prevailing opinion, one that we share, is that myxoma is a true neoplasm and not a thrombus (33). Myxomas rarely if ever occur in regions of the heart that predispose to thrombus formation, namely the atrial appendages and ventricular apices. There is a subset of histologically typical myxomas that embolize to distant arterial sites, and, unlike thrombi, extend into the arterial wall forming aneurysms. Chromosomal abnormalities have been found in some cardiac myxomas, which suggest that myxomas are neoplasms rather than reactive proliferations (18,51). Myxomas occur as a constellation of inherited conditions in the myxoma syndrome in young individuals who have no predisposition to thrombosis. Cell cultures of myxomas result in a mixture of mononuclear and multinuclear polygonal cells similar to those of the original tumor, whereas cultures of organized thrombi are overgrown by fibroblasts (55).

The second facet of the debate regarding cardiac myxoma is the nature of the cell of origin.

There have been many attempts to identify the cellular derivation by immunohistochemical means (5,14,23,24,28–30,38,39,49,55). These studies have led to conflicting theories, partly because of discrepant results and partly because of the interpretation of the significance of positive staining for a given antigen. It has been suggested that myxomas are endothelial, epithelial, smooth muscle, and even neuroendocrine tumors, based on positivity for a variety of cellular markers. A current, widely held theory combines these discrepancies by postulating that the cell of origin is a pluripotential cell capable of many types of differentiation (33,54). Cells of the embryonic endocardial cushion ultrastructurally resemble myxoma cells and may represent myxoma precursors (see chapter 1) (36). The term "subendothelial vasoform reserve cells" has been used to designate these cells (54). A histologic study of normal endocardial tissue of the fossa ovalis has demonstrated minute proliferations of endothelial cells resembling the vascular structures of myxomas (43). The stimulus for persistence and proliferation of these cells along many cell lines, including the glandular structures present in some myxomas, is unknown. A theory has been advanced that the glandular structures occasionally present in cardiac myxoma (see below) are related to endodermal rests budding from foregut tissues (28). These foregut structures are also thought to represent precursors of cystic tumors of the atrioventricular nodal region. However, glandular structures are rare components of myxoma; therefore, this theory is not a comprehensive explanation for the histogenesis of myxoma. Whatever the etiology of cardiac myxoma, there is likely a genetic influence resulting in cases of familial myxoma. Undoubtedly the debate concerning the histogenesis of myxoma, which is far from over (29), will continue until the molecular basis for the development of myxoma is discovered. At this time, the best evidence supports the concept that myxomas are true neoplasms, derived from a primitive cell which resides in the fossa ovalis and surrounding endocardium.

Clinical Features. *Patient Characteristics.* Myxomas occur more often in women than men, but the degree of female predominance is unclear. The female to male ratio is close to 3 to 1 in some series (1,16), and approximately 1 to 1 in others (8,35). The average patient age at presentation is 50 years; 90 percent of patients are 30 to 60 years of age. Myxomas, especially sporadic myxomas, rarely occur in children under age 10, although there have been reports of myxomas occurring in infants (12,61). In some pediatric cases, the histologic appearance is more consistent with a myxoid sarcoma than a myxoma (12). There may be a lesser incidence in blacks than in whites (35), but an imbalance in racial distribution was not found in a recent series (8).

Symptoms. Patients have such a variety of symptoms that myxoma could be termed a "great masquerader." Although the diagnosis can be easily made with imaging studies, some patients are symptomatic for long periods before the diagnosis is clinically considered (8). There is a symptom triad consisting of constitutional symptoms, sequelae of valvular obstruction, and embolic phenomena (35). Constitutional symptoms include fever, malaise, and weight loss, and are associated with laboratory abnormalities such as anemia, increased sedimentation rate, and hypergammaglobulinemia. Although constitutional symptoms and laboratory abnormalities are not typically the initial problems that lead to the diagnosis, they occur in most patients during the course of illness (42). Obstruction of the mitral valve by myxoma leads to a clinical syndrome similar to chronic rheumatic mitral valve disease. Embolic myxomas lead to ischemia of extremities, viscera, or brain (53,61). In most series of cardiac myxomas, symptoms of mitral stenosis are more common than those of embolic phenomena (32,35,53,61).

It is best to consider right-sided and left-sided myxomas separately when considering clinical manifestations. Of the 83 patients with left atrial myxoma referred to the Armed Forces Institute of Pathology (AFIP) since the writing of the last Fascicle, 35 percent presented with embolic phenomena, 22 percent presented with symptoms of mitral stenosis, and in 19 percent, the myxoma was an incidental finding. Less common modes of presentation were cardiac arrhythmias (10 percent), sudden unexpected death (4 percent), chest pain or angina (4 percent), syncope (4 percent), and fever of unknown origin (one patient).

Myxoma emboli to the brain may cause strokes, transient ischemic attacks, seizures, or hemianopsia. Emboli to iliac arteries and distal vessels cause claudication, gangrene, or Lariche's syndrome if located at the iliac bifurcation. Renal emboli result in renal failure, hematuria, or, rarely, rhabdomyolysis.

Typical symptoms of mitral stenosis result from pulmonary hypertension and include dyspnea, orthopnea, and fatigue. Sudden death occurs either because of coronary embolization of tumor fragments or sudden obstruction of the mitral valve orifice. Patients with left atrial myxoma may have supraventricular tachycardias, and, infrequently, atrial flutter and fibrillation. Tumors found incidentally during life are discovered because of heart murmurs, an enlarged cardiac silhouette on chest X ray, or a filling defect during cardiac catheterization for coronary artery disease.

Right atrial myxomas are less frequently symptomatic than those on the left. Of the last 22 cases in the AFIP files, the largest group (41 percent) was discovered incidentally at X ray, auscultation, or autopsy; one of these was in a patient with multiple nevi and the myxoma syndrome (see below). Twenty-three percent of patients presented with syncope, 18 percent with ankle edema or Budd-Chiari syndrome, and 14 percent with pulmonary embolism. One patient presented with sick sinus syndrome. Anemia, weight loss, hypergammaglobulinemia, and bacterial endocarditis occurred with similar frequency in right- and left-sided tumors. One patient with an unsuspected tumor at autopsy had evidence of chronic embolic pulmonary hypertension; long-term severe pulmonary hypertension has been rarely described in patients with right atrial myxoma (25,60).

Auscultatory Findings. Initial auscultatory findings are normal in up to half of patients, even if performed by a cardiologist (8). Abnormal findings include systolic ejection murmur, holosystolic murmur of mitral insufficiency, diastolic murmur of mitral stenosis, loud S1, opening click, loud S2, S4, tumor "plop," and to-and-fro murmurs.

Clinical Differential Diagnosis. Clinically, left atrial myxoma must be differentiated from mitral stenosis, which is usually rheumatic in origin.

Unlike myxoma, rheumatic mitral disease commonly results in atrial enlargement with atrial fibrillation or flutter. Also in the clinical differential diagnosis of cardiac myxoma is subacute bacterial endocarditis, which, unlike myxoma, is often associated with splenomegaly. Cases of infected myxoma are especially difficult to clinically diagnose and require careful imaging studies to distinguish vegetations from tumor. The aneurysms of polyarteritis nodosa can radiographically resemble those caused by embolic myxoma, and the constitutional symptoms of both entities can overlap.

Recurrence and Clinical Course. Approximately 2 percent of cardiac myxomas recur after surgical excision. In a compilation of a series of 20 or more cardiac myxomas with long-term follow-up (4,17,32,40,56), the recurrence rate was 12 of 630 (1.9 percent). The sites of recurrence within the heart are often distant from the site of the original tumor, indicating that recurrence is not usually related to incomplete excision. Patients with recurrent tumors are younger at age of presentation than patients with tumors that do not recur (8), and are more likely to have the myxoma syndrome (see below).

The existence of "malignant" cardiac myxoma is controversial (47). From series of cardiac myxomas with follow-up data (4,17,32,40,56), there were two cases of sudden death, one death related to multiple recurrences, and only one case of possible "malignant transformation" (4) in 630 patients. We agree with a recent review (47) that malignant myxomas have been over-reported and many are myxoid sarcomas that have been misdiagnosed as myxoma (3).

Embolic myxomas have the capacity to grow into the arterial wall in embolic sites, resulting in skin lesions (44) and fusiform cerebral aneurysms that are discovered on angiography (6,7,15,22,46,57). Long-term clinical follow-up in many patients with embolic myxoma is lacking, but these aneurysms can cause symptoms after removal of the primary tumor (46). Embolic myxomas can persist as aneurysms in cerebral vessels or as nodules in pulmonary arteries for months or even years after excision of the primary tumor, or may regress. There are two convincing reports with adequate histologic confirmation of embolic cardiac myxoma with bony deposits that resemble benign myxoma (47,52). However, these lesions did not cause the death of the patient and disseminated tumor was not present. Because embolic myxomas do not have the histologic characteristics of malignant neoplasms, and do not cause tumor deposits in viscera or lymph nodes, we do not interpret these deposits as true metastases.

Myxoma Syndrome. Most cases of cardiac myxoma are sporadic; in less than 5 percent of patients there is a familial history of atrial tumors and extracardiac lesions. In 1980, Atherton et al. (2) described a patient with skin pigmentation, neurofibromas, and cardiac myxomas; this was designated NAME syndrome (nevi, atrial myxoma, myxoid neurofibroma, ephelides). The association between cardiac myxoma and adrenal cortical hyperplasia was made in 1982 in Europe (50), at which time the familial nature of the syndrome was noted. In 1984, the acronym was modified to LAMB (lentigines, atrial myxoma, mucocutaneous myxomas, blue nevi), when it was recognized that the myxoid skin lesions were better classified as myxomas than myxoid neurofibromas (45). One year later, Carney et al. (9) defined the myxoma syndrome as the constellation of skin pigmentation, Sertoli cell tumors of the testis, cutaneous myxoma, myxoid fibroadenoma of the breast, adrenal cortical hyperplasia, and pituitary hyperactivity (gigantism). Several recent reports have confirmed these associations (11,34,37,59). Recently, psammomatous melanotic schwannoma (10,58) has been added to the list of associated entities. The genetic mode of transmission of myxoma syndrome has not been determined, but autosomal dominant transmission is favored in most cases (19). It has been shown by several investigators that familial cardiac myxomas are more often multiple, recurrent, and right sided than sporadic myxomas. In the largest series of cases of myxoma syndrome, the female to male predominance was similar to sporadic cases (9), although a male predominance has been reported (16). On the average, the patients are 20 to 27 years younger than those with sporadic myxoma, with a mean age of approximately 25 years. Screening two-dimensional echocardiography has been recommended for first-degree relatives of patients with cardiac myxoma, particularly for relatives of younger patients with right-sided or bilateral tumors (19). There are several reports of cardiac myxoma diagnosed by echocardiography in asymptomatic relatives, one found in an individual with a normal echocardiogram 1 year earlier (8,19).

Radiologic Diagnosis. The first premortem diagnosis of cardiac myxoma occurred with the use of cardiac catheterization. However, this technique is not particularly safe for left atrial masses because of the risk of peripheral embolization due to dislodgement of the tumor or of a thrombus. Also, false positive results may occur in cases of thrombi of the left atrium. Unless there is significant mitral regurgitation, pulmonary artery injections with left atrial follow-through or transseptal catheterization is required for diagnosis by cardiac catheterization.

If coronary angiography is performed in a patient with cardiac myxoma, a vascular tumor blush may be demonstrated (8). If right heart catheterization is performed, moderate pulmonary hypertension is noted in about one third of patients. Carotid injections performed in patients with cerebral symptoms occasionally demonstrate fusiform aneurysms that are characteristic of embolic myxoma.

Two-dimensional echocardiography is considered nearly 100 percent sensitive for diagnosing cardiac myxoma (8). It provides information regarding tumor size, attachment, and location, and facilitates in the differentiation of left atrial thrombi from myxomas, since the latter have areas of echolucency. The typical echocardiographic finding in cardiac myxoma is an atrial lesion attached to the interatrial septum which moves with diastole, usually through the atrioventricular valve. Calcification, which occurs more often in right-sided myxomas, can occasionally be identified. Mitral or tricuspid insufficiency is uncommon, except for trace degrees noted on color flow Doppler techniques.

There are rare cases of myxomas missed by two-dimensional echocardiography. In addition, the distinction between myxoma and thrombus, myxoma and interatrial lipomatous hypertrophy, and myxoma and vegetation is not always possible. Transesophageal echocardiography is useful, and often superior to transthoracic echoardiography, for resolution of tumor attachment and visualization of right atrial tumors.

Computerized tomography (CT) and magnetic resonance imaging (MRI) with gating are capable of precise localization, and are helpful in the distinction between fat and other tissue, and

between circumscribed and infiltrative processes. In typical cases, however, two-dimensional echocardiography is sufficient preoperatively, and angiography is performed to determine coronary sufficiency in older patients.

The radiologic distinction between cardiac myxoma and cardiac sarcoma is not always possible. Many types of cardiac sarcoma can be found in the left atrium, and sarcomas can, like myxoma, be attached to the atrial wall by a stalk. Infiltrative growth is more common in sarcomas than myxoma. When this feature is identified using MRI or CT, sarcoma should be favored over myxoma. In a series of cardiac sarcomas at the AFIP, nearly 50 percent of those arising in the left atrium were initially clinically and radiologically diagnosed as myxoma. Furthermore, several of these were misdiagnosed as myxomas pathologically, because of myxoid areas, and the true diagnosis suspected only upon recurrence.

Gross Findings. Seventy-five percent of cardiac myxomas are cavitary left atrial masses attached to the fossa ovalis (Table 3-1). Right atrial myxomas, which represent most of the remainder, are less often attached to the fossa ovalis, although this is still the most common location. About 5 percent of cardiac myxomas grow on both sides of the fossa and are biatrial tumors that form a single mass. A small proportion of cardiac myxomas are truly multiple. These rare examples, which are typical of the myxoma syndrome, often occur in sites other than the fossa ovalis in both atria, and occasionally in the ventricles. Single myxomas occurring in the right or left ventricles are distinctly rare, as are myxomas attached to the atrioventricular valves or chordae tendineae.

Cardiac myxomas are attached to the interatrial septum by either a broad base or a narrow pedicle. Broad-based lesions may be more friable and prone to embolism than pedunculated ones. Cardiac myxoma varies from a gelatinous mass with frond-like excrescences that are likely to embolize (figs. 3-1–3-3) to a tumor with a smooth, firm surface that is unlikely to embolize (figs. 3-4–3-6). There are often organized thrombi on the surface. On cut section, tumors are variegated in appearance, and may contain gritty calcified areas. Although small cysts are occasionally noted on gross inspection, myxoma rarely presents as a cystic endocardial mass (27).

Table 3-1

CARDIAC MYXOMA: SITES IN 114 CASES*

Chamber	Total (%)	Specific Site	Number	Recurrences
Left atrium	83 (73%)	Fossa ovalis	73	
		Multiple sites	4	1
		Anterior MV**	2	
		Roof of atrium	3	
		Medial commissure, MV	1	1
Right atrium	22 (19%)	Fossa ovalis	16	
		Multiple sites	3	
		Right lateral wall	1	
		Right atrial appendage	1	
		Coronary sinus	1	
Biatrial	2 (2%)	Fossa ovalis	2	
Left ventricle	2 (2%)	Inflow beneath MV	1	
		Unknown	1	
Right ventricle	2 (2%)	Septal leaflet TV	1	
		RVOT	1	1
Multiple chambers	3 (3%)	LV and RV	1	
		LA, RA, MV	1	1
		LV, LA	1	1

*Adapted from reference 8.
**MV = mitral valve; LA = left atrium; LV = left ventricle; RVOT = right ventricular outflow tract;
RA = right atrium; RV = right ventricle; TV = tricuspid valve.

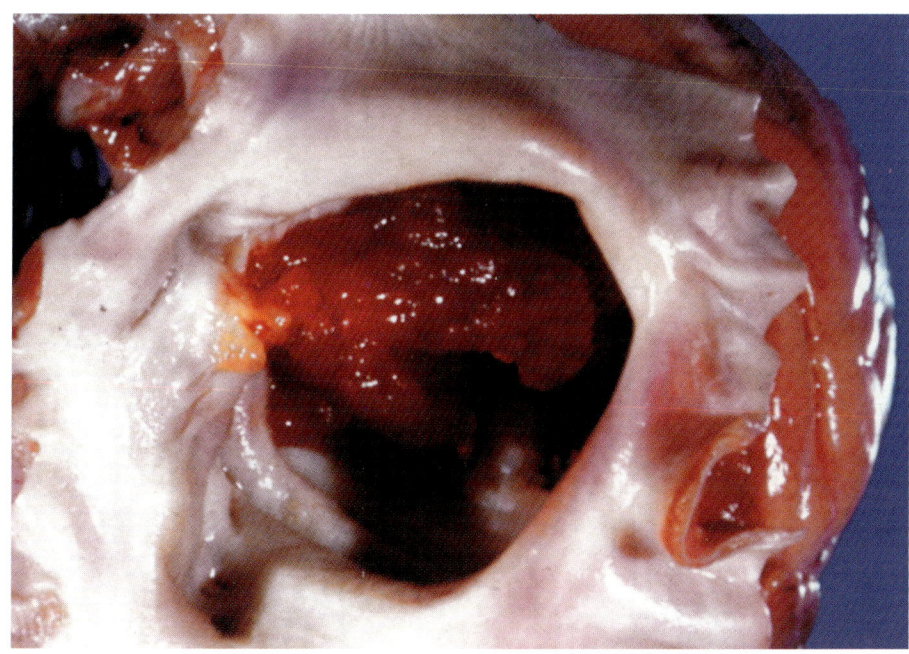

Figure 3-1
CARDIAC MYXOMA
A gelatinous tumor is attached by a narrow pedicle to the atrial septum. The myxoma has an irregular surface and nearly fills the left atrium.

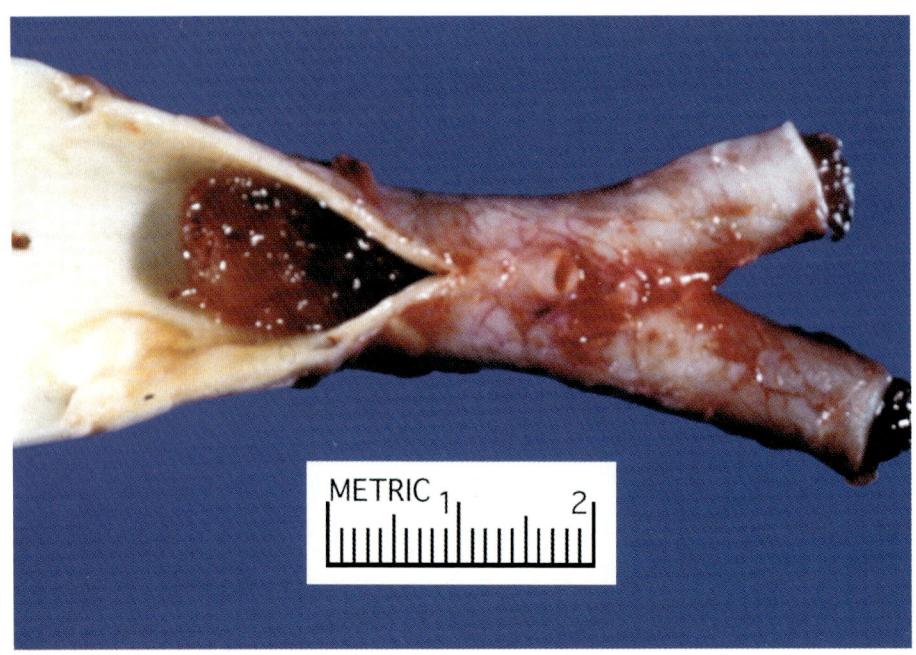

Figure 3-2
MYXOMA EMBOLUS: ILIAC BIFURCATION
An embolized fragment of the tumor illustrated in figure 3-1.

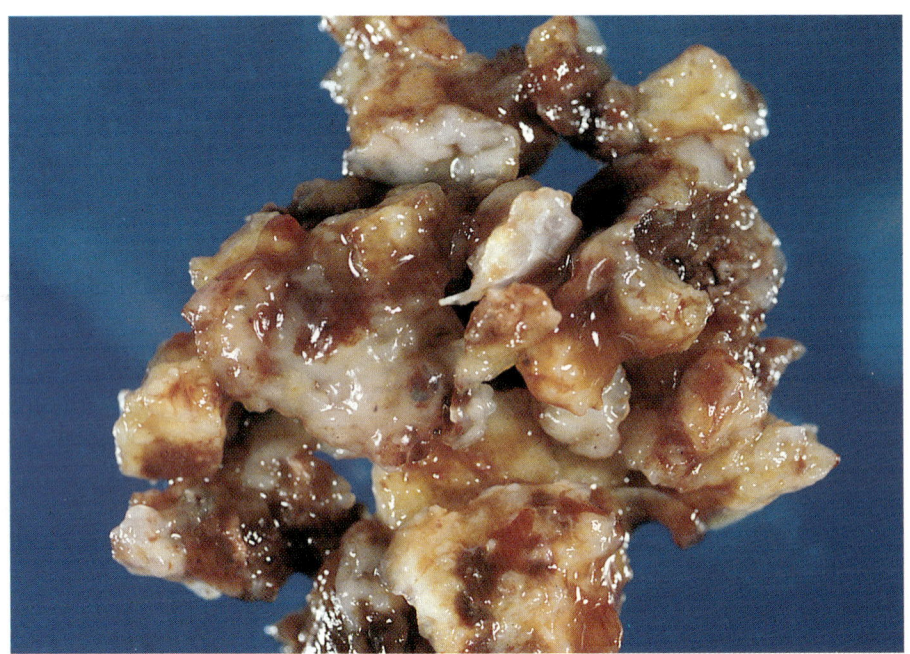

Figure 3-3
CARDIAC MYXOMA
A 71-year-old man had transient ischemic attacks; transesophageal echocardiogram showed a left atrial mass. Note the irregular surface, a feature associated with embolism.

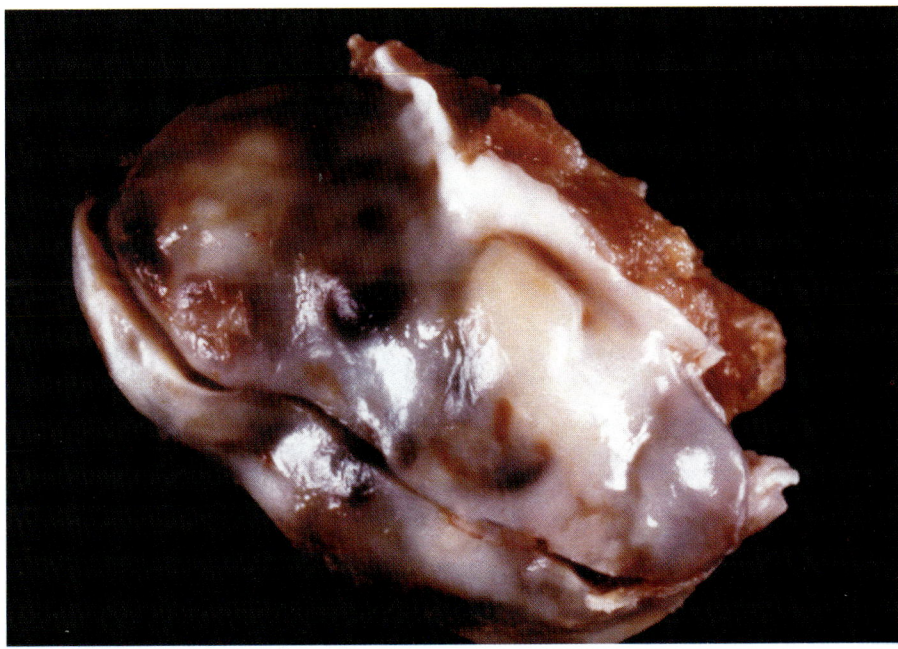

Figure 3-4
CARDIAC MYXOMA
A resected specimen of right atrial myxoma with a smooth surface and a portion of the atrial septum. The patient was a 73-year-old woman with congestive heart failure.

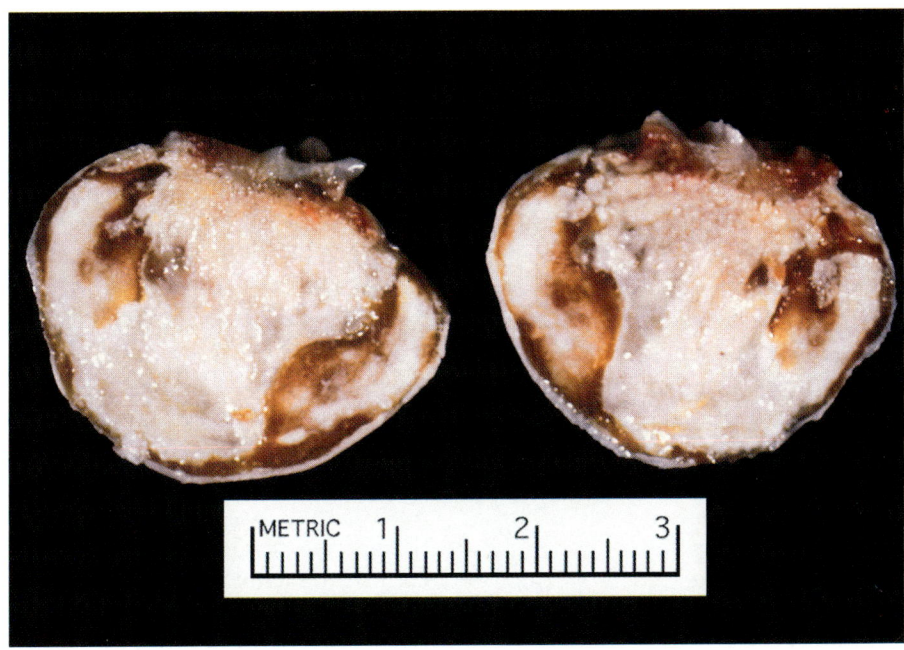

Figure 3-5
CARDIAC MYXOMA
There was a calcified right atrial mass on the X ray of a 47-year-old man. Resection demonstrated a smooth-surfaced tumor. The gritty material seen microscopically on cut section was calcified and ossified myxoma.

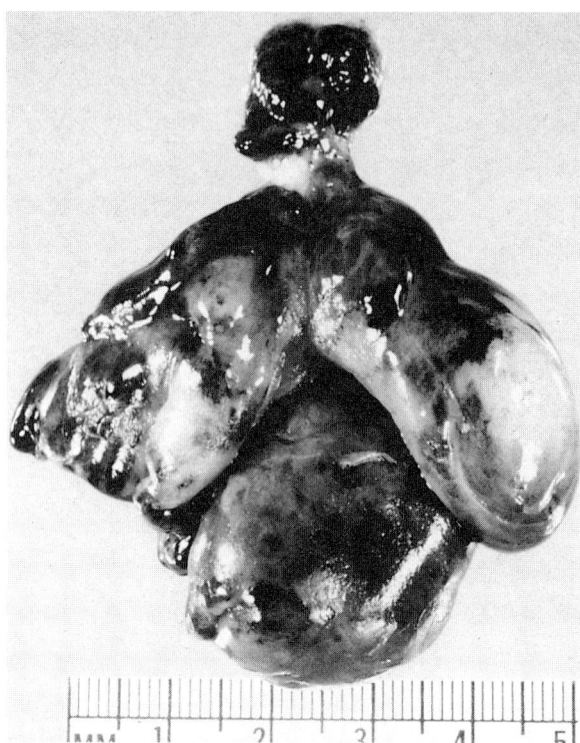

Figure 3-6
CARDIAC MYXOMA
A 58-year-old woman with supraventricular tachycardia and a smooth-surfaced left atrial myxoma. The tumor was completely excised with a stalk and a portion of interatrial septum. In contrast to the tumors in figures 3-4 and 3-5, the stalk is narrow.

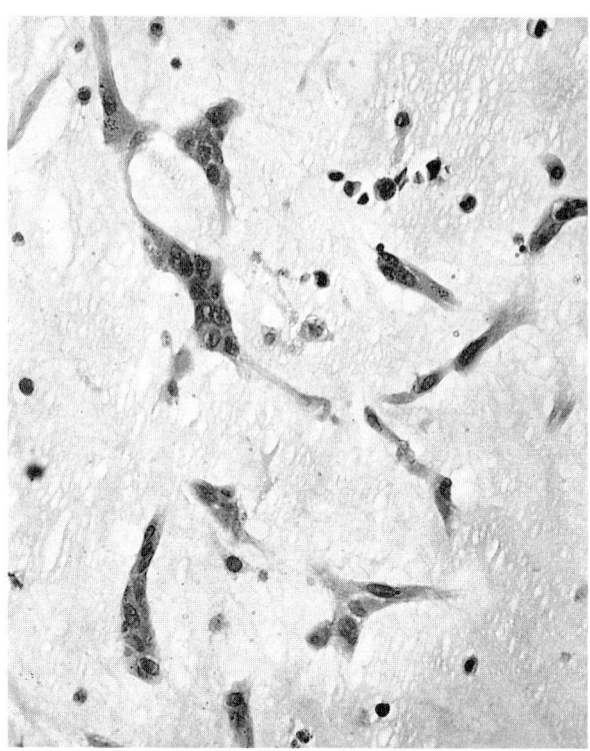

Figure 3-7
CARDIAC MYXOMA
Myxoma cells appear as short cords or syncytia embedded in a myxoid matrix.

Microscopic Findings. The microscopic diagnosis of cardiac myxoma depends on the identification of the myxoma cell, which has occasionally been called "lepidic cell." The classic myxoma cell possesses an oval nucleus with an open chromatin pattern and inconspicuous nucleoli (fig. 3-7), and is different from the tapered, spindled cell of soft tissue myxomas. The myxoma cell has abundant eosinophilic cytoplasm and indistinct cell borders, and may occur singly within a myxoid background, in which case the cytoplasmic outline has a stellate appearance. More often, myxoma cells form complex structures (fig. 3-8). The most common structure is a ring, one or several layers thick, surrounding a blood vessel, and often infiltrated by mononuclear inflammatory cells (figs. 3-9–3-11). The demarcation between the endothelium of the vessel and the myxoma cells is sometimes blurred, imparting the impression that the myx-

oma cells are derived from the vessel itself. Myxomas also form branching cords and tufts on the surface of the tumor (fig. 3-12). The surface tufts can be quite cellular (fig. 3-13), and rare mitotic figures occur near the surface of the tumor (fig. 3-14). Cellularity and mitotic activity, in our experience, are not related to recurrence.

The presence of a myxoid matrix rich in proteoglycans is variable, and is not diagnostic of myxoma but may be found in any intravascular neoplasm. Secondary changes of fibrosis, thrombosis, and calcification often obscure the underlying nature of the lesion (fig. 3-15). Hemosiderin-laden macrophages are virtually always present. Calcification is much more common than is appreciated radiographically, and is more prevalent in right-sided tumors. Fibrosis is more extensive in older patients, and symptoms in these patients are usually present for long periods. Other degenerative changes include ossification (fig. 3-16), which can include bone marrow, and gamna gandy bodies (fig. 3-17). The latter, which are identical to those

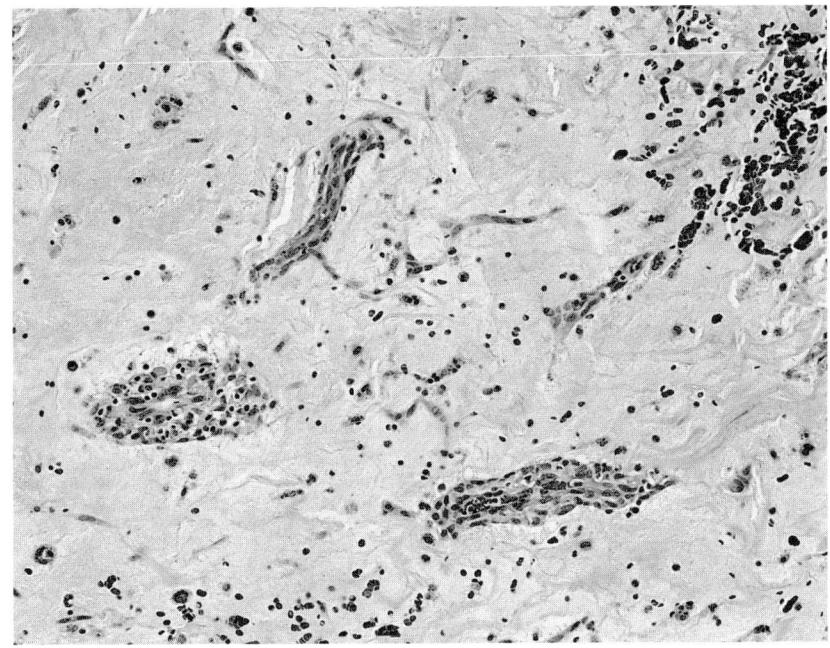

Figure 3-8
CARDIAC MYXOMA
Myxoma cells characteristically form multilayered rings around blood vessels and are often infiltrated by lymphocytes. Note hemosiderin-laden cells (upper right corner) that may be either macrophages or myxoma cells.

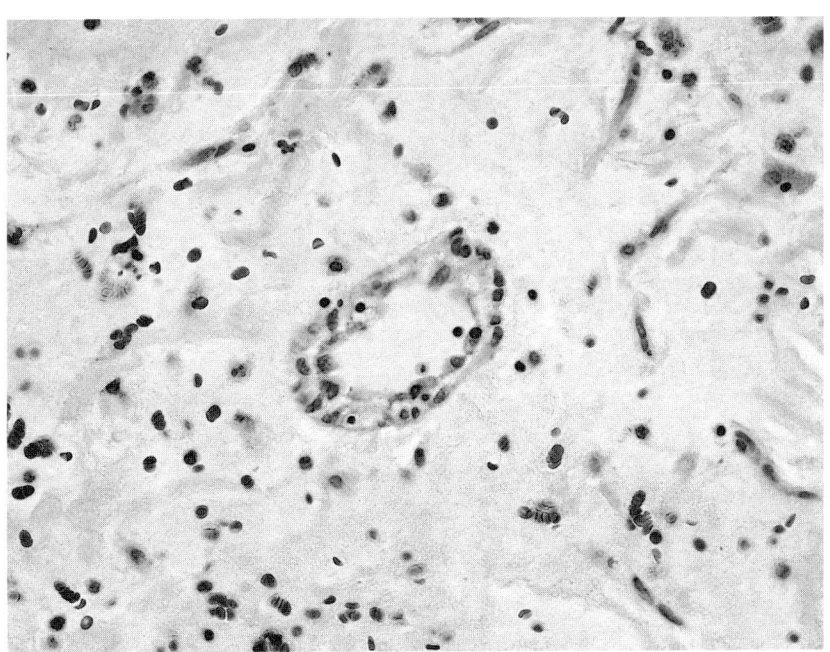

Figure 3-9
RING STRUCTURE, MYXOMA
In this example there are only two cell layers, and the distinction between endothelium and tumor cells is difficult to make.

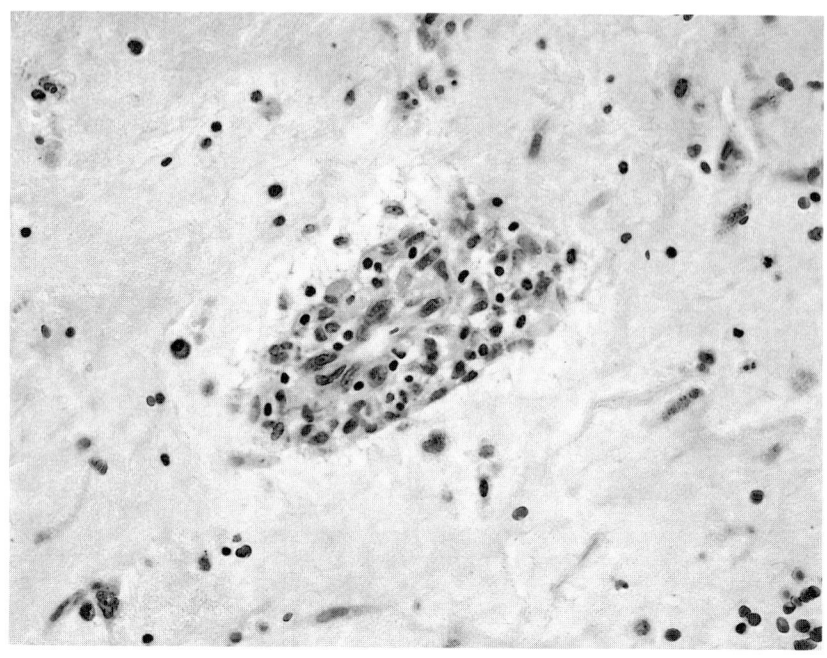

Figure 3-10
RING STRUCTURE, MYXOMA
Higher magnification of figure 3-8 shows more cell layers and a more pronounced inflammatory infiltrate.

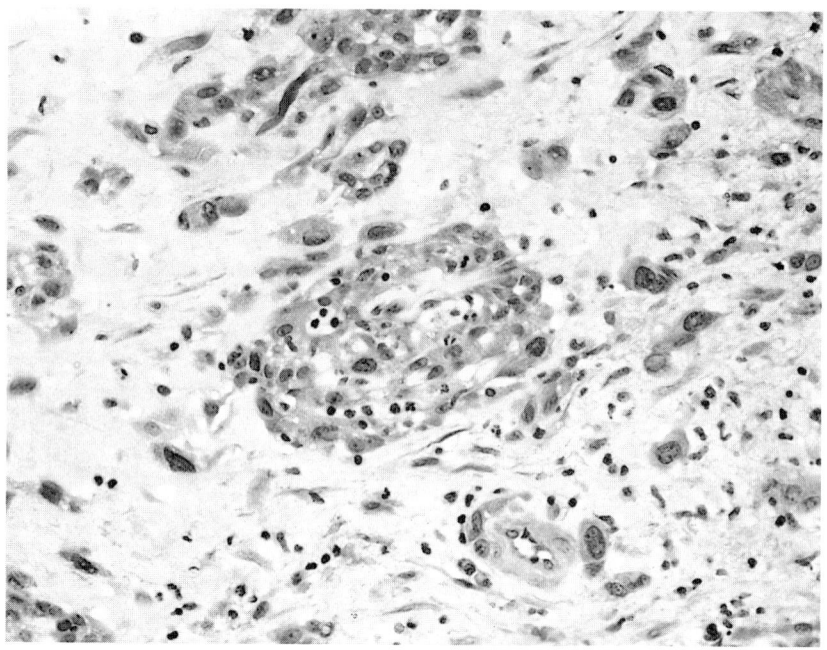

Figure 3-11
RING STRUCTURE, MYXOMA
There is mild cellular pleomorphism and atypia. In contrast to myxoid sarcoma, however, the characteristic cellular arrangement of myxoma is present and mitotic figures are absent.

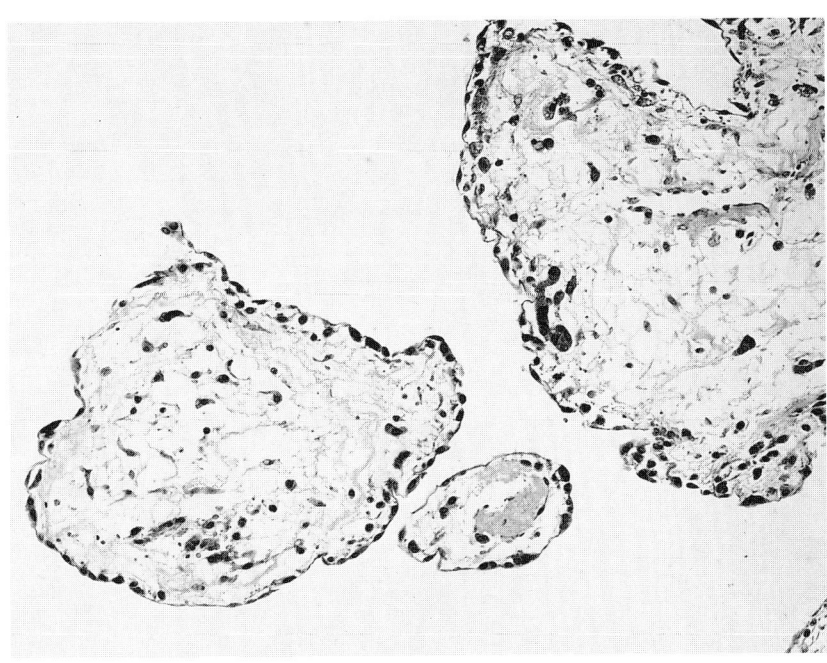

Figure 3-12
CARDIAC MYXOMA
Myxomas with irregular fronds on the surface are likely to embolize and occur in younger individuals.

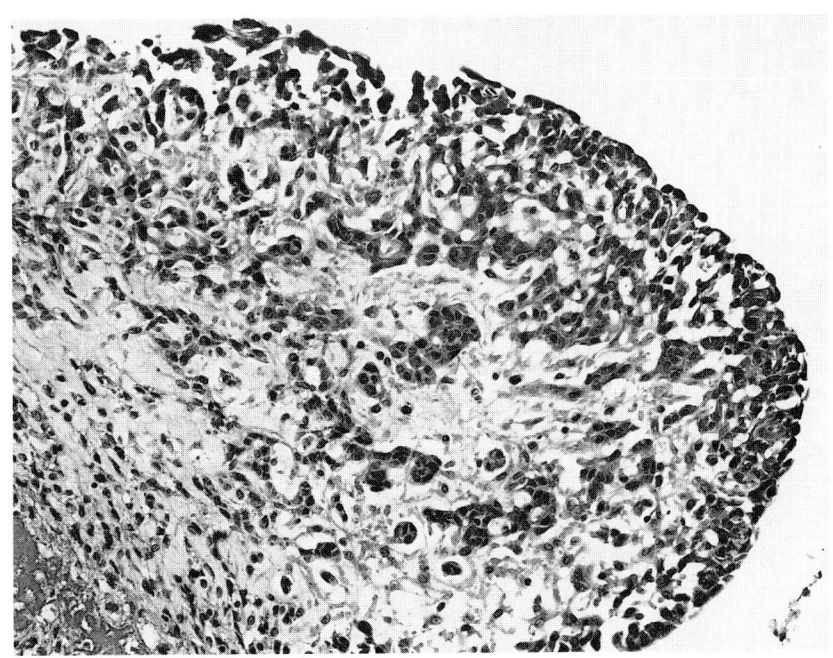

Figure 3-13
CARDIAC MYXOMA
There are cellular areas at the surface that are not indicative of recurrence or aggressive behavior.

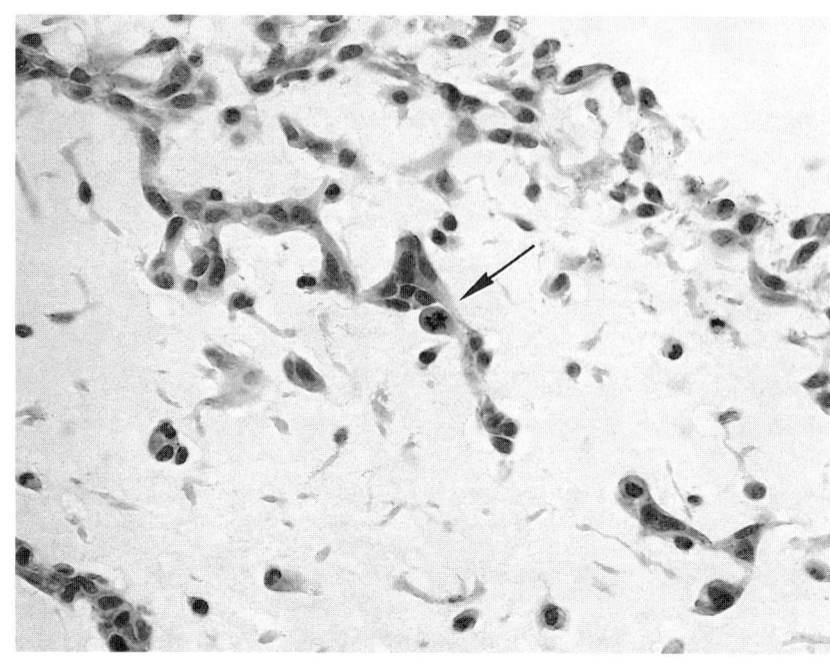

Figure 3-14
CARDIAC MYXOMA

Mitotic figures in myxoma are quite rare. They may occur near the tumor surface (arrow). (Figure 1 from Burke AP, Virmani R. Cardiac myxoma. A clinicopathologic study. Am J Clin Pathol 1993;100:671–80.)

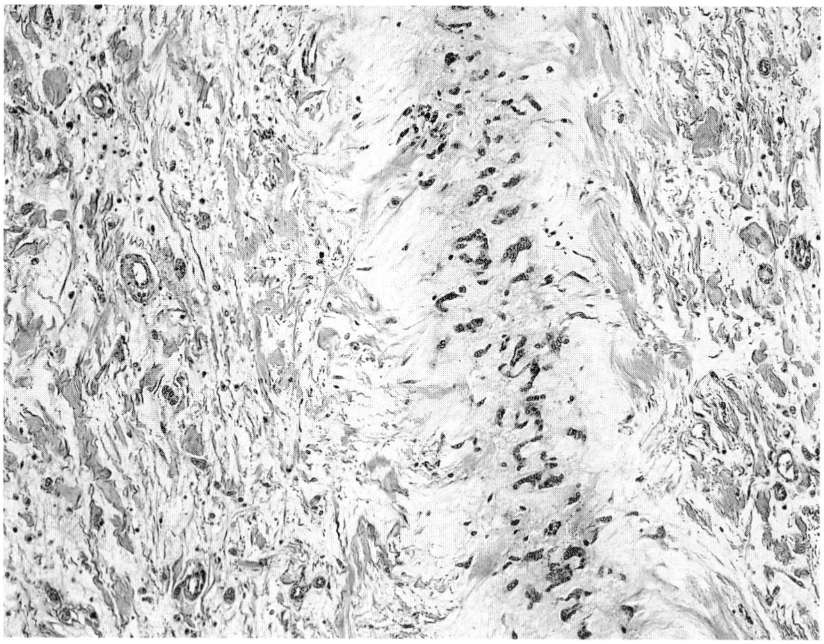

Figure 3-15
CARDIAC MYXOMA

Fibrosis is common. Note the central swath of myxoma cells within a myxoid matrix flanked by areas with collagen bundles. (Fig. 2 from Burke AP, Virmani R. Cardiac myxoma. A clinicopathologic study. Am J Clin Pathol 1993;100:671–80.)

seen in spleens from patients with sickle cell disease, may compose the majority of the tumor, explaining reports in the literature of so-called gamna body of the heart (13). Cardiac myxomas with extensive fibrosis are much less likely to embolize than those with predominantly myxoid backgrounds (8).

Mononuclear inflammatory infiltrates are common in cardiac myxomas and are focally aggregated, infiltrated within the ring structures of myxoma cells, or diffuse within the myxoid matrix. Occasionally, so-called mesothelial/monocytic incidental cardiac excrescences (MICE) occur on the surface of myxomas (see chapter 9). The junction

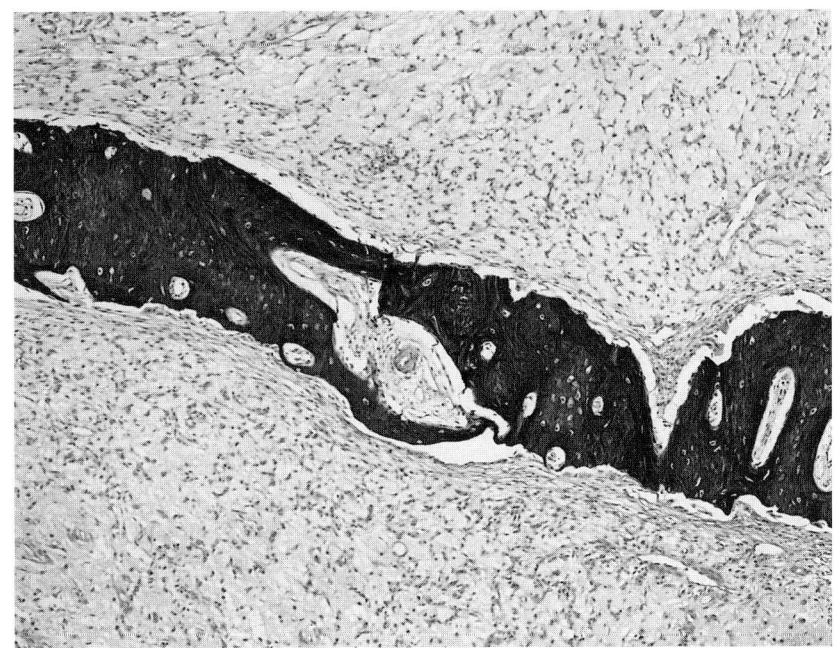

Figure 3-16
CARDIAC MYXOMA
WITH OSSIFICATION
Note central area of bone sur-
rounded by myxoma.

Figure 3-17
CARDIAC MYXOMA:
GAMNA BODIES
A peculiar form of fibrosis with deposition of iron pigment, identical to
that seen in the spleens of patients with
sickle cell anemia, is not uncommon in
myxoma.

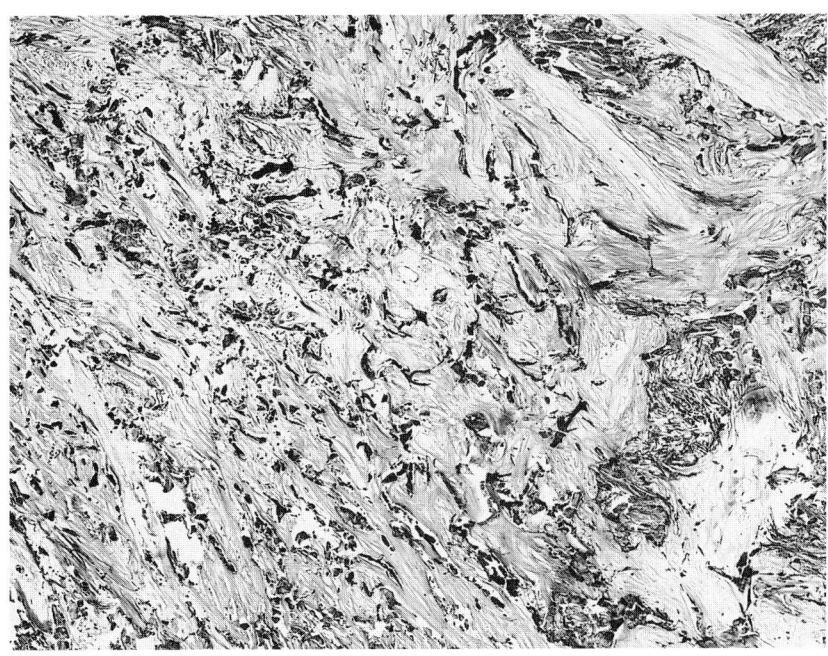

of the tumor and the interatrial septum is often
characterized by lymphoid aggregates with or
without germinal centers, smooth muscle bundles, occasional granuloma formation, and
prominent thick-walled vessels (fig. 3-18).

Extramedullary hematopoiesis is readily identified in about 7 percent of cases (fig. 3-19). The
significance of this finding is unknown. However,

extramedullary hematopoiesis is extremely rare
in tumors of adults, especially in patients without agnogenic myeloid metaplasia (31).

Approximately 1 percent of cardiac myxomas
contain glandular structures lined by mucin-laden
cells that resemble goblet cells of the gastrointestinal tract (figs. 3-20–3-22). The mucin is periodic
acid–Schiff (PAS) positive, diastase resistant,

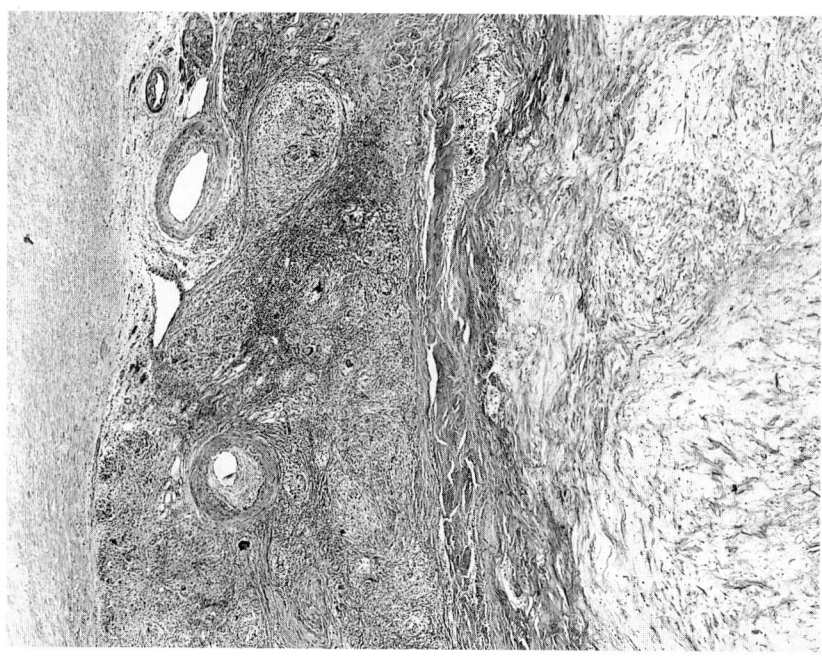

Figure 3-18
CARDIAC MYXOMA
Common features at the interface with the atrial septum include lymphoid aggregates, smooth muscle bundles, and thick walled vessels which angiographically may look like neovascularization.

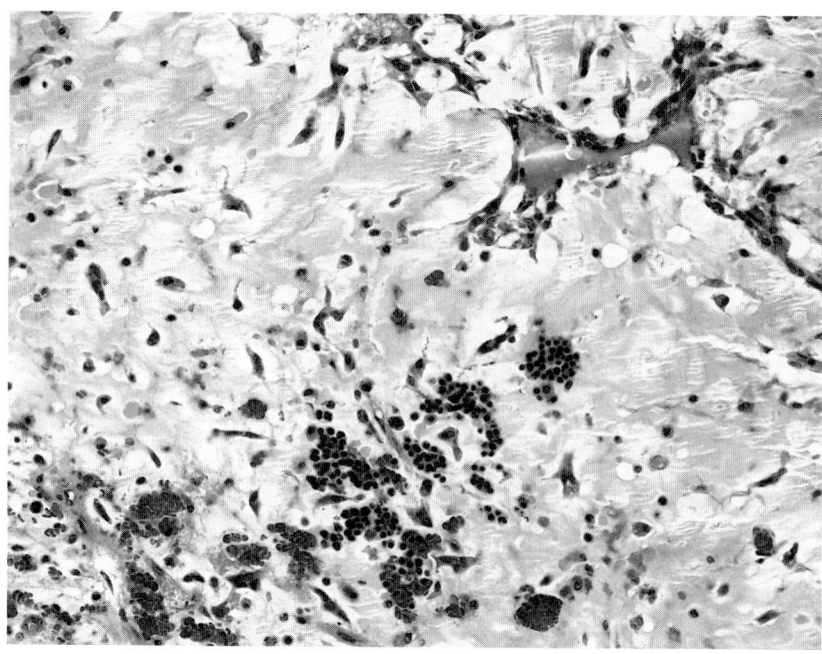

Figure 3-19
CARDIAC MYXOMA
The extramedullary hematopoiesis seen here is present in about 7 percent of cardiac myxomas.

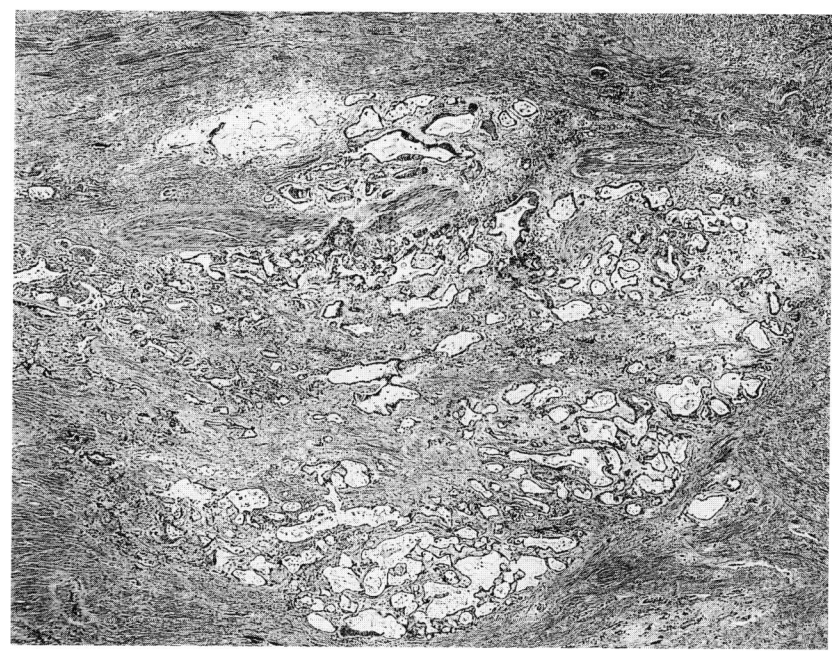

Figure 3-20
CARDIAC MYXOMA
Glandular structures are seen in less than 5 percent of cases. In this example, they were limited to the base of the myxoma.

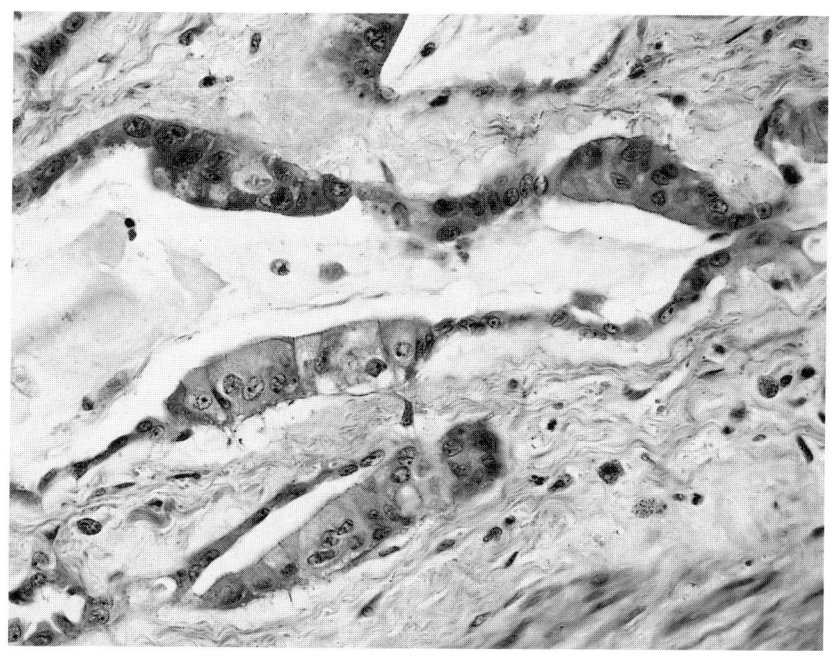

Figure 3-21
CARDIAC MYXOMA
In this higher magnification of figure 3-20 the glandular structures are lined by ciliated mucin-forming cells. (Fig. 4B from Burke AP, Virmani R. Cardiac myxoma. A clinicopathologic study. Am J Clin Pathol 1993;100:671–80.)

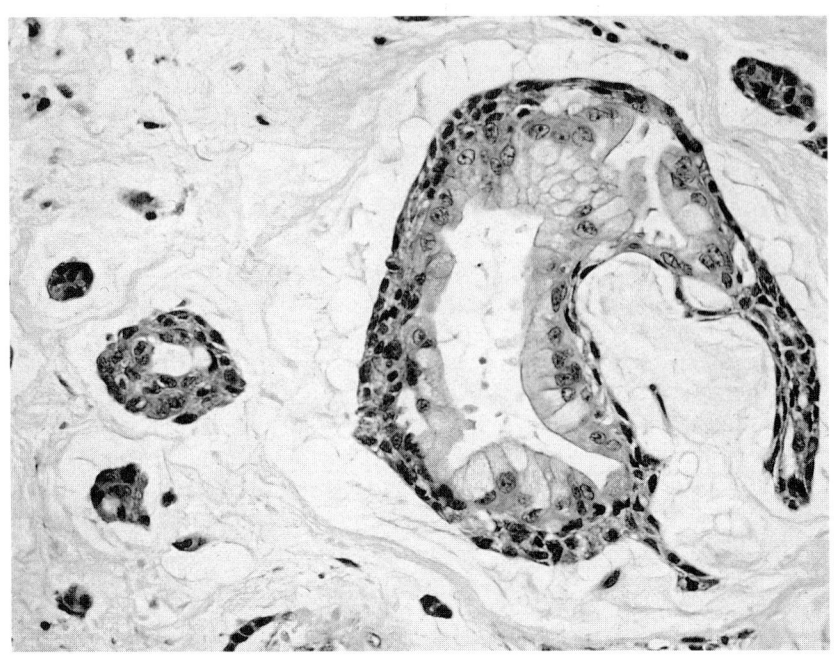

Figure 3-22
CARDIAC MYXOMA
In this myxoma, glandular structures compose the majority of the lesion. Typical myxoma nests merge imperceptibly with glands. The differential diagnosis includes metastatic carcinoma; however, atypia and mitoses are absent.

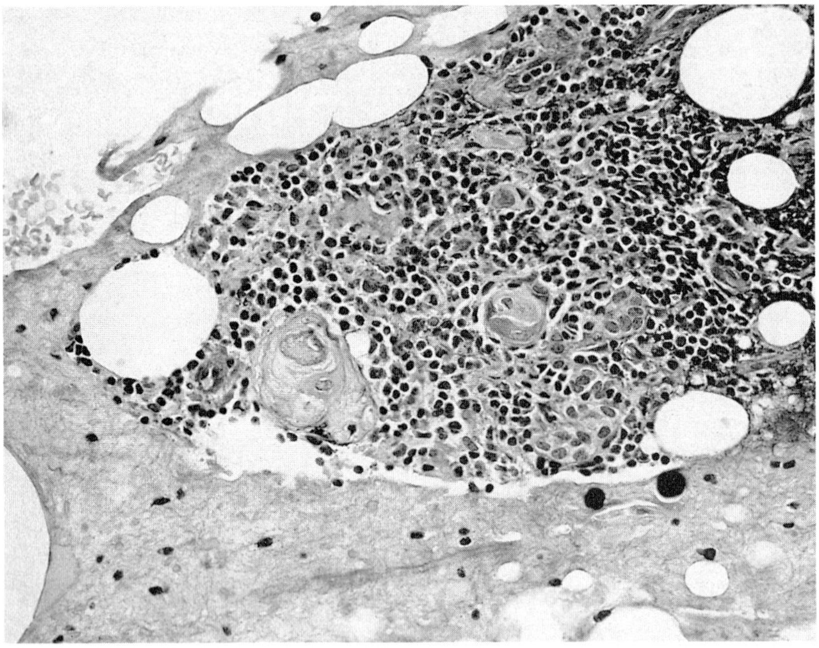

Figure 3-23
CARDIAC MYXOMA:
THYMIC REST
Structure resembling Hassall's corpuscle with lymphoid infiltrate is present within an otherwise typical myxoma.

and the glands stain for cytokeratin and carcinoembryonic antigen by immunohistochemical techniques. The differential diagnosis of myxoma with glandular structures includes metastatic carcinoma, but there is no nuclear anaplasia or mitotic activity within the glands of myxoma. The first reported glandular myxoma was diagnosed as cystic glandular heterotopia of the atrium (26), and

the myxomatous component mentioned descriptively. We have encountered thymic rests in a single case of cardiac myxoma that were present within the tumor itself (fig. 3-23).

Histopathology of Myxoma Emboli. The pathologist may receive a myxoid mass removed from a peripheral artery in a patient without a history of a cardiac mass. In most cases, typical

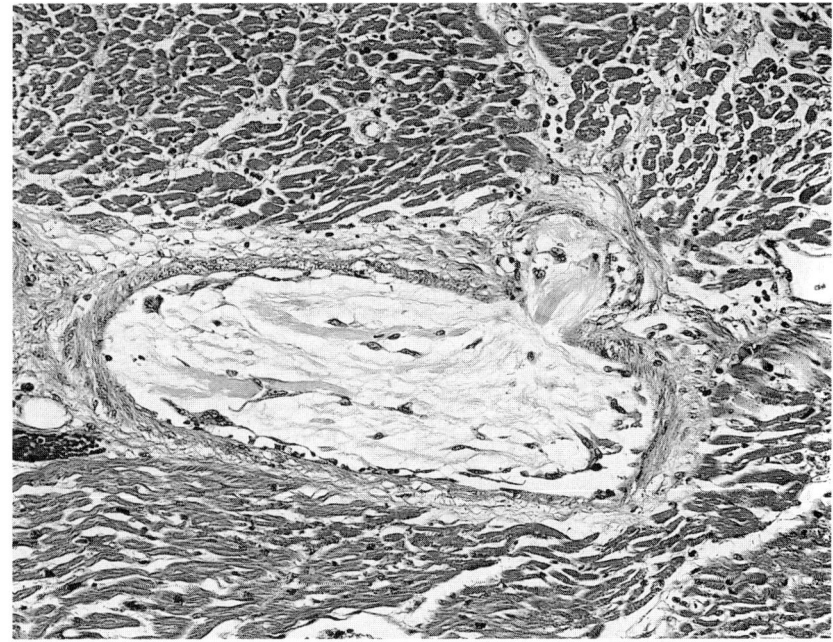

Figure 3-24
MYXOMA EMBOLUS
WITHIN INTRAMYOCARDIAL
CORONARY ARTERY
Histologic section of tumor illustrated in figure 3-1.

Figure 3-25
MYXOMA EMBOLUS:
PULMONARY ARTERY
Myxomas in the right atrium embolize less frequently than those in the left. Pulmonary embolism and chronic pulmonary hypertension can, however, occur.

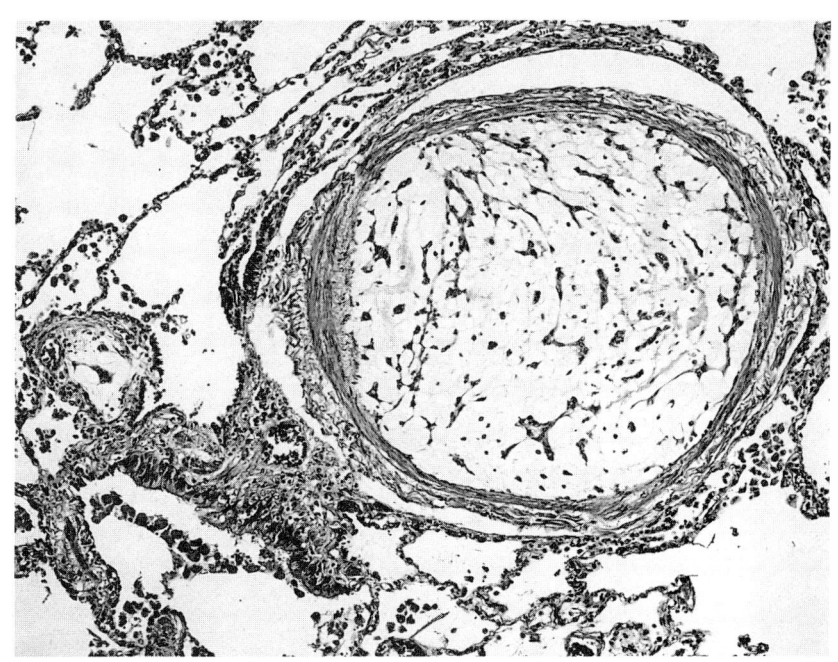

myxoma cells within a myxoid background are seen (figs. 3-24, 3-25), and an echocardiogram demonstrates an atrial tumor. However, myxomas can embolize in toto. Therefore, large embolic fragments with the histologic appearance of cardiac myxoma are best diagnosed as such, even if a subsequent echocardiogram is normal.

Histopathology of the Myxoma Syndrome. As mentioned above, extracardiac lesions in patients with the myxoma syndrome are lentigines of the skin, adrenal cortical hyperplasia, myxoid fibroadenomas (fig. 3-26), psammomatous melanotic schwannoma, and cutaneous myxomas (Table 3-2). Recurrent myxomas and those that

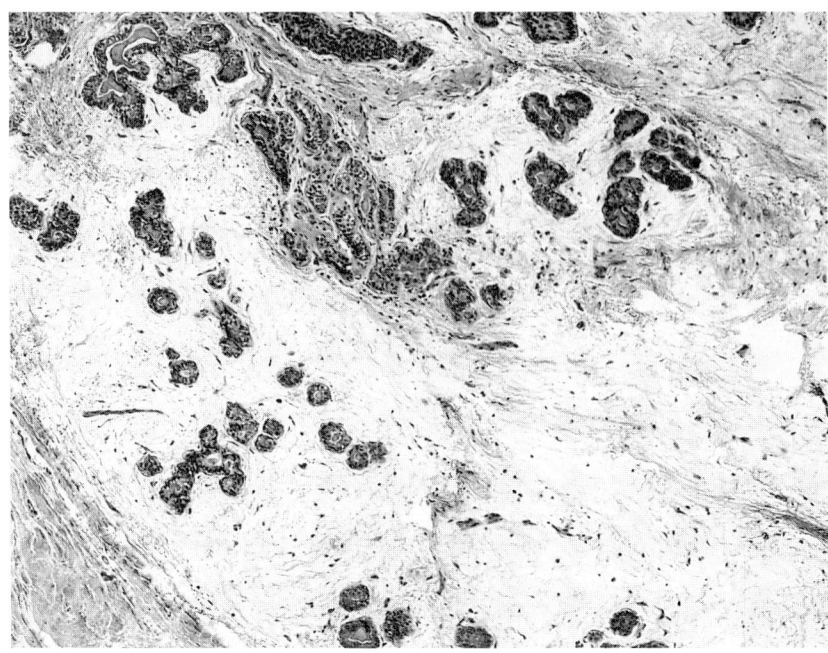

Figure 3-26
MYXOID FIBROADENOMA:
MYXOMA SYNDROME

A section of a breast mass removed from a young woman with recurrent myxomas and a family history of cardiac myxoma. (Fig. 9 from Burke AP, Virmani R. Cardiac myxoma. A clinicopathologic study. Am J Clin Pathol 1993;100:671–80.)

occur in the myxoma syndrome are usually diffusely myxoid with little fibrotic degenerative change, and are grossly friable and gelatinous.

Immunohistochemical Findings. In general, immunohistochemistry is of little use in the differential diagnosis of cardiac myxoma, but helps to explain its histogenesis. The immunohistochemical profile of these tumors has been debated (5,14,21,23,24,28–30,38,39,49,55), and a summary of the extensive publications on this subject is presented in a review (28) (Table 3-3). It has been reported that factor VIII–related antigen is uniformly positive (30,39) and uniformly negative (5,14) in cardiac myxoma. We believe that there is variable expression of surface cells: tumor cells are usually negative (fig. 3-27), although surface cells may be preferentially stained by endothelial markers. There is also disagreement about the expression of cytokeratins: we agree with several reports (24,49) that cytokeratin is generally absent except for rare glandular elements. Likewise, there is discrepancy regarding the detection of neural markers: S-100 protein has been reported as uniformly negative (8) and largely positive (29) in tumor cells, and other neural antigens, such as synaptophysin and neuron-specific enolase have been reported as positive (29). In our recent experience, we have found that S-100 protein is expressed in a subpopulation

Table 3-2

COMPONENTS OF THE MYXOMA SYNDROME

1. Skin and mucous membrane lesions
   Ephelides (spotty pigmentation/lentiginosis)
   Blue nevi
   Myxoma
2. Cardiac myxoma, often multiple or recurrent
3. Mammary myxofibroadenomas
4. Endocrine lesions
   Nodular adrenal cortical hyperplasia
   Acromegaly/pituitary adenomas
   Sertoli cell tumors, testis
   Psammomatous melanotic schwannoma

of myxoma cells in most tumors, but the significance of this finding is unclear. There is general, but not uniform agreement that myxoma cells express vimentin, but results of staining with antismooth muscle antigens have been variable (5,8,14,24). Myxoma cells are positive for nonspecific histiocytic markers, such as lysozyme, alpha-1-antichymotrypsin, and alpha-1-antitrypsin, but do not express specific markers for histiocytic differentiation, such as Kp-1 (CD68).

Table 3-3
IMMUNOHISTOCHEMICAL PROFILE OF CARDIAC MYXOMA

Antigen	General Results Myxoma Cells	Percent Positive*	Remarks
Cytokeratin	Negative	21%	Positive in glandular structures when present
Vimentin	Positive	88%	Generally diffusely positive
Endothelial markers			
Factor VIII	Variable	37%	Surface tumor cells preferentially positive;
UEA**	Variable	55%	capillaries always positive
CD34	Variable	80%	
Muscle markers			
Desmin	Negative	42%	Marked discrepancy among authors
SMA	Variable	50%	
Neural markers			
NSE	Variable	50%	
S-100 protein	Variable	54%	Marked discrepancy among authors
Synaptophysin	Variable	41%	
Histiocyte markers			
Kp-1	Negative	0%	
AAC	Positive	100%	Specificity of AAC is questionable

*From cases reported by Boxer (5), Burke and Virmani (8), Curschellas et al. (14), Govoni et al (24), Johansson (28), Krikler et al. (29), Landon et al. (30), McComb (38), Morales et al. (39), Schuger et al. (49), and Tanimura et al. (55).
**UEA = *Ulex europaeus*; SMA = smooth muscle actin; NSE = neuron-specific enolase; AAC = alpha-1-antichymotrypsin.

These contradictory immunohistochemical findings corroborate the concept that myxomas arise from primitive stromal cells that have the capacity to differentiate along many cell lines. However, the wide disagreement among various reports is difficult to explain fully.

Ultrastructural Findings. Ultrastructural studies of cardiac myxomas reflect the immunohistochemical findings, and demonstrate primitive mesenchymal cells (fig. 3-28) with variable numbers of intermediate filaments (fig. 3-29) and cytoplasmic organelles (20). The cells are present either as single or groups of stellate cells, as is evident by light microscopy. Typical myxomas have primitive tight intracellular junctions (fig. 3-30) but lack desmosomes. Definite evidence of smooth muscle cell or endothelial differentiation is lacking, and the cells are best characterized as pluripotent embryonic cells that occasionally show features of myofibroblasts. The ground substance contains fine electron-dense granules which have been described as identical to the proteoglycan granules seen in the ground substance of cartilage.

As mentioned above, there are rare myxomas that contain mucin-forming glands. Ultrastructural examination of such tumors has demonstrated true desmosomes, villi, and gland-like structures (23).

Differential Diagnosis. *Malignant Tumors.* Sarcomas of the heart often occur in the left atrium and can be extensively myxoid, so-called myxoid imitators (3). There have been several examples of recurrent left atrial sarcomas that were initially erroneously diagnosed, radiologically and histologically, as myxoma (61). Many of these tumors have chondroid differentiation, which is rarely, if ever, present in myxoma. Most importantly, myxoid sarcomas lack ovoid or polygonal myxoma cells that form rings and cords, but are composed of atypical spindled cells. Hemosiderin-laden macrophages are usually absent in sarcomas and plentiful in myxomas. With sufficient sampling of the lesion, areas diagnostic of

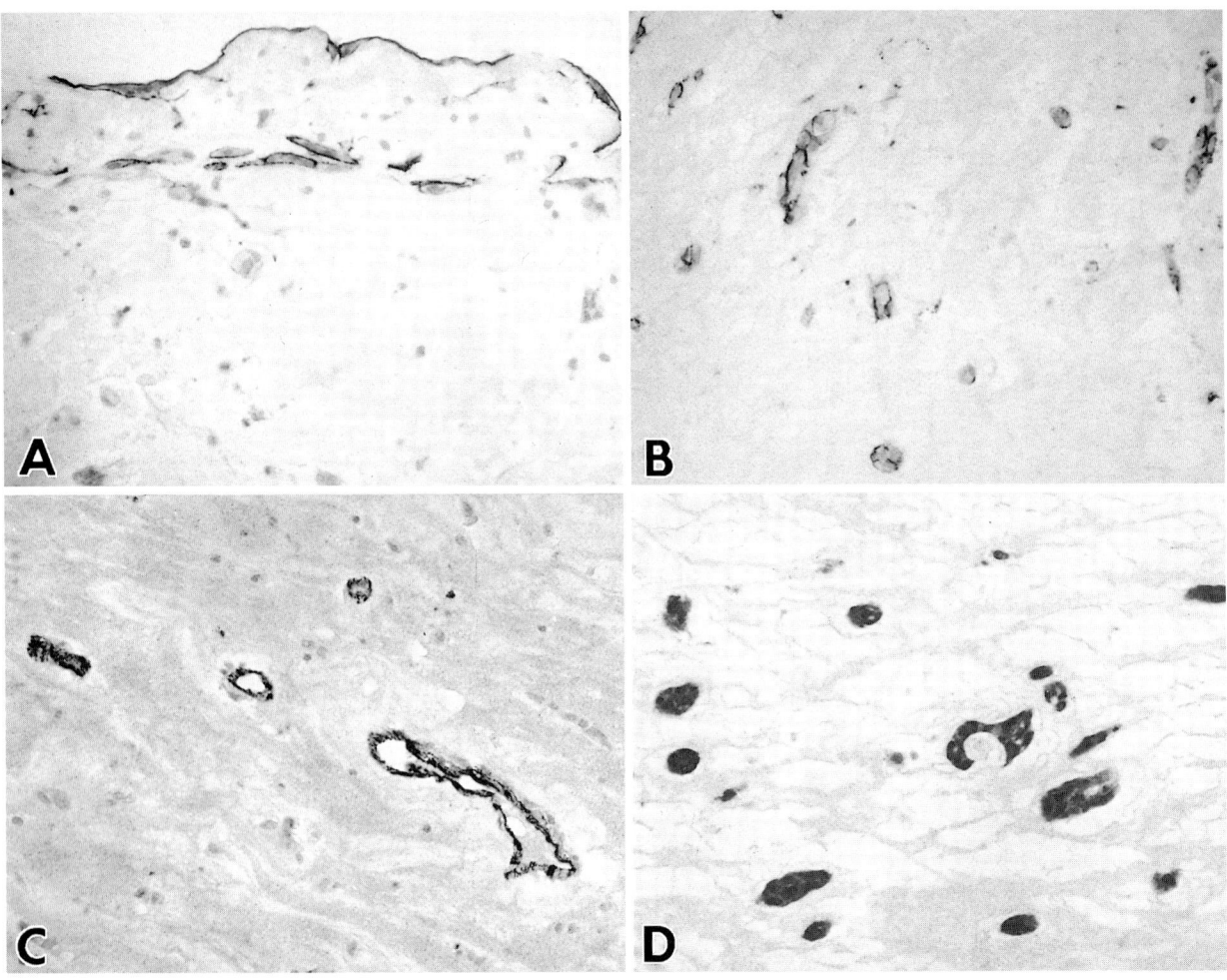

Figure 3-27
CARDIAC MYXOMA
A: There is surface positivity for CD34; myxoma cells under the surface are negative.
B: Myxoma cells under the surface of this tumor are positive for CD34.
C: Myxoma cells are negative for factor VIII–related antigen in this tumor. Note positive endothelial cells in vessels.
D: Smooth muscle actin is diffusely positive in this tumor.

myxoid fibrosarcoma, chondrosarcoma, or myxoid malignant fibrous histiocytoma are found in most myxoid sarcomas. Mitotic figures are rare in myxomas and are confined to the surface of the tumor when present.

Although myxoid sarcomas are frequently misdiagnosed as myxoma, it is rare that myxomas are misdiagnosed as malignancies. Occasionally, myxomas may have cellular areas on the tumor surface, and rarely, mitotic figures may be found that suggest aggressive behavior. These findings are not indicative of future recurrence (8,51). We have seen two cases of myxoma with densely cellular areas suggestive of malignancy (figs. 3-31, 3-32). These patients were without evidence of recurrence years after surgery (8), indicating that there may be pseudomalignant changes in a small subset of cardiac myxomas. The diagnosis of myxoma in both of these cases was made because there were areas of tumor typical of myxoma and cellular areas devoid of mitotic figures.

Papillary Fibroelastoma. Both myxoma and papillary fibroelastoma are endocardial lesions with a myxoid matrix. In contrast to myxoma, papillary fibroelastomas are generally located on

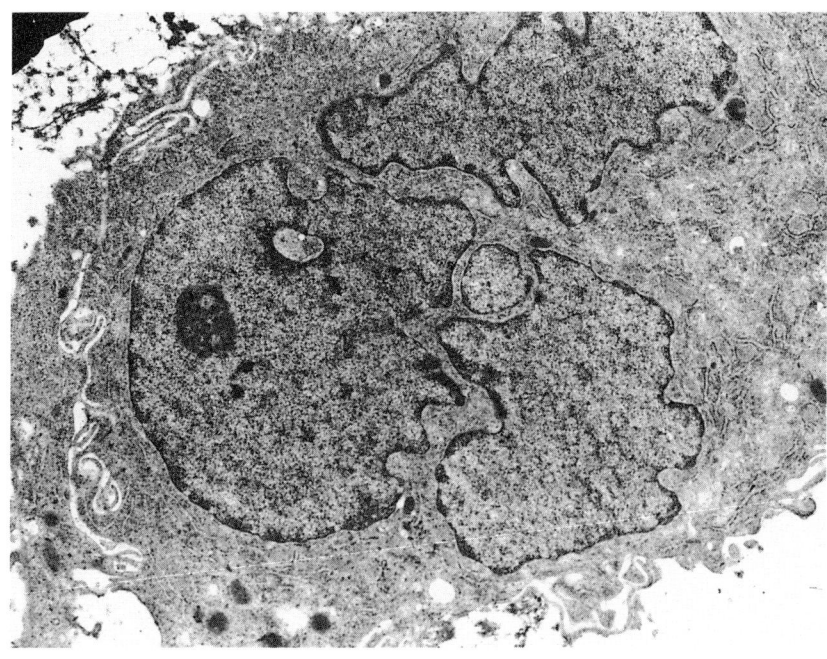

Figure 3-28
CARDIAC MYXOMA
Ultrastructurally, nuclei often appear multiple. There is little ultrastructural differentiation noted in most myxomas.

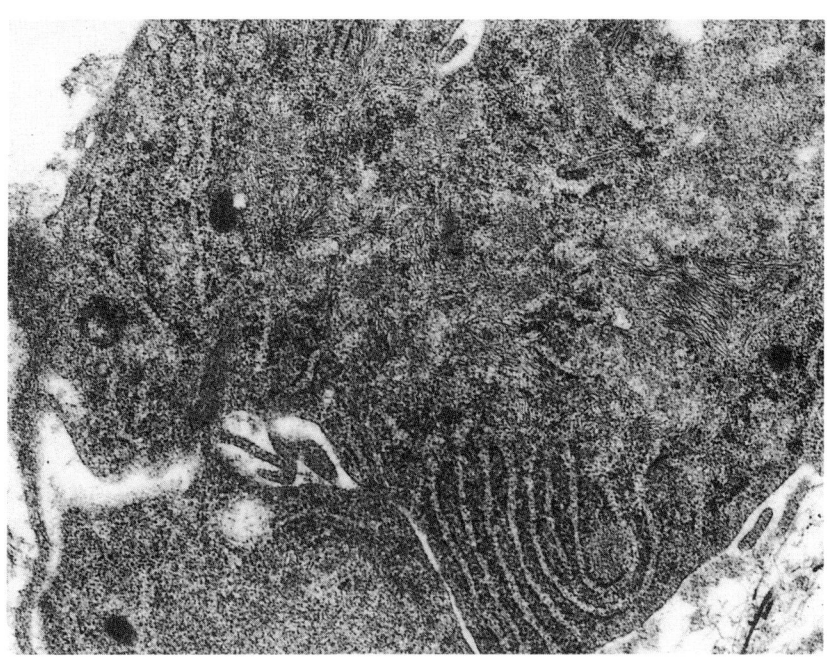

Figure 3-29
CARDIAC MYXOMA
This tumor demonstrates bundles of intermediate filaments and a prominent rough endoplasmic reticulum.

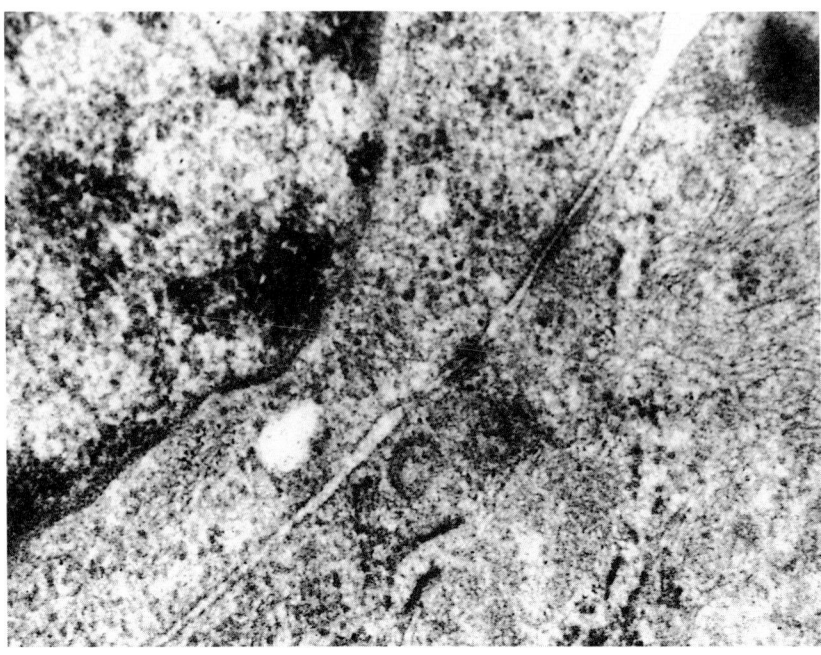

Figure 3-30
CARDIAC MYXOMA
Note the primitive intercellular junction. Desmosomes are absent, and are only seen if the tumor is composed of glandular structures.

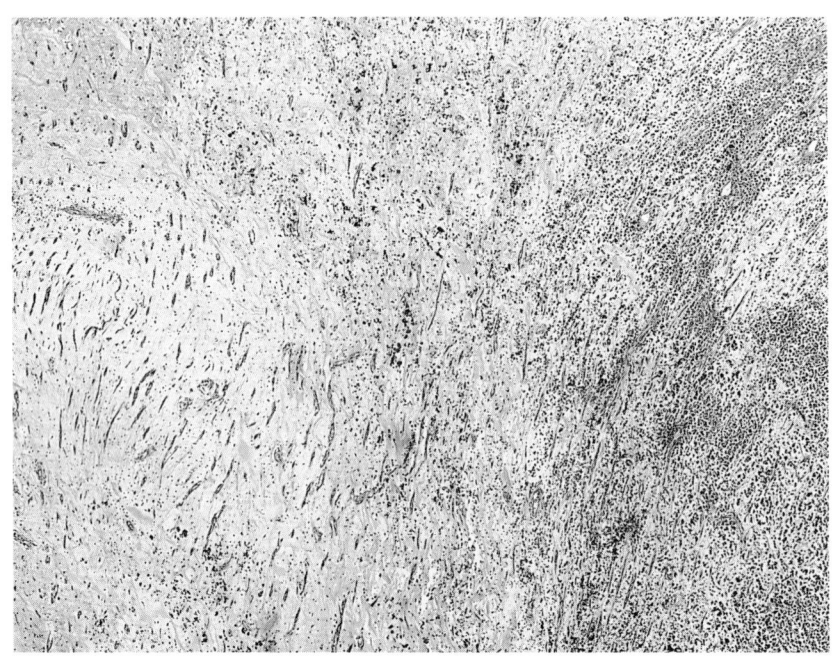

Figure 3-31
CARDIAC MYXOMA WITH PSEUDOMALIGNANT CELLS
Typical myxoma (left) shows cords of myxoma cells, identifiable at higher power (not shown). (Fig. 5A from Burke AP, Virmani R. Cardiac myxoma. A clinicopathologic study. Am J Clin Pathol 1993;100:671–80.)

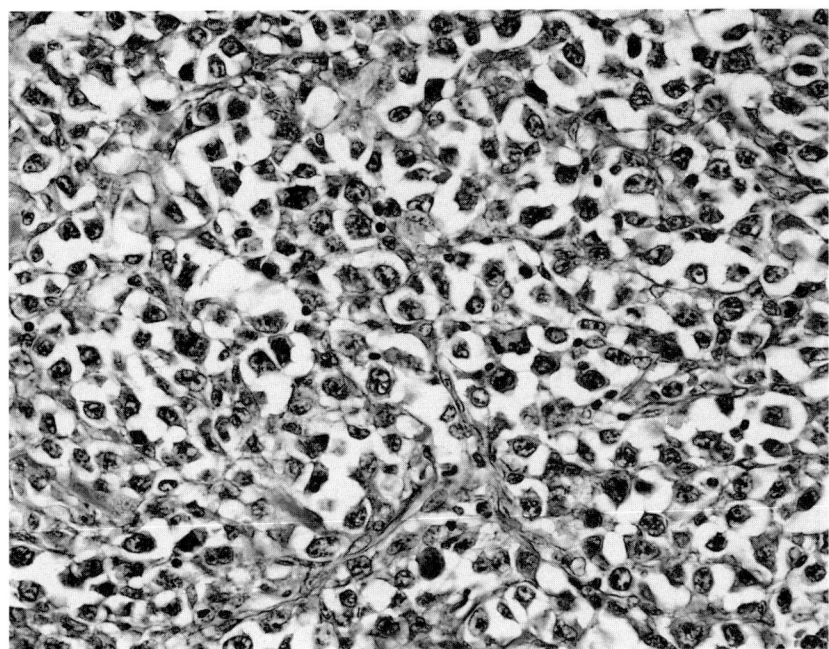

Figure 3-32
CARDIAC MYXOMA WITH
PSEUDOMALIGNANT CELLS
A higher magnification of figure 3-31 (right of field) demonstrates an infiltrate suggestive of an aggressive hematopoietic infiltrate. The patient was alive and well 12 years after removal of the myxoma without evidence of any neoplasm. (Fig. 5B from Burke AP, Virmani R. Cardiac myxoma. A clinicopathologic study. Am J Clin Pathol 1993;100:671–80.)

a valve cusp. The papillary fronds of papillary fibroelastoma are avascular, whereas a capillary network is always present in myxoma. Polygonal "myxoma" cells are absent in papillary fibroelastoma. The myxoid matrix of myxoma is diffuse, in areas that are not hyalinized, whereas the myxoid matrix of papillary fibroelastoma is located on the outer surfaces. Laminated elastic fibers are generally, but not always, present in papillary fibroelastoma, and absent in myxoma.

Mural Thrombus. Occasionally, a cardiac mural fibrous mass is seen without diagnostic areas of myxoma despite multiple sections (fig. 3-33). The distinction between an organized thrombus and myxoma cannot be made, and a descriptive diagnosis is all that can be rendered. Because fibrotic myxomas rarely, if ever, recur, the distinction is probably not critical.

Myxoma Emboli. In the differential diagnosis of embolic myxoma is myxoid thrombus. Intraluminal organizing thrombi can elaborate myxoid ground substance from proliferating mesenchymal cells (fig. 3-34). However, myxoma cells forming cords and rings are absent.

Embolic sarcomas may also resemble embolic myxoma on histologic examination. We have seen examples of embolic chondrosarcoma, one originating in the aortic intima, which were initially misdiagnosed in an embolic site as cardiac myxoma. Again, the characteristic structures formed by myxoma cells are absent in embolic sarcoma, and the occasional mitotic figures and chondroid differentiation favored a malignant diagnosis.

Treatment. Most patients with cardiac myxoma are cured by simple surgical excision. A biatrial approach with full-thickness excision of septum, necessitating repair of the resulting septal defect with a synthetic graft, is favored in some centers. The routine removal of septum is not, however, necessary in all cases (40), and primary closure of the septum can be performed without significant risk of recurrence. It was previously believed that the risk of recurrence is increased if surgical excision is incomplete; however, currently it is believed that the major factor in recurrence is the genetic predisposition to multiple and recurrent tumors (19,37). In approximately 5 percent of cases, the mitral valve must be replaced or repaired because of tumor encroachment (4). Surgical mortality is currently less than 1 percent (4,17,40,56) and long-term prognosis is excellent; the recurrence rate, as estimated above, is approximately 2 percent.

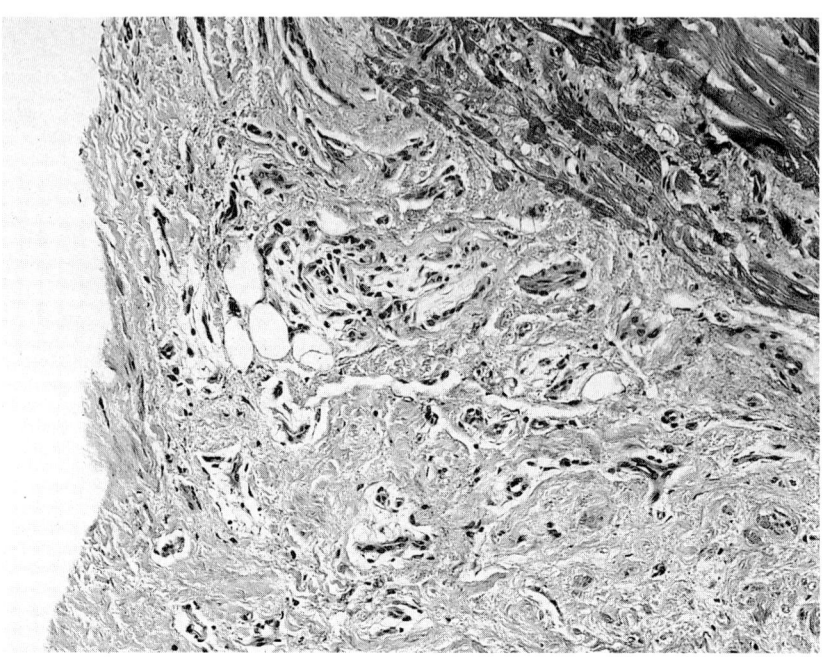

Figure 3-33
POSSIBLE CARDIAC MYXOMA

Occasionally, fibrotic masses are found attached to the endocardium. The diagnosis of myxoma can only be suggested, as in this case of a right ventricular mass which contained areas of myxoma-like cells entrapped in fibrous tissue. Myocardium is in the upper right.

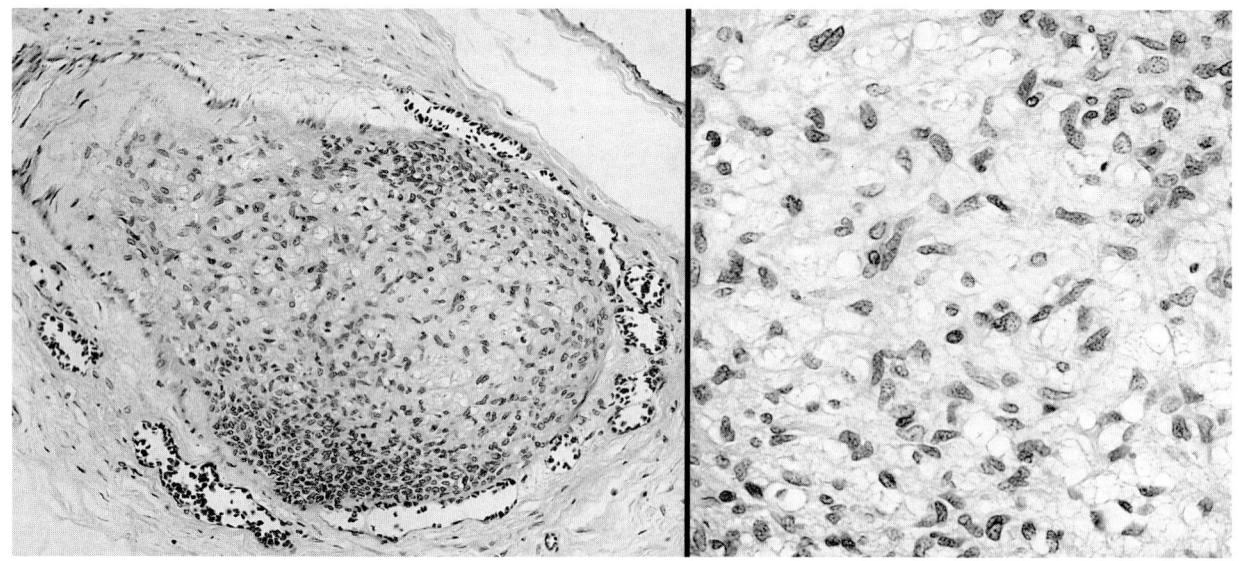

Figure 3-34
MYXOID THROMBUS

Intravascular thrombi may accumulate a myxoid matrix and resemble a myxoid embolus. Unlike myxoma, there are no myxoma cells arranged in nests, cords, or rings; rather, there is a population of spindled mesenchymal cells. Note the difference in cellular appearance from figures 3-24 and 3-25. This patient died and had no evidence of cardiac myxoma at autopsy.

REFERENCES

1. Aldrige HE, Greenwood WF. Myxoma of the left atrium. Br Heart J 1960;22:189–200.
2. Atherton DJ, Pitcher DW, Wells RS, MacDonald DM. A syndrome of various cutaneous pigmented lesions, myxoid neurofibromata and atrial myxoma: the NAME syndrome. Br J Dermatol 1980;103:421–9.
3. Attum AA, Johnson GS, Masri Z, Girardet R, Lansing AM. Malignant clinical behavior of cardiac myxomas and myxoid imitators. Ann Thorac Surg 1987;44:217–22.
4. Blondeau P. Primary cardiac tumors—French studies of 533 cases. Thorac Cardiovasc Surg 1990;38:192–5.
5. Boxer ME. Cardiac myxoma: an immunoperoxidase study of histogenesis. Histopathol 1984;8:861–72.
6. Branch CL Jr, Laster DW, Kelly DL Jr. Left atrial myxoma with cerebral emboli. Neurosurgery 1985;16:675–80.
7. Budzilovich G, Aleksic S, Greco A, Fernandez J, Harris J, Finegold M. Malignant cardiac myxoma with cerebral metastases. Surg Neurol 1979;11:461–9.
8. Burke AP, Virmani R. Cardiac myxomas. A clinicopathologic study. Am J Clin Pathol 1993;100:671–80.
9. Carney JA. Differences between nonfamilial and familial cardiac myxoma. Am J Surg Pathol 1985;9:53–5.
10. _____. Psammomatous melanotic schwannoma. A distinctive, heritable tumor with special associations, including cardiac myxoma and the Cushing syndrome. Am J Surg Pathol 1990;14:206–22.
11. _____, Gordon H, Carpenter PC, Shenoy BV, Go VL. The complex of myxomas, spotty pigmentation, and endocrine overactivity. Medicine (Baltimore) 1985;64:270–83.
12. Chan HS, Sonley MJ, Moes CA, Daneman A, Smith CR, Martin DJ. Primary and secondary tumors of childhood involving the heart, pericardium, and great vessels. A report of 75 cases and review of the literature. Cancer 1985;56:825–36.
13. Coard KC, Silver MD. Gamna body of the heart. Pathology 1984;16:459–61.
14. Curschellas E, Toia D, Borner M, Mihatsch MJ, Gudat F. Cardiac myxomas: immunohistochemical study of benign and malignant variants. Virchows Arch [A] 1991;418:485–91.
15. Damasio H, Seabra-Gomes R, da Silva JP, Damasio AR, Antunes JL. Multiple cerebral aneurysms and cardiac myxoma. Arch Neurol 1975;32:269–70.
16. Danoff A, Jormark S, Lorber D, Fleischer N. Adrenocortical micronodular dysplasia, cardiac myxomas, lentigines, and spindle cell tumors. Report of a kindred. Arch Inter Med 1987;147:443–8.
17. Dein JR, Frist WH, Stinson EB, et al. Primary cardiac neoplasms. Early and late results of surgical treatment in 42 patients. J Thorac Cardiovasc Surg 1987;93:502–11.
18. Dewald GW, Dahl RJ, Spurbeck JL, Carney JA, Gordon H. Chromosomally abnormal clones and nonrandom telomeric translocations in cardiac myxomas. Mayo Clin Proc 1987;62:558–67.
19. Farah MG. Familial cardiac myxoma. A study of relatives of patients with myxoma. Chest 1994;105:65–8.
20. Feldman PS, Horvath E, Kovacs K. An ultrastructural study of seven cardiac myxomas. Cancer 1977;40:2216–32.
21. Ferrans VJ, Roberts WC. Structural features of cardiac myxomas. Histology, histochemistry, and electron microscopy. Hum Pathol 1973;4:111–46.
22. Frank RA, Shalen PR, Harvey DG, Berg L, Ferguson TB, Schwarz HG. Atrial myxoma with intellectual decline and cerebral growths on CT scan. Ann Neurol 1979;5:396–400.
23. Goldman BI, Frydman C, Harpaz N, Ryan SF, Loiterman D. Glandular cardiac myxomas. Histologic, immunohistochemical, and ultrastructural evidence of epithelial differentiation. Cancer 1987;15:1767–75.
24. Govoni E, Severi B, Cenacchi G, et al. Ultrastructural and immunohistochemical contribution to the histogenesis of human cardiac myxoma. Ultrastruct Pathol 1988;12:221–33.
25. Heck HA Jr, Gross CM, Houghton JL. Long-term severe pulmonary hypertension associated with right atrial myxoma. Chest 1992;102:301–3.
26. Honey M, Axelrad MA. Intracardiac endodermal heterotopia. Brit Heart J 1962;24:667–70.
27. Hwang JJ, Lien WP, Kuan P, Hung CR, How SW. Atypical myxoma. Chest 1991;100:550–1.
28. Johansson L. Histogenesis of cardiac myxomas. An immunohistochemical study of 19 cases, including one with glandular structures, and review of the literature. Arch Pathol Lab Med 1989;113:735–41.
29. Krikler DM, Rode J, Davies MJ, Woolf N, Moss E. Atrial myxoma: a tumour in search of its origins. Br Heart J 1992;67:89–91.
30. Landon G, Ordonez NG, Guarda LA. Cardiac myxomas. An immunohistochemical study using endothelial, histiocytic, and smooth-muscle cell markers. Arch Pathol Lab Med 1986;110:116–20.
31. Lara JF, Rosen PP. Extramedullary hematopoiesis in a bronchial carcinoid tumor. An unusual complication of agnogenic myeloid metaplasia. Arch Pathol Lab Med 1990;114:1283–5.
32. Larsson S, Lepore V, Kennergren C. Atrial myxomas: results of 25 years' experience and review of the literature. Surgery 1989;105:695–8.
33. Lie JT. The identity and histogenesis of cardiac myxomas. A controversy put to rest [Editorial]. Arch Pathol Lab Med 1989;113:724–6.
34. Manthos CL, Sutherland RS, Sims JE, Perloff JJ. Carney's complex in a patient with hormone-producing Sertoli cell tumor of the testicle. J Urol 1993;150:1511–2.
35. Markel ML, Waller BF, Armstrong WF. Cardiac myxoma. A review. Medicine (Baltimore) 1987;66:114–25.
36. Markwald RR, Fitzharris TP, Manasek FJ. Structural development of endocardial cushions. Am J Anat 1977;148:85–119.
37. McCarthy PM, Piehler JM, Schaff HV, et al. The significance of multiple, recurrent and complex cardiac myxoma. J Thorac Cardiovasc Surg 1986;91:389–96.
38. McComb RD. Heterogeneous expression of factor VIII/von Willebrand factor by cardiac myxoma cells. Am J Surg Pathol 1984;8:539–44.
39. Morales AR, Fine G, Castro A, Nadji M. Cardiac myxoma (endocardioma). An immunocytochemical assessment of histogenesis. Hum Pathol 1981;12:896–9.
40. Murphy MC, Sweeney MS, Putnam JB Jr., et al. Surgical treatment of cardiac tumors: a 25-year experience. Ann Thorac Surg 1990;49:612–7.

41. Nolan J, Carder PJ, Bloomfield P. Atrial myxoma: tumour or trauma? Br Heart J 1992;67:406–8.

42. Price DL, Harris JL, New PF, Cantu RC. Cardiac myxoma. A clinicopathologic and angiographic study. Arch Neurol 1970;23:558–67.

43. Prichard RW. Tumors of the heart: review of the subject and report of one hundred and fifty cases. AMA Arch Pathol 1951;51:98–128.

44. Reed RJ, Utz MP, Terezakis N. Embolic and metastatic cardiac myxoma. Am J Dermatopathol 1989;11:157–65.

45. Rhodes AR, Silverman RA, Harrist TJ, Perez-Atayde AR. Mucocutaneous lentigines, cardiomucocutaneous myxomas, and multiple blue nevi. The "LAMB" syndrome. J Am Acad Dermatol 1984:10:72–82.

46. Roeltgen DP, Weimer GR, Patterson LF. Delayed neurologic complications of left atrial myxoma. Neurology 1981;31:8–13.

47. Rupp GM, Heyman RA, Martinez AJ, Sekhar LN, Jungreis CA. The pathology of metastatic cardiac myxoma. Am J Clin Pathol 1989;91:221–7.

48. Salyer WR, Page DL, Hutchins GM. The development of cardiac myxomas and papillary endocardial lesions from mural thrombus. Am Heart J 1975;89:4–17.

49. Schuger L, Ron N, Rosenmann E. Cardiac myxoma: a retrospective immunohistochemical study. Pathol Res Pract 1987;182:63–6.

50. Schweizer-Cagianut M, Salomon F, Hedinger CE. Primary adrenocortical nodular dysplasia with Cushing's syndrome and cardiac myxomas, a peculiar familial disease. Virchows Arch [A] 1982;397:183–92.

51. Seidman JD, Berman JJ, Hitchcock CL, et al. DNA analysis of cardiac myxomas: flow cytometry and image analysis. Hum Pathol 1991;22:494–500.

52. Seo IS, Warner TF, Colyer RA, Winkler RF. Metastasizing atrial myxoma. Am J Surg Pathol 1980;4:391–8.

53. St. John Sutton MG, Mercier LA, Giuliani ER, Lie JT. Atrial myxomas. A review of clinical experience in 40 patients. Mayo Clin Proc 1980;55:371–6.

54. Stein AA, Mauro J, Thibodeau L, Alley R. The histogenesis of cardiac myxomas: relation to other proliferative diseases of subendothelial vasoform reserve cells. Pathol Annu 1969;4:293–312.

55. Tanimura A, Kitazono M, Nagayama K, Tanaka S, Kosuga K. Cardiac myxoma: morphologic, histochemical, and tissue culture studies. Hum Pathol 1988;19:316–22.

56. Tazelaar HD, Locke TJ, McGregor CG. Pathology of surgically excised primary cardiac tumors. Mayo Clin Proc 1992;67:957–65.

57. Todo T, Usui M, Nagashima K. Cerebral metastasis of malignant cardiac myxoma. Surg Neurol 1992;37:374–9.

58. Utiger CA, Headington JT. Psammomatous melanotic schwannoma. A new cutaneous marker for Carney's complex. Arch Dermatol 1993;129:202–4.

59. Van Gelder HM, O'Brien DJ, Staples ED, Alexander JA. Familial cardiac myxoma. Ann Thorac Surg 1992;53:419–24.

60. Virmani R, Posey DM, Clark MA, McAllister HA. Right atrial myxoma causing pulmonary emboli and pulmonary hypertension. Am J Forens Med Pathol 1982;3:249–52.

61. Wold LE, Lie JT. Cardiac myxomas: a clinicopathologic profile. Am J Pathol 1980;101:219–40.

✧ ✧ ✧

4
PAPILLARY FIBROELASTOMA

Definition. Papillary fibroelastomas are benign avascular papillomas of the endocardium that are related to Lambl excrescences. There are numerous synonyms, including *fibroelastic papilloma, papilloma of valves, giant Lambl's excrescence, myxofibroma, myxoma of valves, hyaline fibroma,* and *fibroma of valves.*

Histogenesis. Because papillary fibroelastomas resemble Lambl excrescences both grossly and microscopically, a shared histogenesis is probable. Lambl excrescences are filiform fronds that occasionally occur on cardiac valves of elderly patients (figs. 4-1–4-3). In semilunar valves, they are most common at the nodules of Aranti and along the lines of closure and free cuspal edges. (Nodules of Aranti are age-related areas of thickening in the center of semilunar valves at the junction between the lines of closure and the free edge.) In atrioventricular valves, Lambl excrescences are found at the site of valve closure on the atrial surface. In either site, they are thought to be age-related changes and may be organized mural thrombi at the site of minor endothelial damage.

It is not always possible to distinguish Lambl excrescences and papillary fibroelastoma based exclusively on microscopic findings (3). Differences between the two entities are based largely on size and site (3,4). Papillary fibroelastomas are larger and more gelatinous than Lambl excrescences, and are present on valves away from the lines of closure and free edges and on the endocardial surfaces of the atria or ventricles. Lambl excrescences are, by definition, at the sites of valve closure.

Because Lambl excrescences are believed to be unusual organizing thrombi, a similar histogenesis has been advocated for papillary fibroelastoma. The presence of fibrin, hyaluronic acid, and laminated elastic fibers within the papillae supports this view (1,10,24,29). Fibrin has also been detected within the papillary cores by immunohistochemistry (9).

Because papillary fibroelastomas are often present where there is little hemodynamic stress, it is likely that processes other than, or perhaps in addition to, organizing thrombosis play a role in their histogenesis. Evidence in favor of a hamartoma (26) includes the histologic appearance, which suggests a proliferation of miniature chordae tendineae rather than an organizing thrombus, as well as the observation

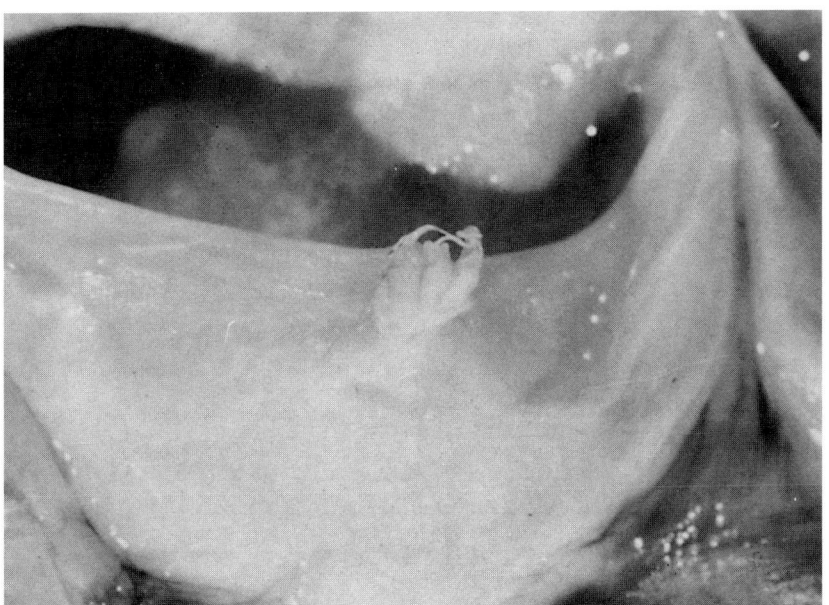

Figure 4-1
PAPILLARY FIBROELASTOMA OR
GIANT LAMBL'S EXCRESCENCE
This tumor is located midline at the site of closure of the aortic valve cusp (nodules of Aranti). At this location, the term papillary fibroelastoma or Lambl's excrescence may be used; the distinction is based on the size of the tumor. (Fig. 4 from Edwards FH, Hale D, Cohen A, Thompson L, Pezella T, Virmani R. Primary cardiac valve tumors. Ann Thorac Surg 1991;52:1127–31.)

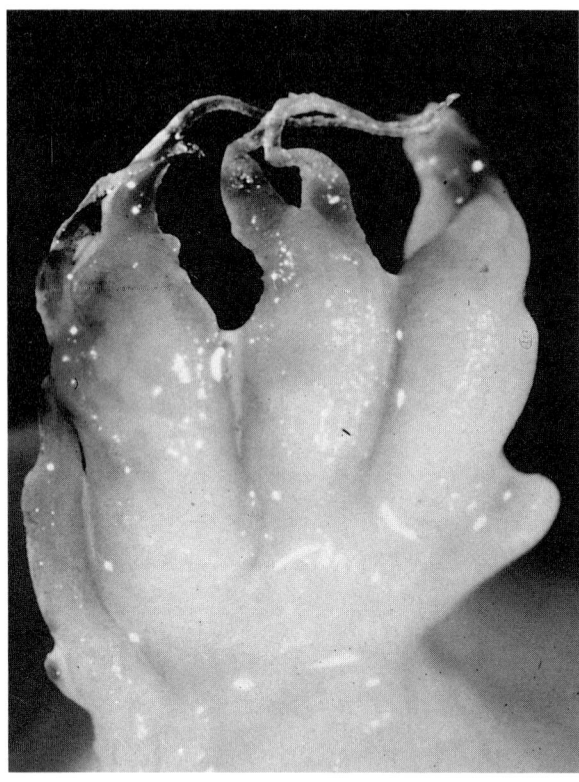

Figure 4-2
PAPILLARY FIBROELASTOMA
OR GIANT LAMBL'S EXCRESCENCE

Higher magnification of figure 4-1. (Fig. 5 from Edwards FH, Hale D, Cohen A, Thompson L, Pezella T, Virmani R. Primary cardiac valve tumors. Ann Thorac Surg 1991;52:1127–31.)

that some cases may be congenital (11,24). The congenital nature of some papillary fibroelastomas is supported by an early age at onset of symptoms, and an association with other congenital anomalies (11,24). We have recently seen papillary fibroelastomas arising on endocardial surfaces thickened by radiation therapy and prosthetic valves, suggesting a reactive process in some cases.

The histogenesis of both papillary fibroelastoma and Lambl excrescences remains elusive. It appears that endocardial tissue may, in response to shear stresses or possible congenital factors, proliferate in a unique way, resulting in avascular fronds that resemble disorganized chordae tendineae. In exaggerated cases, especially those away from normal areas of stress, these proliferations are classified as papillary fibroelastoma; the more common, smaller lesions near lines of closure are considered Lambl excrescences.

Incidence. The true incidence of papillary fibroelastoma is unknown because it can be easily overlooked at autopsy and only rarely causes symptoms. It is considered rare: by 1991, only 132 cases had been published in the medical literature (2). The tumors are easily detected by echocardiography and surgically excised (32,35). In many series of surgically resected cardiac tumors, there are few or no examples, possibly

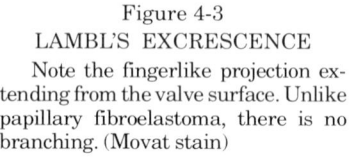

Figure 4-3
LAMBL'S EXCRESCENCE

Note the fingerlike projection extending from the valve surface. Unlike papillary fibroelastoma, there is no branching. (Movat stain)

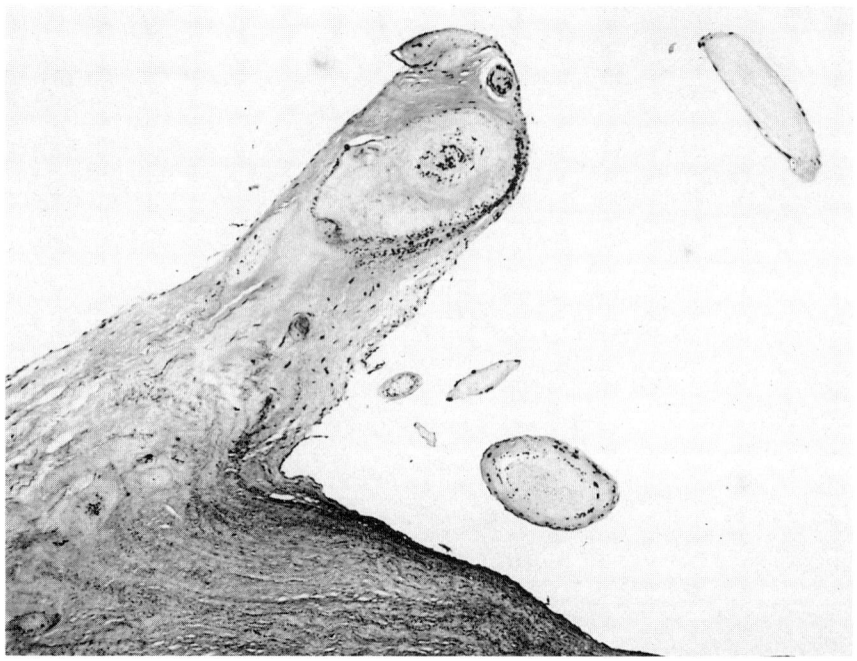

because of imprecise terminology and because papillary fibroelastomas are occasionally classified as myxomas. Among 102 benign tumors excised at the Mayo Clinic, 7 were papillary fibroelastomas, representing the second most common nonmyxomatous benign tumor after fibroma (31). In a surgical series from Stanford University Hospital, 2 of 34 benign cardiac tumors were papillary fibroelastomas (7). In the files at the Armed Forces Institute of Pathology (AFIP), papillary fibroelastoma is the second most common cardiac tumor after myxoma (see chapter 1), representing 10 percent of tumors, excluding mesothelial cysts.

Clinical Features. Papillary fibroelastomas occur equally in adults of both sexes. The mean age at detection is approximately 60 years (2,8, 10,17,21), although they have been described in teenagers (2,5). Some series note the association of papillary fibroelastoma and preexisting heart disease (1), and there have been reports of patients with this tumor and coexisting rheumatic valvular disease (18). In larger series, however, most patients had no cardiac symptoms. In a series of 41 cases reported by Edwards et al. (8), 9 patients had congestive heart failure from unrelated causes, 2 had neurologic symptoms, 2 died suddenly, and the remainder were asymptomatic. In 1991, 22 reports of papillary fibroelastoma causing symptoms were compiled from the literature (34). All involved the left side of the heart, specifically the mitral valve (10 cases), aortic valve (9 cases), left ventricular papillary muscle (2 cases), or free wall (1 case). Symptoms were caused by coronary occlusion (acute myocardial infarct, 13 cases), cerebral vascular occlusion (8 cases), and renal vascular occlusion (1 case). Sudden death and ischemic heart disease are generally attributed to embolization or prolapse of tumors that are located on either the ventricular or sinus surfaces of the right or left coronary cusps of the aortic valve (2,6,16,27,28). At least one illustration of a "myxoma" resulting in sudden death by embolism appears to represent a papillary fibroelastoma of the aortic valve (25). The cause of peripheral vascular occlusion is usually embolization of attached fibrin clots. It is unlikely that papillary fibroelastoma causes valvular insufficiency or congestive heart failure; however, one report of an unusually large tumor suggests this possibility (11).

The diagnosis is readily made clinically by two-dimensional echocardiography (30); tumors may be detected either as incidental findings (13), during an investigation for neurologic symptoms (12,19,22), or during echocardiography for cardiac disease (11,27). Transthoracic echocardiography may be helpful in precise diagnosis (23). If the diagnosis of papillary fibroelastoma is made prior to surgery, the tumor can be removed by simple excision without removing the underlying valve (20). Uchida (33) described a case of papillary fibroelastoma that lacked the typical frond-like appearance on echocardiography, indicating that differentiating between papillary fibroelastoma and myxoma is not always possible by imaging studies.

Since the writing of the last Fascicle on cardiac tumors (21), the AFIP files show 29 cases of papillary fibroelastoma: 20 were in men, 9 in women, and the mean age at time of presentation was 59 years. Five of these tumors caused symptoms: 2 tumors on the aortic valve caused sudden death by embolization into the right and circumflex coronary arteries, respectively; 2 left atrial tumors caused transient ischemic attacks and were removed surgically; and 1 additional tumor caused transient ischemic attacks and was detected by echocardiography and removed from the anterior papillary muscle of the left ventricle. An additional 4 asymptomatic tumors were surgically removed.

Gross Findings. Papillary fibroelastomas are invariably located on the endocardial surface, with 90 percent located on valve surfaces. Tumors of cardiac valves are relatively rare; 73 percent are papillary fibroelastoma, the remainder representing sarcomas, myxomas, lipomatous hamartomas, and hemangiomas (8). Grossly, papillary fibroelastomas resemble large Lambl excrescences. However, Lambl excrescences, as discussed previously, are specifically located at the lines of closure of the valve, whereas papillary fibroelastomas may occur anywhere on the valvular surface. When they occur on the atrioventricular valves, they have a predilection for the atrial surface, but there is no predilection between one side or the other for semilunar valves (figs. 4-4–4-6) (2,8, 21). The most common site is the aortic valve (Table 4-1). Unusual nonvalvular sites include the papillary muscles, the ostium of the right coronary artery (4), ventricular septum (11), right atrium

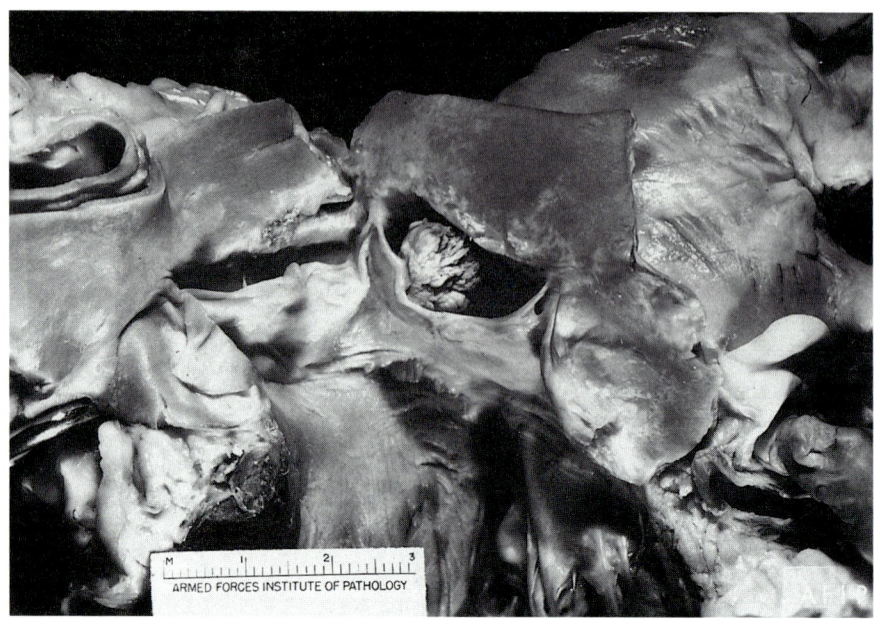

Figure 4-4
PAPILLARY
FIBROELASTOMA
Unlike Lambl excrescences, papillary fibroelastomas are often on the arterial surface and may project into the coronary ostium, causing ostial occlusion. This tumor is in the noncoronary sinus.

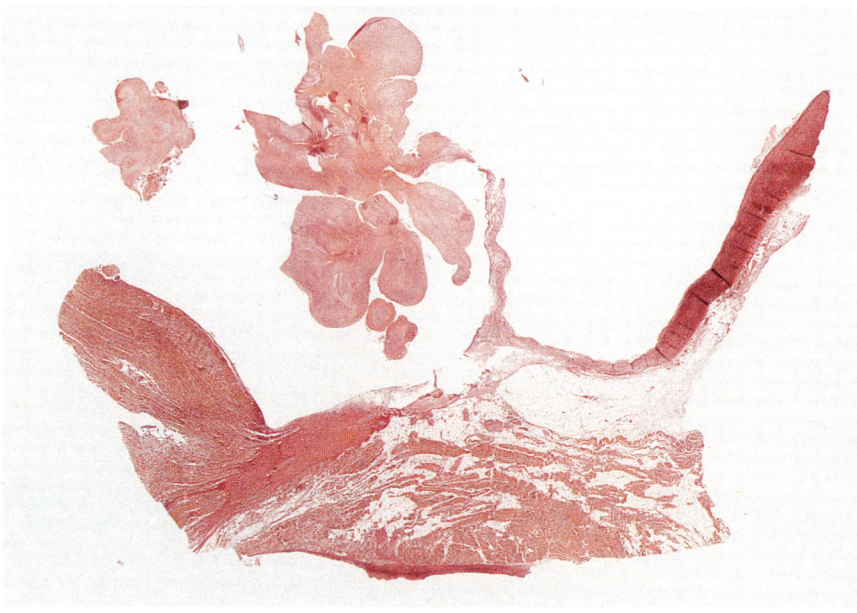

Figure 4-5
PAPILLARY
FIBROELASTOMA
This whole mount shows the papilloma arising from the aortic valve cusp.

(14,29), left ventricular outflow tract (33), and Chiari network (34). We have recently seen a papillary fibroelastoma with two attachments by separate stalks on the anterior leaflet of the mitral valve and left ventricular outflow tract.

Papillary fibroelastomas have a characteristic flower-like appearance that has been likened to that of a sea anemone and is best appreciated by immersing the specimen in water. Cystic spaces are occasionally present (5) and approximately 13 percent are multiple (8). Although the majority of tumors are 1 cm or less in largest diameter, tumors as large as 5 cm have been reported (11). The gross appearance may be obscured by attached organizing thrombi, in which case the characteristic papillary structure is not appreciated.

Histologic Findings. The papillary fronds of papillary fibroelastoma are narrow, elongated, and branching. The papillae resemble chordae tendineae and are longer than those seen in

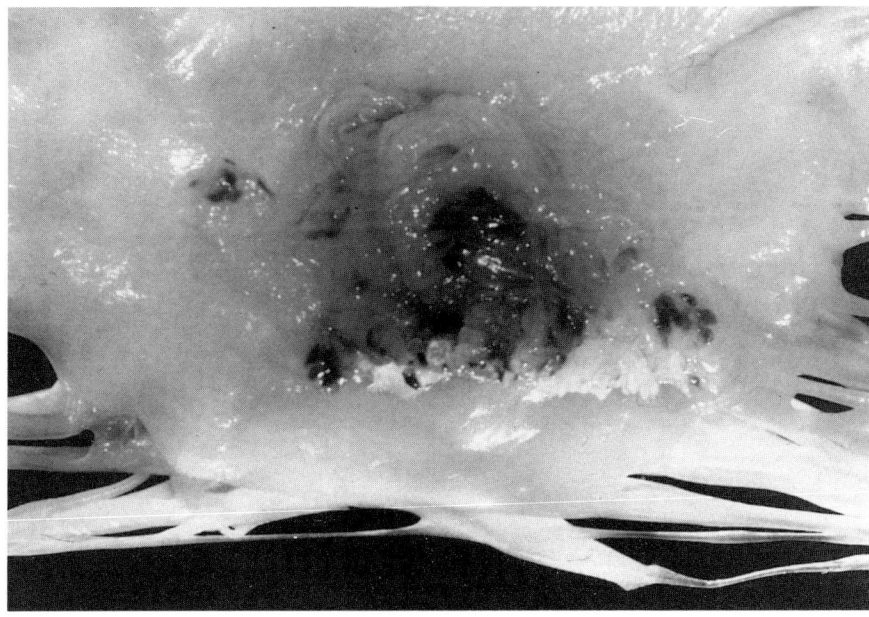

Figure 4-6
PAPILLARY FIBROELASTOMA
When located on the mitral valve, these tumors are usually on the anterior leaflet of the atrial surface.

Table 4-1

LOCATION OF PAPILLARY FIBROELASTOMA

Site	AFIP 1900–1976 (42 patients)*	AFIP 1976–1994 (29 patients)**	Total
Aortic valve	15	13	28 (37%)
Tricuspid valve	9	4	13 (17%)
Mitral valve	7	4	11 (14%)
Pulmonary valve	8	2	10 (13%)
Right atrium	2	3	5 (7%)
Left atrium	1	4	5 (7%)
Right ventricle	2	0	2 (2%)
Left ventricle septum	1	0	1 (1%)
Left ventricle, papillary muscle	0	1	1 (1%)
Total	**45**	**31**	**76**

* Multiple tumors were present in 3 patients. These data are derived from reference 21.
** Multiple tumors were present in 2 patients.

nodules of Aranti (fig. 4-3). The matrix consists of mucopolysaccharides, elastic fibers, and rare spindle cells resembling smooth muscle cells or fibroblasts. Movat's pentachrome stain is especially useful for delineating these components (figs. 4-7, 4-8). The presence of elastic fibers is variable, and some sections of tumor may fail to demonstrate them. The papillary surface is covered by a single layer of endothelial cells.

Ultrastructural Findings. The connective tissue of papillary fibroelastoma contains mature collagen with irregular elastic fibers that are longitudinally oriented (10,11). Fibroblasts and more primitive mesenchymal cells are present within the matrix. The surface endothelial cells are hyperplastic and possess numerous organelles and pinocytotic vesicles. Because the surface cells of papillary fibroelastoma ultrastructurally resemble endothelial cells, in contrast to atrial myxoma, Fishbein et al. (10) recommended the use of the term "endocardial papillary elastofibroma" for these tumors.

Differential Diagnosis. There are few entities that can histologically be mistaken for papillary fibroelastoma. Myxomas are rarely located on the valve surface. Papillary fibroelastoma differs histologically from myxoma (29) by the absence of vessels within papillae (these are always present in myxoma), the absence of polygonal "myxoma" cells within the papillae and on the surface of the tumor, the outer localization of myxoid matrix (diffuse in myxoma), and the presence of laminated elastic fibers. It should be stressed that the last finding is variable: elastic tissue may be absent in papillary fibroelastoma,

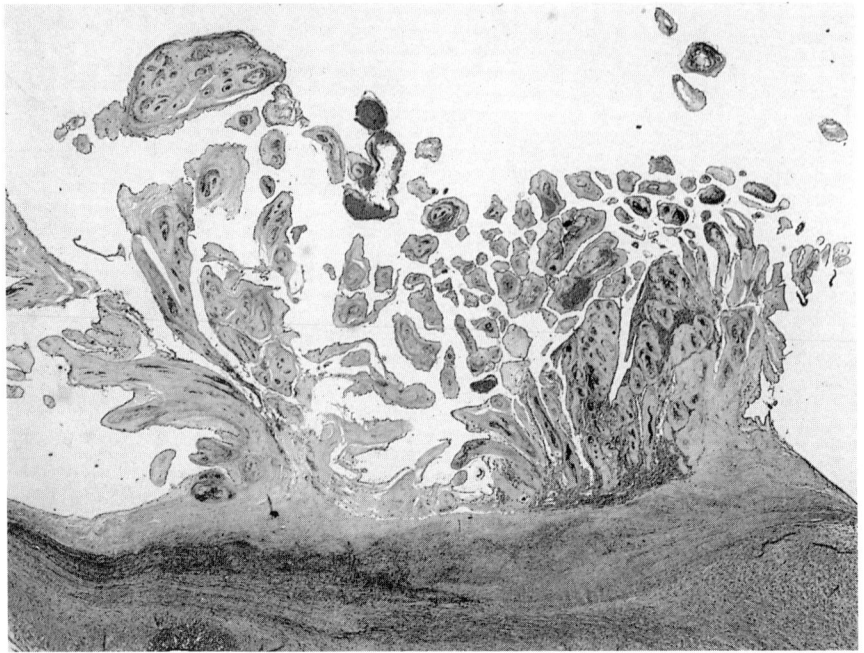

Figure 4-7
PAPILLARY FIBROELASTOMA
There are avascular fronds lined by endothelial cells. (Movat pentachrome stain)

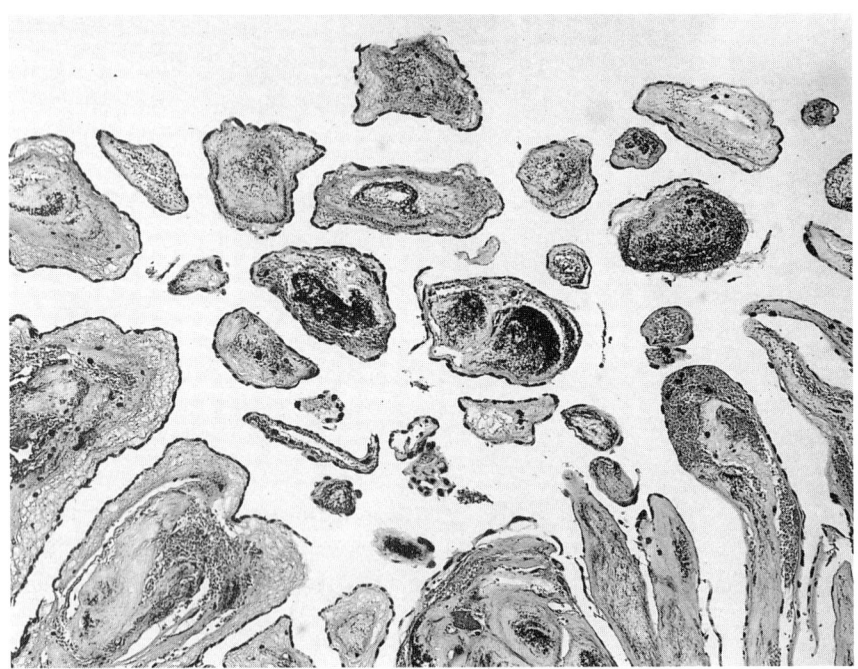

Figure 4-8
PAPILLARY FIBROELASTOMA
This is a higher magnification of figure 4-7. The fronds contain varying amounts of elastin, stained black, surrounded by myxoid ground substance.

especially if only superficial portions of the tumor are sampled.

Another diagnostic problem is the overgrowth of papillary fibroelastoma by attached fibrin thrombi (marantic endocarditis). These vegetations may cause embolic symptoms, and the un-derlying tumor may be obscured by an organizing thrombus (fig. 4-9). The gross appearance of papillary fibroelastoma can therefore mimic marantic endocarditis. For this reason, valvular excrescences should be routinely evaluated histologically.

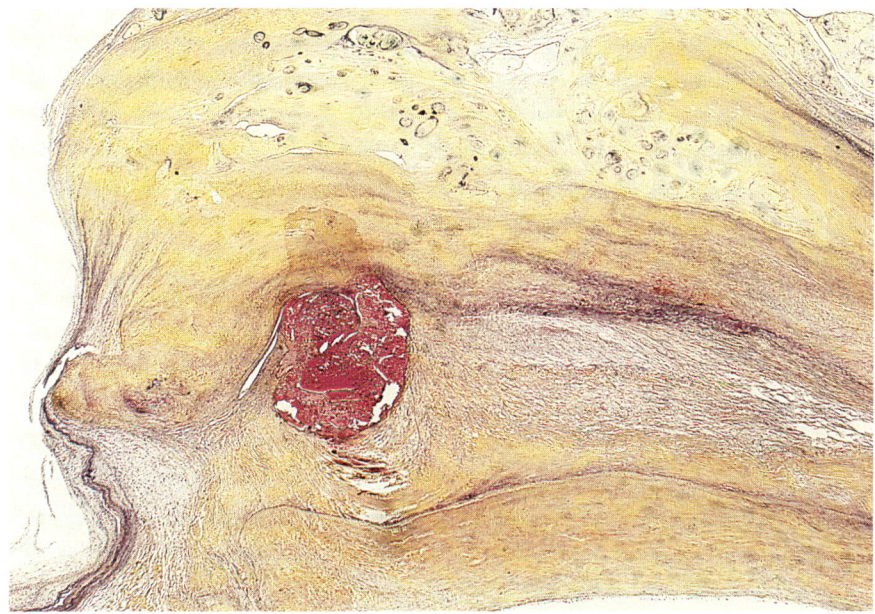

Figure 4-9
PAPILLARY FIBROELASTOMA
Scarring may obliterate the papillary configuration. The diagnosis is made on the basis of entrapped cores of elastic tissue.

Treatment. The treatment is simple excision, which is curative (15,20,31,32). We are not aware of a report of recurrent papillary fibroelastoma. Most often, the tumor can be removed without excision of significant areas of surrounding endocardium or valve (20). In a few cases with large attached thrombi, aortic valve removal with implantation of a prosthetic valve was necessary (20).

REFERENCES

1. Almagro UA, Perry LS, Choi H, Pinar K. Papillary fibroelastoma of the heart. Report of six cases. Arch Pathol Lab Med 1982;106:318–21.
2. Amr SS, Abu al Ragheb SY. Sudden unexpected death due to papillary fibroma of the aortic valve. Report of a case and review of the literature. Am J Forensic Med Pathol 1991;12:143–8.
3. Boone SA, Campagna M, Walley VM. Lambl's excrescences and papillary fibroelastomas: are they different? Can J Cardiol 1992;8:372–6.
4. _____, Higginson LA, Walley VM. Endothelial papillary fibroelastomas arising in and around the aortic sinus, filling the ostium of the right coronary artery. Arch Pathol Lab Med 1992;116:135–7.
5. Braile DM, Rossi MA, Jacob JL, Thevenard RS, Suzigan S, Ramos SG. Cystic fibroelastoma of the mitral valve: report of a case [Letter]. J Thorac Cardiovasc Surg 1993;106:1128–30.
6. Butterworth JS, Poindexter CA. Papilloma of cusp of the aortic valve: report of a patient with sudden death. Circulation 1973;48:213–5.
7. Dein JR, Frist WH, Stinson EB, et al. Primary cardiac neoplasms. Early and late results of surgical treatment in 42 patients. J Thorac Cardiovasc Surg 1987;93:502–11.
8. Edwards FH, Hale D, Cohen A, Thompson L, Pezzella AT, Virmani R. Primary cardiac valve tumors. Ann Thorac Surg 1991;52:1127–31.
9. Fekete PS, Nassar VH, Talley JD, Boedecker EA. Cardiac papilloma. A case report with evidence of thrombotic origin. Arch Pathol Lab Med 1983;107:246–8.
10. Fishbein MC, Ferrans VJ, Roberts WC. Endocardial papillary elastofibromas. Arch Pathol 1975;99:335–41.
11. Flotte T, Pinar H, Feiner H. Papillary elastofibroma of the ventricular septum. Am J Surg Pathol 1980;4:585–8.
12. Fowles RE, Miller DC, Egbert BM, Fitzgerald JW, Popp RL. Systemic embolization from a mitral valve papillary endocardial fibroma detected by two dimensional echocardiography. Am Heart J 1981;102:128–30.
13. Frumin H, O'Donnell L, Kerin NZ, Levine F, Nathan LE Jr, Klein SP. Two dimensional echocardiographic detection and diagnostic features of tricuspid papillary fibroelastoma. J Am Coll Cardiol 1983;2:1016–8.
14. Gallas MT, Reardon MJ, Reardon PR, DeFelice CA, Raizner AE, Mody DR. Papillary fibroelastoma. A right atrial presentation. Tex Heart Inst J 1993;20:293–5.
15. Gorton ME, Soltandeh H, Mitral valve fibroelastoma. Ann Thorac Surg 1989;47:605–7.

16. Harris LS, Adelson L. Fatal coronary embolism from a myxomatous polyp of the aortic valve: an unusual cause of sudden death. Am J Clin Pathol 1965;43:61–4.

17. Heath D, Best PV, Davis BT. Papilliferous tumors of the heart valves. Br Heart J 1961;23:20–4.

18. Kalman JM, Lubicz S, Brennan JB, Vernon-Roberts E, Calafiore P. Multiple cardiac papillary fibroelastomas and rheumatic heart disease. Aust N Z J Med 1991;21:744–6.

19. Mann J, Parker DJ. Papillary fibroelastoma of the mitral valve: a rare cause of transient neurological defects. Br Heart J 1994;71:6.

20. Marvasti MA, Obeid AT, Cohen PS, et al. Successful removal of papillary endocardial fibroma. Thorac Cardiovasc Surg 1983;31:254–7.

21. McAllister HA, Fenoglio JJ Jr. Tumors of the cardiovascular system. Atlas of Tumor Pathology, 2nd Series, Fascicle 15. Washington, D.C.: Armed Forces Institute of Pathology, 1977;20–5.

22. McFadden PM, Lacy JR. Intracardiac papillary fibroelastoma: an occult cause of embolic neurologic deficit. Ann Thorac Surg 1987;43:667–9.

23. Narang J, Neustein S, Israel D. The role of transesophageal echocardiography in the diagnosis and excision of a tumor of the aortic valve. J Cardiothorac Vasc Anesth 1992;6:68–9.

24. Pomerance A. Papillary "tumours" of the heart valves. J Pathol Bact 1961;81:135–40.

25. Puff M, Taff ML, Spitz WU, Eckert WG. Syncope and sudden death caused by mitral valve myxomas. Am J Forensic Med Pathol 1986;7:84–6.

26. Raeburn C. Papillary fibro-elastic hamartomas of the heart valves. J Pathol 1953;65:371–3.

27. Richard J, Castello R, Dressler FA, et al. Diagnosis of papillary fibroelastoma of the mitral valve complicated by non-Q-wave infarction with apical thrombus: transesophageal and transthoracic echocardiographic study. Am Heart J 1993;126:710–2.

28. Rona G, Feeney N, Kahn DS. Fibroelastic hamartoma of the aortic valve producing ischemic heart disease. Associated pulmonary glomus bodies. Am J Cardiol 1963;12:869–74.

29. Schiller AL, Schantz A. Papillary endocardial excrescence of the right atrium: report of two cases. Amer J Clin Pathol 1970;42:617–21.

30. Shub C, Tajik AJ, Seward JB, et al. Cardiac papillary fibroelastomas. Two-dimensional echocardiographic recognition. Mayo Clin Proc 1981;56:629–33.

31. Tazelaar HD, Locke TJ, McGregor CG. Pathology of surgically excised primary cardiac tumors. Mayo Clin Proc 1992;67:957–65.

32. Topol EJ, Biern RO, Reitz BA. Cardiac papillary fibroelastoma and stroke: echocardiographic diagnosis and guide to excision. Am J Med 1986;80:129–32.

33. Uchida S, Obayashi N, Yamanari H, Matsubara K, Saito D, Haraoka S. Papillary fibroelastoma in the left ventricular outflow tract. Heart Vessels 1992;7:164–7.

34. Valente M, Basso C, Thiene G, et al. Fibroelastic papilloma: a not-so-benign cardiac tumor. Cardiovasc Pathol 1992;1:161–6.

35. Wasdahl DA, Wasdahl WA, Edwards WD. Fibroelastic papilloma arising in a Chiari network. Clin Cardiol 1992;15:45–7.

5

BENIGN TUMORS OF CARDIAC MYOCYTES

CARDIAC RHABDOMYOMA

Definition. Cardiac rhabdomyoma is a hamartoma that occurs exclusively in the heart, often as multiple nodules composed of altered cardiac myocytes with large vacuoles and abundant glycogen. There is a strong association with tuberous sclerosis (3,10,13).

Histogenesis. Although it was once considered a glycogen storage defect (14) or a true neoplasm (15), current opinion is that rhabdomyoma is most likely a form of hamartoma (9,10,21). Unlike most neoplasms, they are often multiple, lack mitotic activity, and are congenital rather than acquired (10). The focal nature of the lesions, absence of biochemical evidence of an enzyme deficiency, and lack of extracardiac involvement are incompatible with a glycogen storage disease.

There is debate regarding the precise cell type of cardiac rhabdomyoma. Electron microscopic studies have favored a growth of developmentally arrested contractile myocytes (10), based on the presence of abundant myofilaments. The theory that rhabdomyomas are tumors of Purkinje cells ("Purkinjeomas") was originally put forth by Heath (13), and is still favored by some investigators (21). Studies have suggested the presence of primitive T-tubules in rhabdomyoma; these structures are indicative of cardiac muscle, as opposed to Purkinje cells. Leptomeric fibers, which are plentiful in Purkinje cells, are occasionally present in rhabdomyomas, but their specificity for Purkinje cell differentiation has been questioned (28). The presence of desmosomes has been used both as an argument for Purkinje cell origin (9) and for myocyte origin (21). Evidence of Purkinje cell origin is not conclusive and current opinion favors a myocyte origin of cardiac rhabdomyoma (3).

Incidence. Although rare, rhabdomyoma is the most common cardiac tumor in infancy and childhood (6,15,23), accounting for half to three quarters of pediatric tumors. There were 7 cases among 11,000 autopsies in Boston Children's Hospital Medical Center (15), and 8 cases at The Hospital for Sick Children in Toronto over a 62-year period (6). It is an extremely rare diagnosis in patients older than 10 years (20). Over 90 percent of intracardiac tumors discovered in intrauterine life are rhabdomyomas (12).

Clinical Features. Cardiac rhabdomyomas can be divided into three groups: those that arise in patients with tuberous sclerosis, sporadic rhabdomyomas, and those associated with structural congenital heart disease.

In 1862, von Recklinghausen (4,10) noted that cardiac rhabdomyomas occur in patients with tuberous sclerosis (4,10). Up to 50 percent of patients with cardiac rhabdomyoma have the tuberous sclerosis syndrome, which is characterized by intracranial hamartomas, facial angiofibromas, subungual fibromas, linear epidermal nevi, renal angiomyolipomas, and other hamartomas. The prevalence of cardiac rhabdomyomas in patients with tuberous sclerosis is dependent on age: most of infants with tuberous sclerosis have cardiac masses consistent with rhabdomyoma, as seen by echocardiography (8,22,23,25); however, only 60 percent of children and less than 25 percent of adults with the syndrome have detectable cardiac masses (22,25). The decrease in incidence of tumors as age progresses is not only a function of better survival of patients without cardiac tumors, but is also because rhabdomyomas have been shown to regress spontaneously (23,25).

There is no sex predilection for patients with cardiac rhabdomyoma and tuberous sclerosis. The presenting symptoms are usually related to the tuberous sclerosis or fetal hydrops (10). Patients who survive the first few weeks of life usually have no cardiac symptoms because tumors in these patients are usually intramural and do not obstruct blood flow (10). The prevalence of asymptomatic rhabdomyomas in patients with tuberous sclerosis has become apparent with the routine use of echocardiography, which usually reveals multiple small rhabdomyomas (23). Occasionally, cardiac rhabdomyoma may result in arrhythmias, cyanosis, right ventricular outflow tract obstruction (11), and murmurs (17). Tumors are multiple in over 90 percent of cases (10); conversely, up to 86 percent of patients with multiple rhabdomyomas have tuberous sclerosis (4). The most common locations are the left ventricle and ventricular septum, although 30 percent have atrial wall or right ventricular involvement (23).

Contrary to older reports of the grim prognosis of cardiac rhabdomyoma (6,14), more recent series of children with cardiac rhabdomyoma and tuberous sclerosis have shown an excellent prognosis, with regression of cardiac lesions the rule (23). Patients with cardiac rhabdomyoma and tuberous sclerosis who survive the first month of life usually die because of other cardiac defects or central nervous system tumors (6).

There have been reports of cardiac rhabdomyoma associated with glomerulocystic disease and megacystic-microcolon-intestinal hypoperistalsis syndrome (7,19), which may be unusual manifestations of tuberous sclerosis.

The next largest group of patients with cardiac rhabdomyoma are those who lack other pathologic lesions or syndromes. Although the age at presentation ranges from birth to 15 years, these patients generally become symptomatic early in life because their tumors are likely to project into the ventricular lumen. There is no sex predilection. Presenting symptoms vary and are related to hydrops fetalis, congestive heart failure, sudden cardiac death (3,20), supraventricular and ventricular arrhythmias (5), and ventricular outflow obstruction (3,17). In contrast to patients with tuberous sclerosis, approximately 50 percent of sporadic cardiac rhabdomyomas are single lesions. These patients often benefit from surgical excision, which can be curative (2,6,16,17).

The smallest group of patients with cardiac rhabdomyoma are those with structural abnormalities of the heart. Hypoplastic left heart syndrome, transposition of the great arteries, ventricular septal defect, endocardial fibroelastosis, subaortic stenosis, Ebstein's anomaly, hypoplastic tricuspid valve, double outlet right ventricle, and pulmonary atresia have all been described in patients with cardiac rhabdomyoma (3,10,15, 18,24). In these cases, tuberous sclerosis is not usually present and the clinical features are dominated by the congenital heart disease.

Gross Findings. Rhabdomyomas are firm, white, well-circumscribed lobulated nodules

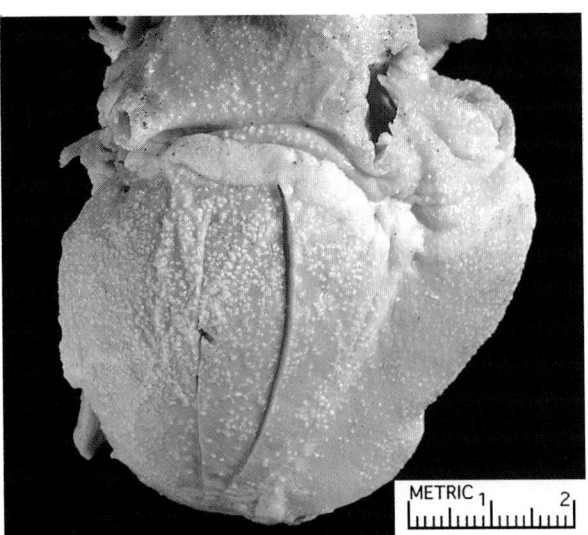

Figure 5-1
CARDIAC RHABDOMYOMA
Note the multiple, minute tumors studding the epicardial surface. This pattern of involvement is typical in patients with tuberous sclerosis. (Fig. 26 from Fascicle 15, 2nd series.)

that occur in any location in the heart, but are more common in the ventricles. When multiple, they can consist of numerous miliary nodules measuring less than 1 mm (fig. 5-1) (20); in these instances, the term *rhabdomyomatosis* has been used. Tumors can become quite large, especially in sporadic cases (figs. 5-2–5-4). Of 14 cases in the Armed Forces Institute of Pathology (AFIP) files in which tumor size was measured, the range was 0.3 to 9 cm, with a mean of 3.4 cm.

Histologic Findings. Cardiac rhabdomyomas are quite distinctive and unlikely to be confused with other entities. Tumors are well demarcated and composed of enlarged cells with clear cytoplasm and occasional spider cells (figs. 5-5, 5-6). There is uniform vacuolization of cells and cytoplasm is relatively sparse, in contrast to adult rhabdomyoma (see below). There is a strong reaction with periodic acid–Schiff (PAS), reflecting the glycogen content of rhabdomyoma cells. Spider cells are so named because of their centrally located nucleus surrounded by cytoplasm with radial extensions from the center of the cell to the periphery.

Immunohistochemical studies document the striated muscle characteristics of rhabdomyoma cells, which express myoglobin, desmin, actin, and vimentin (figs. 5-7, 5-8) (3).

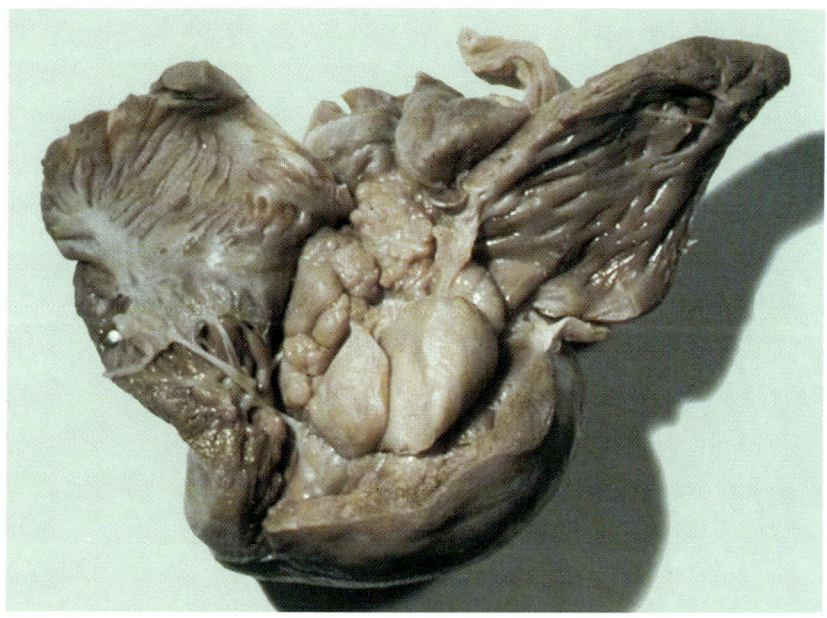

Figure 5-2
CARDIAC RHABDOMYOMA

Occasionally, cardiac rhabdomyomas, especially sporadic cases in patients without tuberous sclerosis, project into the cavity. This particular tumor obstructed the tricuspid valve. (Fig. 1 from Fenoglio JJ, McAllister HA, Ferrans VJ. Cardiac rhabdomyoma: a clinicopathologic and electron microscopic study. Am J Cardiol 1976;38:241–51.)

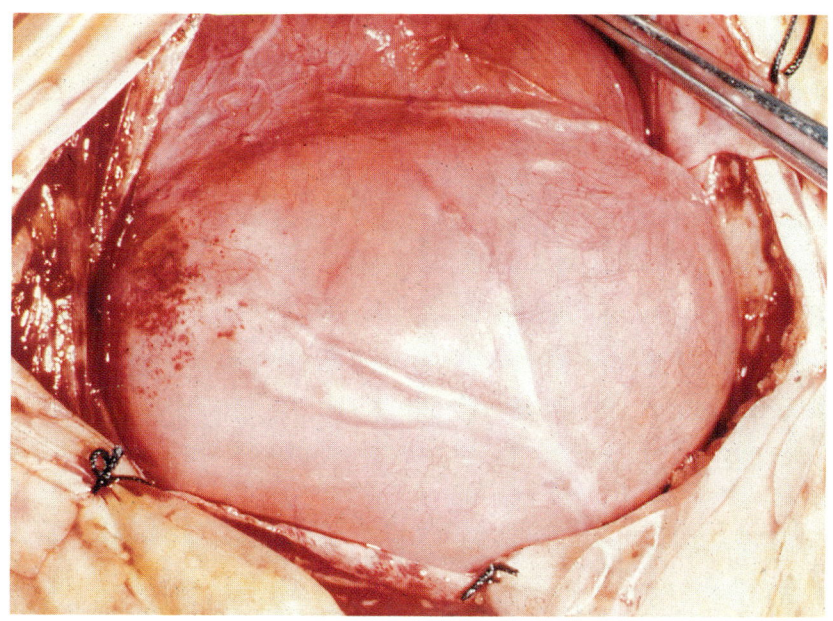

Figure 5-3
CARDIAC RHABDOMYOMA

A well-circumscribed tumor in a 3-year-old girl who presented with a heart murmur. There was a single mass in the right ventricle. There was no indication of tuberous sclerosis.

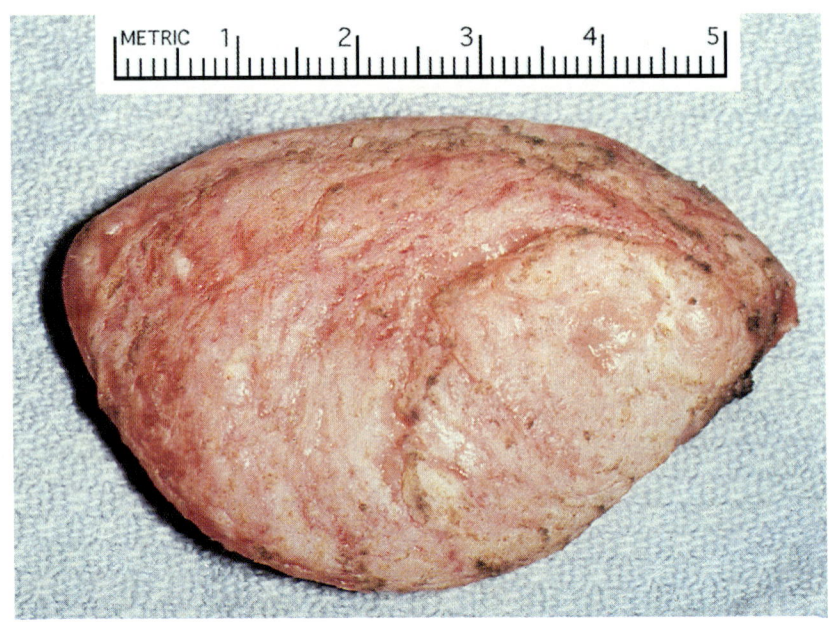

Figure 5-4
CARDIAC RHABDOMYOMA
This is a surgically excised specimen (unfixed) from the tumor illustrated in figure 5-3 showing a whitish tan cut surface.

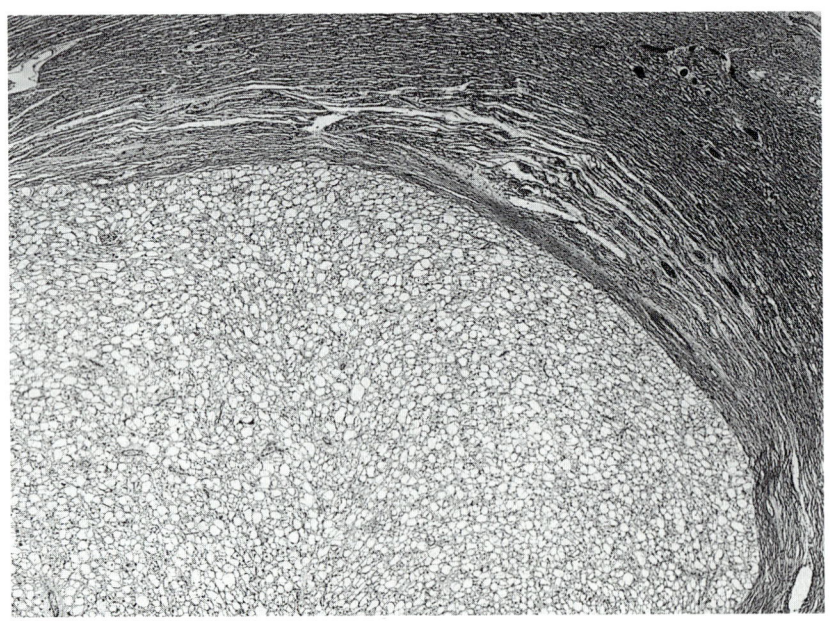

Figure 5-5
CARDIAC RHABDOMYOMA
Low magnification demonstrates demarcation between vacuolated tumor cells and adjacent cardiac muscle. (Fig. 1A from Burke AP, Virmani R. Cardiac rhabdomyoma: a clinicopathologic study. Mod Pathol 1991;4:70–4.)

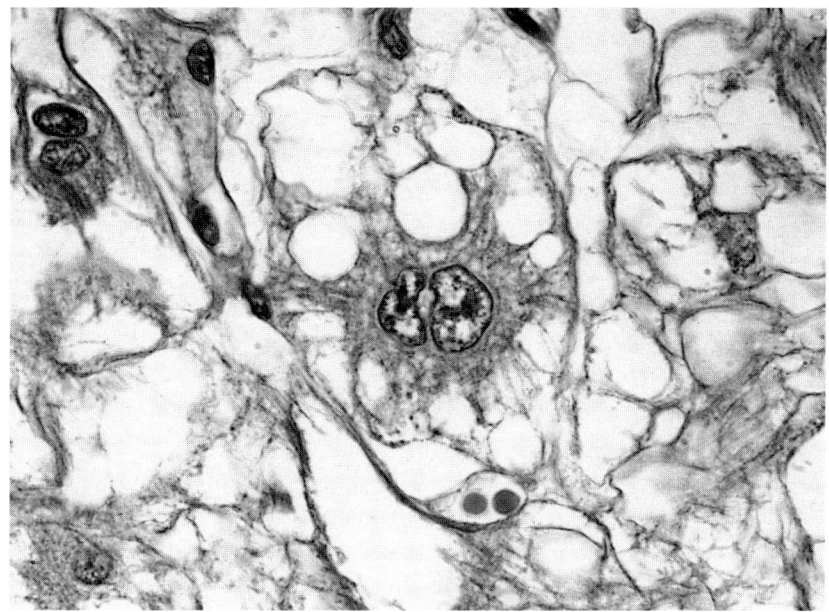

Figure 5-6
CARDIAC RHABDOMYOMA
Oil immersion photomicrograph demonstrates a spider cell (center) and intracellular myofilaments.

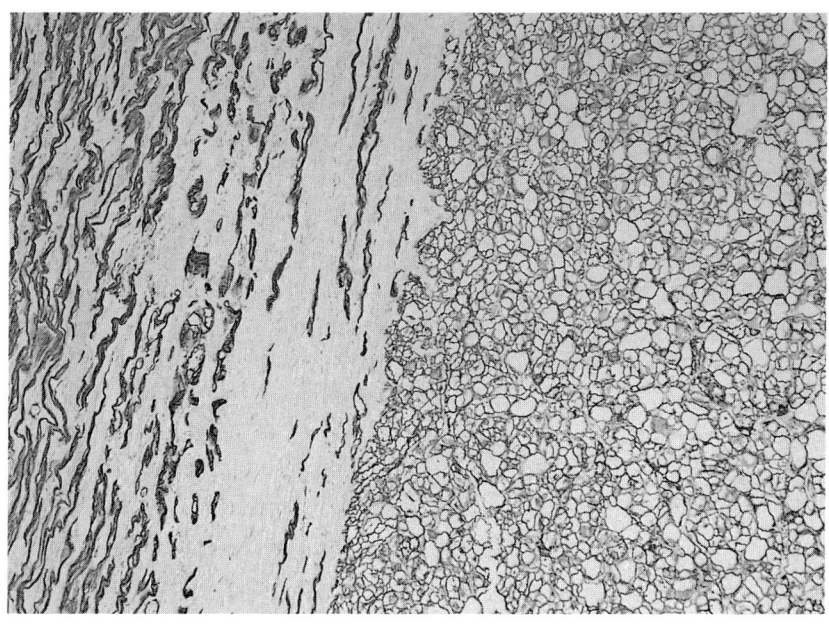

Figure 5-7
CARDIAC RHABDOMYOMA
Immunohistochemical preparation shows staining with antimuscle-specific actin. Tumor cells (right of field) stain, as do cardiac cells (left). (Fig. 2A from Burke AP, Virmani R. Cardiac rhabdomyoma: a clinicopathologic study. Mod Pathol 1991;4:70–4.)

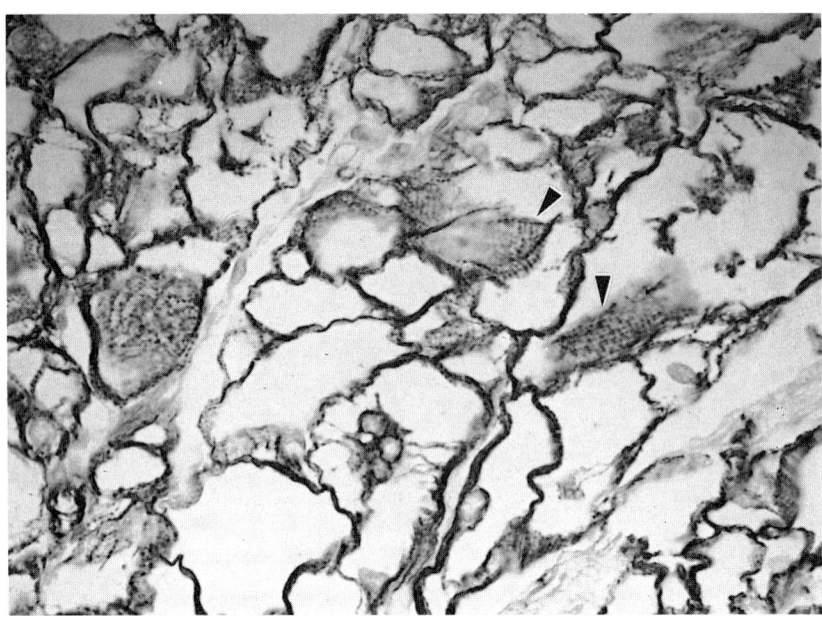

Figure 5-8
CARDIAC RHABDOMYOMA
Cross striations (arrowheads) and a spider cell are visible using immunohistochemical antibodies against muscle-specific actin.

Ultrastructural Findings. By electron microscopy, the cells of cardiac rhabdomyoma resemble altered myocytes (9,21). They possess abundant glycogen (fig. 5-9) and small and sparse mitochondria; cellular junctions resembling intercalated disks surround the periphery of the cell. In contrast, the intercalated disks of differentiated myocytes are located exclusively at the poles of the cell. Intercalated discs and myofibrils or collections of Z-band material are present, and there have been reports of primitive T-tubules in cardiac rhabdomyoma cells. Leptomeric fibers close to the sarcolemma may be identified.

Differential Diagnosis. The diagnosis of cardiac rhabdomyoma is rarely problematic; indeed, in patients with tuberous sclerosis, a tissue diagnosis is considered unnecessary if multiple cardiac masses are present. Histologically, the differential diagnosis includes lipoma, granular cell tumor, glycogen storage diseases, and histiocytoid cardiomyopathy. Lipomas lack myofibers and are located primarily on the epicardial surface. Lipomatous hypertrophy of the interatrial septum is an infiltrative process without clear boundaries, and is composed of brown fat mixed with mature fat and enlarged myocytes. Granu-

lar cell tumors are small lesions that are generally present on the epicardial surface and lack the vacuolated cells of rhabdomyoma. Granular cell tumors do not possess myofibers, and are S-100 positive and desmin and myoglobin negative, unlike rhabdomyomas. Glycogen storage diseases can mimic the vacuolated appearance of cardiac rhabdomyoma and possess similar abundant intracytoplasmic glycogen. However, they do not form well-circumscribed nodules, and ultrastructurally the cells show intact polar intercalated discs of mature myocytes. Histiocytoid cardiomyopathy has been termed a form of rhabdomyomatosis; in contrast to rhabdomyoma, however, tumor nodules are small, and there is fine granularity to the cells without large vacuoles and spider cells.

Treatment. Patients with rhabdomyomas and arrhythmias or cardiac murmurs have been treated surgically with excellent outcome (1–3, 6,16,17). Of the 28 surgical cases of cardiac rhabdomyoma compiled from these reports, most were single tumors; most patients were under 6 months of age, although there was a single 9-year-old (3); there were 3 early deaths, but the remainder of patients survived the procedure

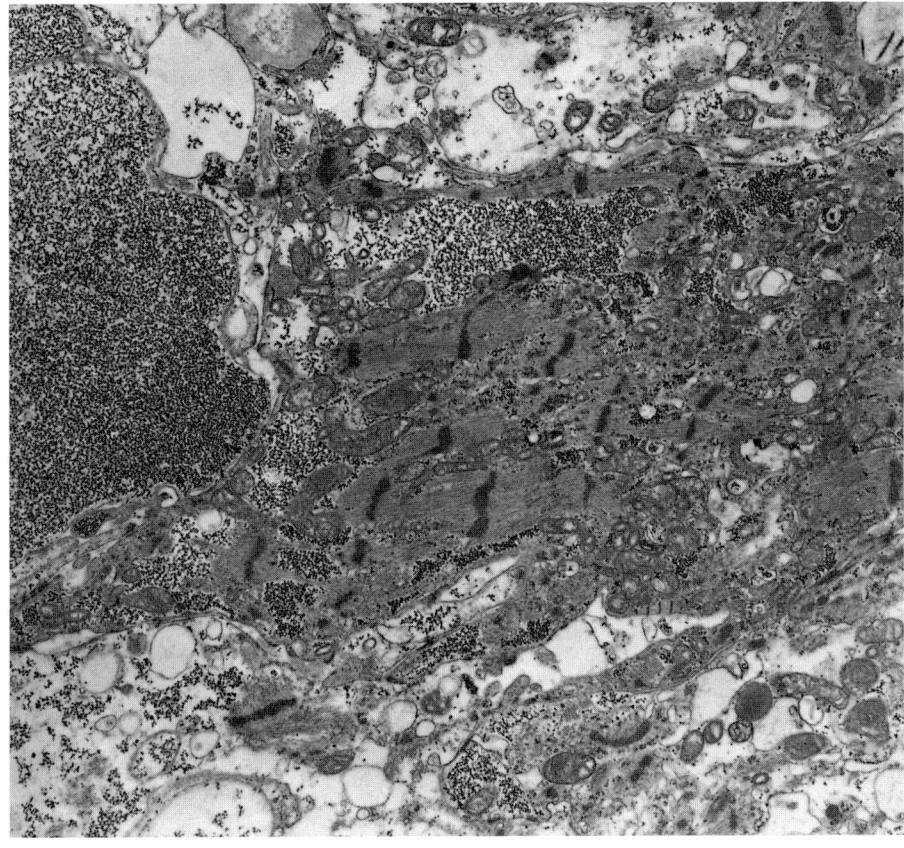

Figure 5-9
CARDIAC RHABDOMYOMA

Ultrastructurally there is an abundance of glycogen; mitochondria are small and sparse. There are fragmented irregular myofilaments with Z-bands. This figure illustrates a single right ventricular tumor resected from a 12-week-old without evidence of tuberous sclerosis.

well and no late deaths were recorded; only 5 patients had documented evidence of tuberous sclerosis, one of whom survived 29 years (6); and 5 patients had ventricular outflow obstruction, with 2 requiring complex surgery with graft placement. In some patients with refractory arrhythmias, electrophysiologic mapping is performed intraoperatively to localize arrhythmogenic tumors (16). These results indicate that surgical treatment is indicated in selected patients with rhabdomyoma, especially sporadic cases of single tumors.

HISTIOCYTOID CARDIOMYOPATHY

Definition. Histiocytoid cardiomyopathy is a multicentric hamartoma of oncocytic cardiac cells of myocyte origin. It occurs in infants and children and results in ventricular tachyarrhythmias. There are numerous synonyms, in-

cluding *Purkinje cell hamartoma, Purkinje cell tumor, infantile cardiomyopathy, oncocytic cardiomyopathy, xanthomatous cardiomyopathy,* and *congenital glycogenic tumor.*

Histogenesis. Although originally considered a form of histiocyte, the cell of origin of histiocytoid cardiomyopathy is currently considered to be either a cardiac myocyte or a Purkinje cell (see below). Because they are multicentric aggregates of modified cells occurring exclusively in infants, the clusters of cells in histiocytoid cardiomyopathy are currently believed to be hamartomas (26,28). Other considerations of histogenesis include a form of mitochondrial cardiomyopathy; however, the focal nature of the affected cells and lack of extracardiac muscle involvement weaken this theory. A sequela of rubella infection has also been considered, but there is little clinical and morphologic evidence for this theory (28).

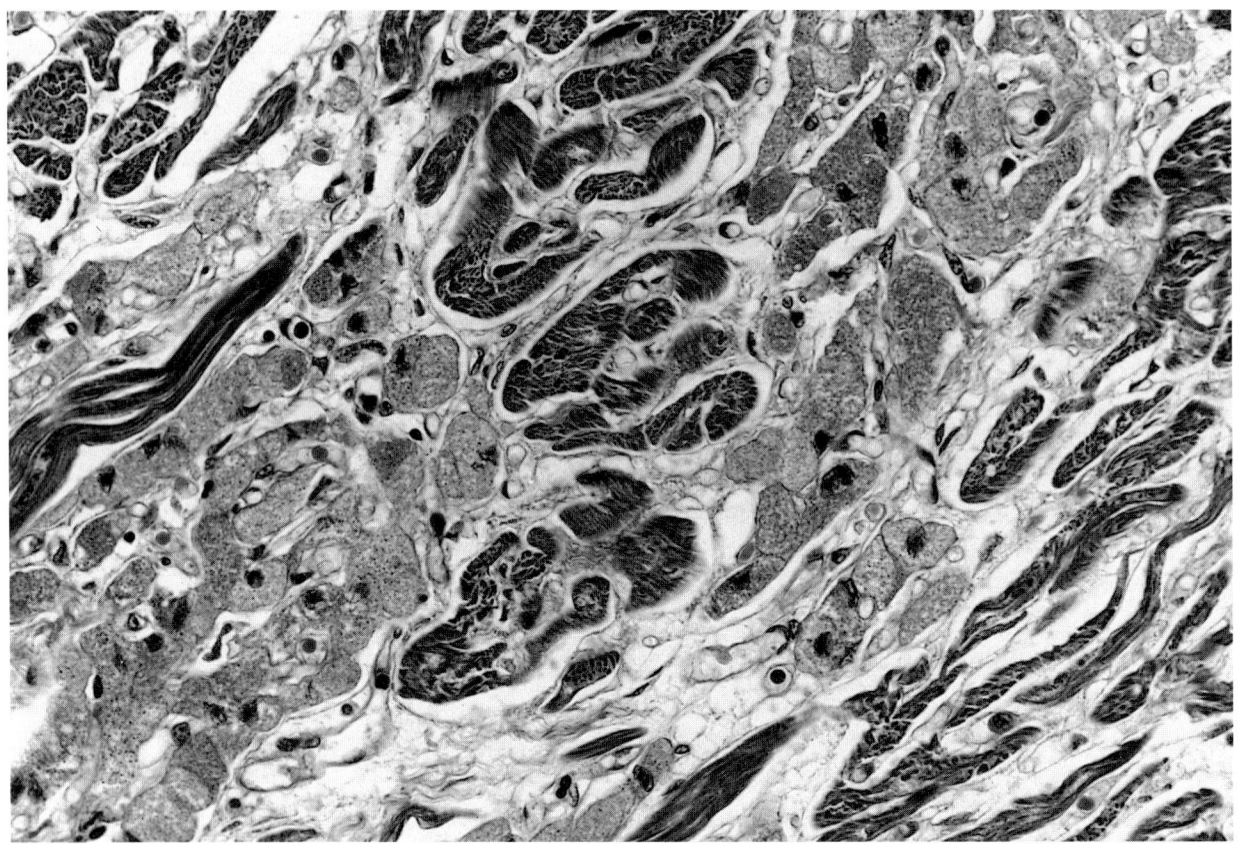

Figure 5-10
HISTIOCYTOID CARDIOMYOPATHY
Clusters of finely granular myocytes with the appearance of histiocytes are present among normal myocytes.

Incidence. Histiocytoid cardiomyopathy is quite rare: 53 cases were reported by 1994 (28). Thirteen cases initially described clinically in a large surgical series (29) were subsequently reported with pathologic documentation (27).

Clinical Features. The age range at presentation is birth to 4 years (mean, 12.5 months) (26, 28). There is female predominance of 4 to 1. The most common presenting features are arrhythmias, followed by seizures, heart failure, cyanosis, dyspnea, and sudden death (28). The arrhythmias and conduction disturbances include ventricular tachycardia and fibrillation, supraventricular tachycardias, premature ventricular contractions, Wolff-Parkinson-White syndrome, heart block, and Lown-Ganong-Levine syndrome.

Associated cardiac and extracardiac anomalies affect approximately 25 percent of patients. These include atrial and ventricular septal defect, hypoplastic left heart syndrome, ovarian cysts, midline defects of the central nervous system, malformations of the eyes, and oncocytic changes in glands (28).

Gross Findings. The nodules of histiocytoid cardiomyopathy are raised and yellowish. They range from 1mm to 1.5 cm, and are usually less than 2 mm in diameter. The left ventricle is always involved, but right ventricular and atrial nodules are also common. There is a predilection for subendocardial regions at the base of the ventricular septum, but subepicardial nodules occur in over 50 percent of cases.

Microscopic Findings. Histiocytoid cardiomyopathy is characterized by clusters of foamy cells that are well demarcated from adjacent normal myocardium (fig. 5-10). The abnormal cells are large, pale, and round to oval, and are often surrounded by thin collagen fibers. They stain faintly with PAS. In contrast to rhabdomyoma, large vacuoles and cytoplasmic streaming are

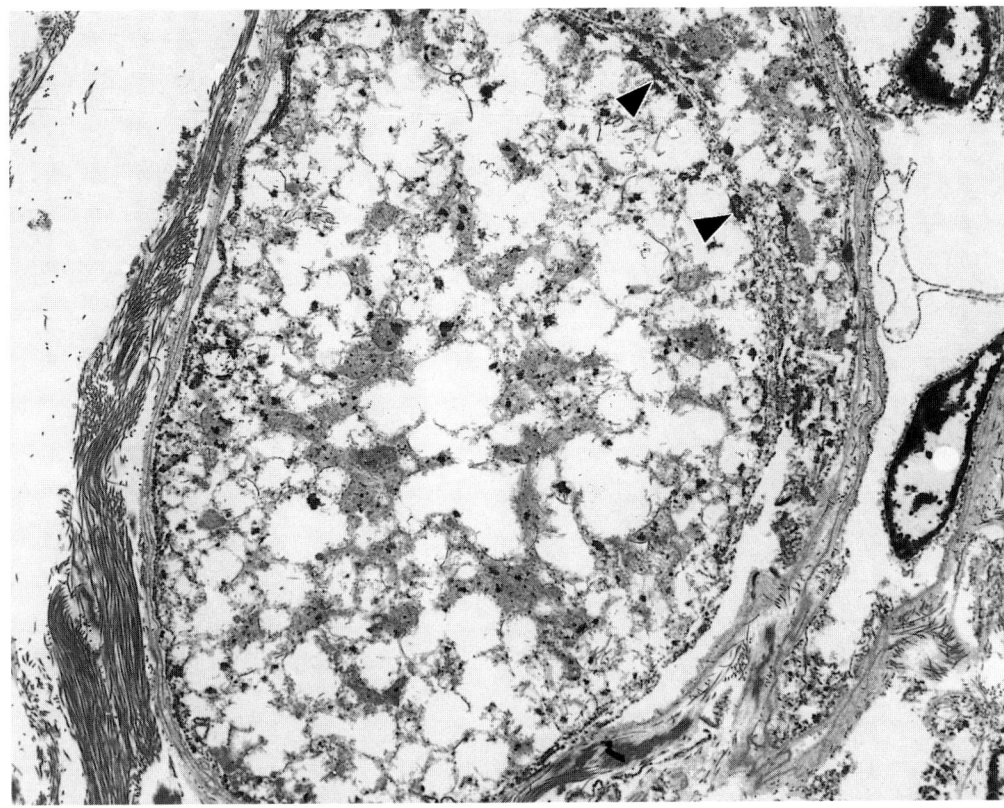

Figure 5-11
HISTIOCYTOID CARDIOMYOPATHY
Ultrastructurally, histiocytoid cells have abundant mitochondria, which replace myofibrils. In this illustration, the mitochondria are in various stages of degeneration, and Z-band–like material is seen towards the periphery of the cell (arrowheads).

absent. By immunohistochemical techniques, the cells are negative for lysozyme and alpha-1-antitrypsin, and weakly positive for myoglobin, desmin, and myosin.

Ultrastructural Findings. Histiocytoid cells show few or no myofibrils, marked mitochondriosis (fig. 5-11), an absence of T-tubules, limited numbers of desmosomes, rare intercalated discs, and occasional leptomeric fibers (fig. 5-12) (28). The findings are similar to rhabdomyoma, except that mitochondria are extremely numerous in histiocytoid cardiomyopathy, glycogen is not increased as in rhabdomyoma, and cellular junctions are less developed. The absence of T-tubules is characteristic of Purkinje cells; however, the lack of glycogenosis, lack of complex intercellular junctions with nexus formation, and increased mitochondria are not characteristic. The lack of T-tubules has been explained by the relative paucity of myofibrils,

and does not necessarily indicate a Purkinje cell origin. A currently held view is that histiocytoid cardiomyopathy represents a focal oncocytic change in cardiac myocytes, rejecting the theory of a Purkinje cell origin (28).

Treatment. In cases of refractory arrhythmias, electrophysiologic mapping with cryoablation or surgical excision has been successful in ameliorating symptoms (29).

MISCELLANEOUS BENIGN TUMORS OF CARDIAC MUSCLE

Hamartomas of Mature Cardiac Myocytes

There are rare hamartomas of cardiac muscle which differ histologically and clinically from cardiac rhabdomyoma of histiocytoid cardiomyopathy. These are demarcated masses of enlarged, hypertrophied, mature myocytes with a variable amount of collagen (figs. 5-13–5-15).

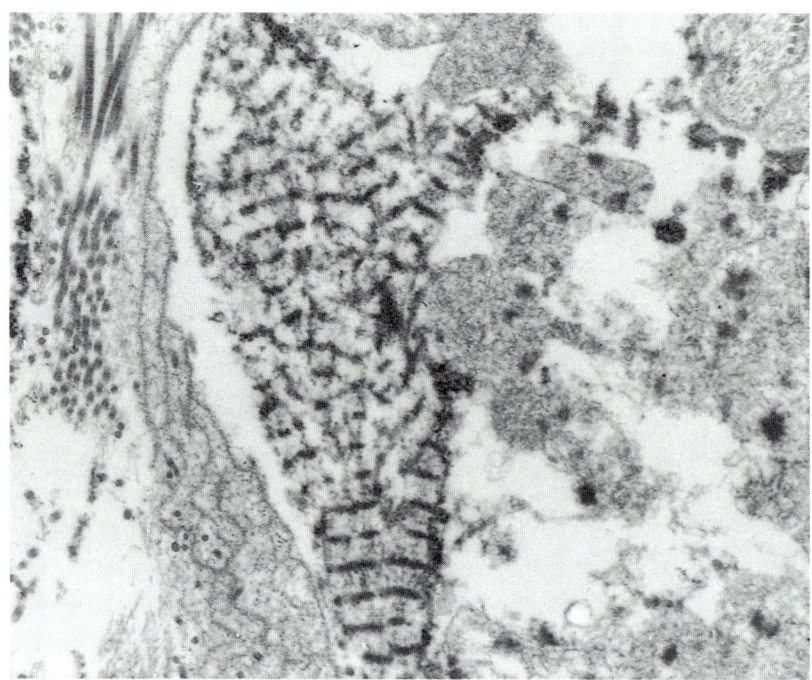

Figure 5-12
HISTIOCYTOID CARDIOMYOPATHY: LEPTOMERIC FIBRIL
Leptomeric fibrils vary in length, measuring several microns, and are 0.2 to 0.5 μm in width. Bundles of thin filaments form cross striations with a periodicity of 100 to 180 nm.

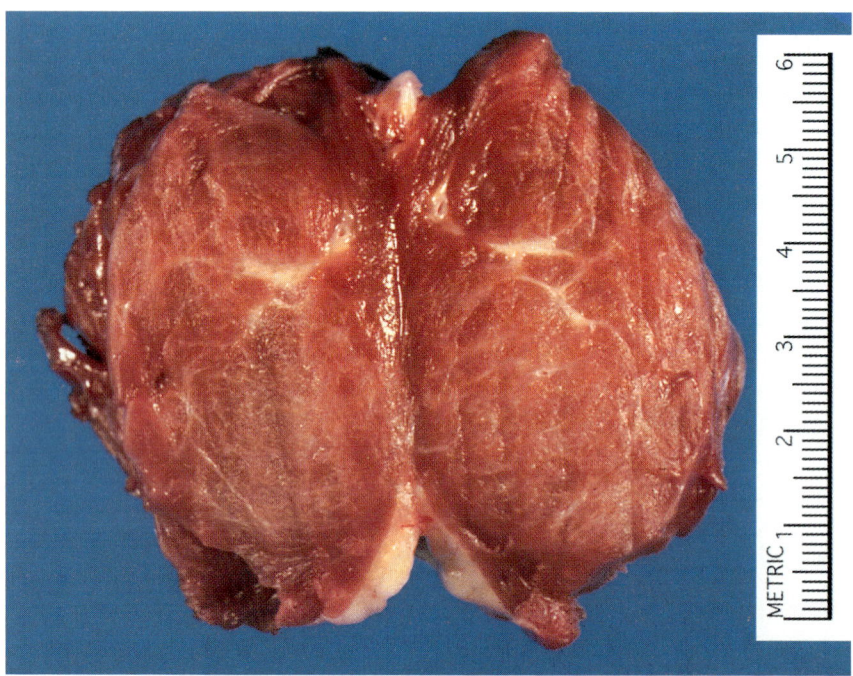

Figure 5-13
CARDIAC HAMARTOMA
This right ventricular mass was resected from an asymptomatic young man with an incidental murmur.

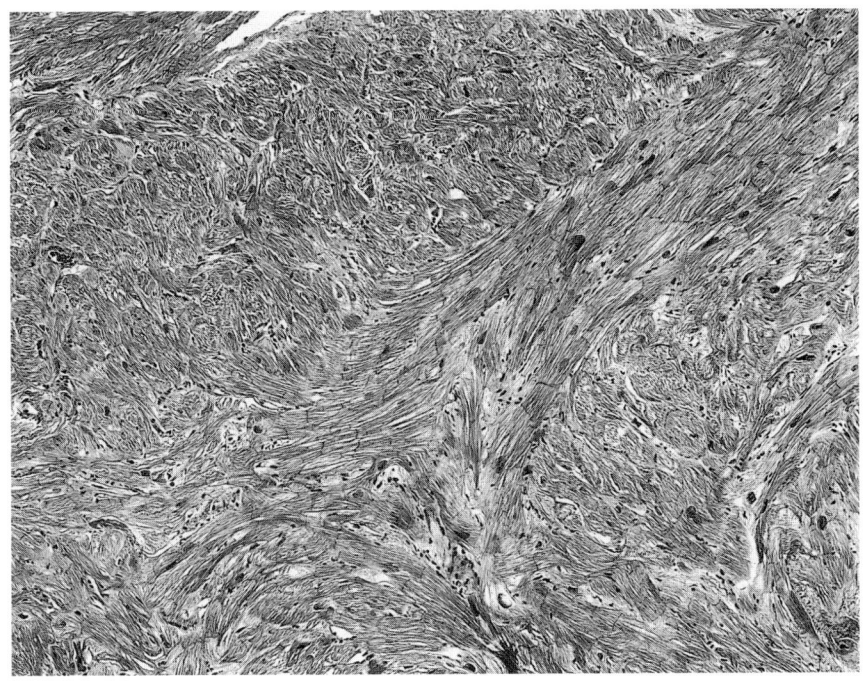

Figure 5-14
CARDIAC HAMARTOMA
Histologic section of the mass illustrated in figure 5-13 shows disorganized cardiac cells with prominent nuclei.

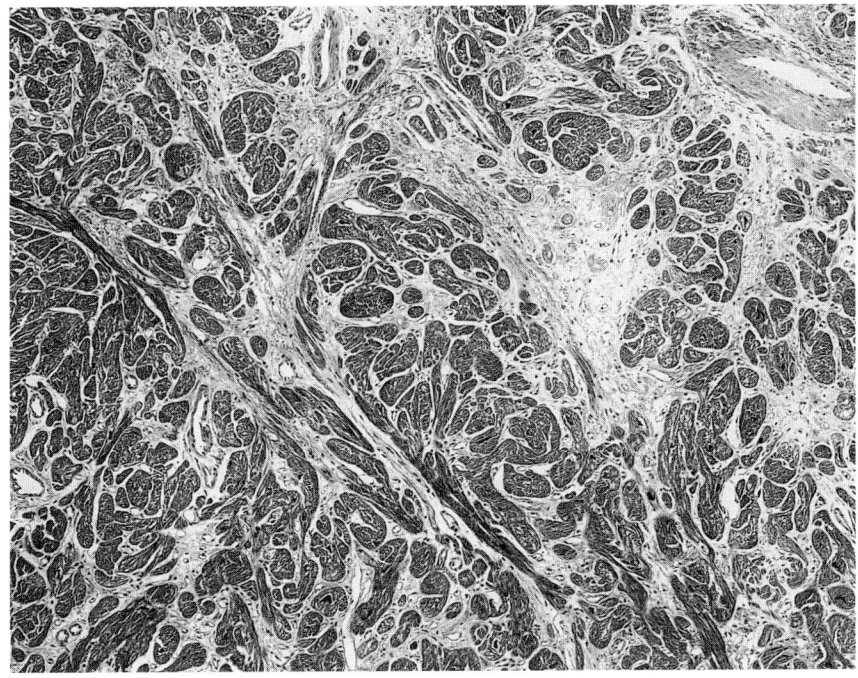

Figure 5-15
CARDIAC HAMARTOMA
These lesions show areas of fibrosis in addition to haphazard, hypertrophied myocytes.

The myofibers in these tumors demonstrate fibromuscular disarray suggestive of hypertrophic cardiomyopathy. In contrast to hypertrophic cardiomyopathy, however, these tumors are usually in the right ventricle or atrium and are circumscribed. Until more cases are reported, it remains unknown whether they are forms of cardiomyopathy or are more related to rhabdomyoma. The myocardial hamartomas reported in the literature as part of larger series (30,31) are not histologically characterized and may represent similar tumors.

Adult (Extracardiac) Rhabdomyoma

The classification of soft tissue rhabdomyomas is based largely on site. Those of the heart are congenital nodules composed of vacuolated striated muscle cells filled with glycogen (see above). Extracardiac rhabdomyomas are histologically distinct from cardiac rhabdomyomas and are separated into three groups: the genital type are polyps, usually in the external genitalia of women, composed of large rhabdomyoblasts in a myxoid matrix; the adult and fetal types are solitary masses, usually in the head and neck region. Adult rhabdomyoma is histologically composed of tightly packed, round to polygonal cells with eosinophilic, finely granular cytoplasm, occasional vacuoles, and spider cells. Unlike cardiac rhabdomyoma, there is abundant eosinophilic cytoplasm.

A single case of a tumor resembling an adult rhabdomyoma has been reported in a 42-year-old woman who presented with palpitations and a right atrial mass (32). Because of the patient's age and histologic features, this tumor was classified as a cardiac rhabdomyoma resembling an extracardiac rhabdomyoma.

REFERENCES

Rhabdomyoma

1. Arciniegas E, Hakimi M, Farooki ZQ, Truccone NJ, Green EW. Primary cardiac tumors in children. J Thorac Cardiovasc Surg 1980;79:582–91.
2. Blondeau P. Primary cardiac tumors—French studies of 533 cases. Thorac Cardiovasc Surg 1990;38:192–5.
3. Burke AP, Virmani R. Cardiac rhabdomyoma, a clinicopathologic study. Mod Pathol 1991;4:70–4.
4. Byard RW, Smith NM, Bourne AJ. Incidental cardiac rhabdomyomas: a significant finding necessitating additional investigation at the time of autopsy. J Forensic Sci 1991;36:1229–33.
5. Case CL, Gillette PC, Crawford FA. Cardiac rhabdomyomas causing supraventricular and lethal ventricular arrhythmias in an infant. Am Heart J 1991;122:1484–6.
6. Chan HS, Sonley MJ, Moes CA, Daneman A, Smith CR, Martin DJ. Primary and secondary tumors of childhood involving the heart, pericardium, and great vessels. A report of 75 cases and review of the literature. Cancer 1985;56:825–36.
7. Couper RT, Byard RW, Cutz E, Stringer DA, Durie PR. Cardiac rhabdomyomata and megacystic-microcolon-intestinal hypoperistalsis syndrome. J Med Genet 1991;28:274–6.
8. Diamant S, Sharaz J, Holtzman M, Lanaido S. Echocardiographic diagnosis of cardiac tumors in symptomatic tuberous sclerosis patients. Clin Pediatr 1983;22:297–9.
9. Fenoglio JJ Jr, Diana DJ, Bowen TE, McAllister HA, Ferrans VJ. Ultrastructure of a cardiac rhabdomyoma. Hum Pathol 1977;8:700–6.
10. _____, McAllister HA, Ferrans VJ. Cardiac rhabdomyoma: a clinicopathologic and electron microscopic study. Am J Cardiol 1976;38:241–51
11. Golding R, Reed G. Rhabdomyoma of the heart. Two unusual clinical presentations. N Engl J Med 1967;276:957–9.
12. Groves AM, Fagg NL, Cook AC, Allan LD. Cardiac tumors in intrauterine life. Arch Dis Child 1992;67:1189–92.
13. Heath D. Pathology of cardiac tumors. Am J Cardiol 1968;21:315–27.
14. Kidder LA. Congenital glycogenic tumor of the heart. AMA Arch Pathol 1950;49:55–60.
15. Nadas AS, Ellison RC. Cardiac tumors in infancy. Am J Cardiol 1968;21:363–6.
16. Murphy MC, Sweeney MS, Putnam JB Jr, et al. Surgical treatment of cardiac tumors: a 25-year experience. Ann Thorac Surg 1990;49:612–7.
17. Reece IJ, Cooley DA, Frazier OH, Hallman GL, Powers PL, Montero CG. Cardiac tumors. Clinical spectrum and prognosis of lesions other than classical benign myxoma in 20 patients. J Thorac Cardiovasc Surg 1984;88:439–46.
18. Russell GA, Dhasmana JP, Berry PJ, Gilbert-Barness EF. Coexistent cardiac tumours and malformations of the heart. Int J Cardiol 1989;22:890–8.

19. Saguem MH, Laarif M, Remadi S, Bozakoura C, Cox JN. Diffuse bilateral glomerulocystic disease of the kidneys and multiple cardiac rhabdomyomas in a newborn. Relationship with tuberous sclerosis and review of the literature. Pathol Res Pract 1992;188:367–73.
20. Shrivastava S, Jacks JJ, White RS, Edwards JE. Diffuse rhabdomyomatosis of the heart. Arch Pathol Lab Med 1977;101:78–90.
21. Silverman JF, Kay S, McCue CM, Lower RR, Brough AJ, Chang CH. Rhabdomyoma of the heart: ultrastructural study of three cases. Lab Invest 1976;35:596–606.
22. Smith HC, Watson GH, Patel RG, Super M. Cardiac rhabdomyomata in tuberous sclerosis: their course and diagnostic value. Arch Dis Child 1989;64:196–200.
23. Smythe JF, Dyck JD, Smallhorn JF, Freedom RM. Natural history of cardiac rhabdomyoma in infancy and childhood. Am J Cardiol 1990;66:1247–9.
24. Watanabe T, Hojo Y, Kozaki T, Nagashima M, Ando M. Hypoplastic left heart syndrome with rhabdomyoma of the left ventricle. Pediatr Cardiol 1991;12:121–2.
25. Watson GH. Cardiac rhabdomyomas in tuberous sclerosis. Ann N Y Acad Sci 1991;615:50–7.

Histiocytoid Cardiomyopathy

26. Gelb AB, Van Meter SH, Billingham ME, Berry GJ, Rouse RV. Infantile histiocytoid cardiomyopathy myocardial or conduction system hamartoma: what is the cell type involved? Hum Pathol 1993;24:1226–31.
27. Kearney DL, Titus JL, Hawkins EP, Ott DA, Garson A. Pathologic features of myocardial hamartomas causing childhood tachyarrhythmias. Circulation 1987; 75:705–10.
28. Malhotra V, Ferrans VJ, Virmani R. Infantile histiocytoid cardiomyopathy: report of three cases and review of literature. Am Heart J, 1994;128:1009-21.
29. Murphy MC, Sweeney MS, Putnam JB, et al. Surgical treatment of cardiac tumors: a 25-year experience. 1990;49:612–7.

Miscellaneous Tumors of Cardiac Muscle

30. Blondeau P. Primary cardiac tumors—French studies of 533 cases. Thorac Cardiovasc Surg 1990;38:192–5.
31. Dein JR, Frist WH, Stinson EB, et al. Primary cardiac neoplasms. Early and late results of surgical treatment in 42 patients. J Thorac Cardiovasc Surg 1987;93:502–11.
32. Yu GH, Kussmaul WG, DiSesa VJ, Lodato RF, Brooks JS. Adult intracardiac rhabdomyoma resembling the extracardiac variant. Hum Pathol 1993;24:448–51.

6
BENIGN TUMORS OF FIBROUS TISSUE

CARDIAC FIBROMA

Definition. Cardiac fibroma is a benign congenital tumor that occurs as a discrete bulging mass composed primarily of fibroblasts and collagen. Synonyms include *fibromatosis* (32), *fibrous hamartoma* (23), and *fibroelastic hamartoma* (10). We discourage use of the term fibromatosis, since this suggests an aggressive, nonlocalized lesion. Cardiac involvement occasionally occurs with congenital generalized fibromatosis (28), and the term is more appropriate there.

Incidence. Cardiac fibromas are rare tumors: 70 were reported by 1976 (10) and fewer than 100 have been reported since then (1–13, 15–17,19,21–22,24–26,29–35). With the exception of the previous Fascicle on cardiac tumors (18) and two recent series of 23 cases and 5 cases (4,5), the literature on cardiac fibromas consists of case reports or series of 4 patients or less (34). After rhabdomyoma, cardiac fibroma is the second most common tumor of childhood in autopsy series (5,18,20), but is the most commonly resected tumor of children (2,10). In surgical series of patients of all ages, fibromas are the second most common benign primary cardiac tumor after myxoma (2,19,25,31).

Histogenesis. The exact nature of cardiac fibroma is unclear. Because many fibromas occur in infants and histologic changes are somewhat age-dependent, cardiac fibromas are most likely congenital lesions. There is some debate whether cardiac fibroma is a hamartoma or benign neoplasm, although these terms are not always considered to be mutually exclusive (10). Because most fibromas of the heart do not appear to recur or grow aggressively (see below), they are probably hamartomatous lesions. There are, however, rare aggressive tumors that do recur, similar to fibromatoses at extracardiac sites (32); these may be, in fact, true neoplasms. Ultrastructurally, the predominant cell type is the fibroblast, although there may be a myofibroblastic component as well (10,12,32).

Clinical Features. Eighty-six percent of cardiac fibromas occur in children, one third of whom are under 1 year of age (10). In a series of 23 patients, the mean age at presentation was 13 years (4). The age range at presentation extends from newborn to 75 years (33). There is no sex or race predominance.

Approximately one third of patients present with heart failure or cyanosis, one third with arrhythmias or syncope, and one third are asymptomatic and tumor discovery is incidental (4,5,13,29,33,35). Incidental lesions are identified either by auscultating murmurs at physical examination (5), noting calcification or mild cardiomegaly on chest radiographs, or at evaluation for Gorlin's syndrome (see below). Sudden death may also be the initial presentation (4). Rarely, cardiac fibromas result in left ventricular outflow obstruction (21,27), pulmonary outflow obstruction (19), unexplained pericardial effusion (4), and coronary insufficiency (26). Because of the predilection for the ventricular septum, fibromas may mimic hypertrophic cardiomyopathy (26).

There is little correlation between the type of presenting symptom and the location of tumor in the heart. Arrhythmias can occur in patients with tumors in any location in the heart, including the right ventricle, left ventricle, and interventricular septum. Patients with heart failure generally have large, bulky tumors in either ventricle that are difficult to treat surgically.

Cardiac fibroma must be considered in the differential diagnosis of a child with unexplained congestive heart failure, arrhythmia, cardiomegaly, murmur, or pericardial effusion. Although rhabdomyomas are more common in the newborn period, they are usually multiple; fibromas are nearly always single lesions. Fibromas are readily delineated by imaging studies (3,4,24). If calcification is noted in a cardiac mass of a child on chest X ray, echocardiography, angiography, magnetic resonance imaging (MRI), or computed tomography (CT), fibroma is a likely diagnosis; rhabdomyomas rarely calcify (26). Other calcified cardiac masses include myxomas and rarely lipomas (26). Calcification is not a sensitive diagnostic marker, since it occurs in less than one third of cases on chest radiography, but it is more readily detected by MRI and CT (4).

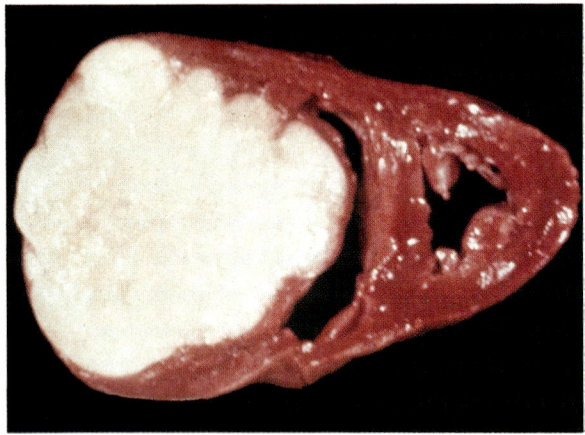

Figure 6-1
CARDIAC FIBROMA
A large circumscribed mass is seen in the lateral right ventricular wall, obliterating the right ventricular cavity.

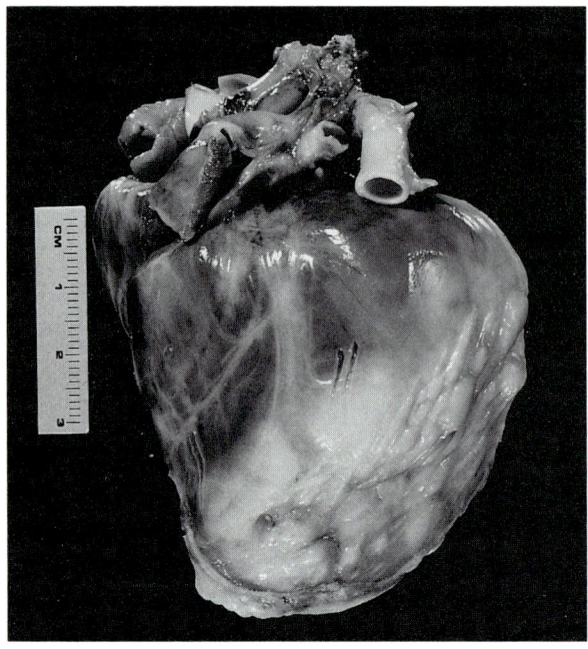

Figure 6-2
CARDIAC FIBROMA
Anterior and right lateral border of the heart shows a large mass in the area of the ventricular septum.

There is an increased risk of cardiac fibroma in patients with Gorlin's syndrome (8,14), also known as the nevoid-basal cell carcinoma syndrome, Gorlin-Goltz syndrome, and basal cell nevus syndrome. Gorlin's syndrome is characterized by an enlarged occipital circumference, odontogenic keratocysts of the jaws, epidermal cysts, rib anomalies, multiple basal cell carcinomas of the skin, and several other manifestations (14). Cardiac fibromas are noted in less than 14 percent of patients with Gorlin's syndrome but the association is not considered random (14). A patient with cardiac fibroma and multiple neural midline defects has also been described (9).

Gross Findings. The cardiac sites of fibromas are, in order of decreasing frequency, the ventricular septum, left ventricular free wall, right ventricle, and atria (4,5). Atrial fibroma is rare (13,32). In some cases, fibromas are massive tumors that obliterate the ventricular cavities. Cardiac fibromas are rounded masses that are fibrous, white, and whorled (figs. 6-1–6-4). They are nearly always mural lesions, although a single polypoid fibroma resulting in subaortic stenosis in an infant has been described (21). Every reported case but one (13) has been single. In a study by the authors (4), the mean diameter was 5 cm, but tumors as large as 8 cm have been reported (33). Cardiac fibromas can be either grossly circumscribed or infiltrating with push-

ing margins. Margins are readily identifiable and can extend beyond what the surgeon believes to be resectable.

Histologic Findings. Cardiac fibroma is a homogeneous proliferation of monomorphic fibroblasts that demonstrate little, if any, atypia. The degree of cellularity decreases with the age of the patient, whereas the amount of collagen increases (figs. 6-5–6-8) (4). Fibromas of adults and children are quite collagenous. Mitoses are generally present only in tumors of patients less than a few months of age. There can be occasional perivascular aggregates of lymphocytes and histiocytes (fig. 6-5) or sparse chronic inflammation at the junction of the tumor and uninvolved myocardium. Variable numbers of elastic fibers can be present; this finding is independent of age (fig. 6-9) (4). The presence of elastic fibers accounts for occasional use of the term *elastofibroma or fibroelastic hamartoma* (10). Calcification is a common finding in fibromas from patients of all ages and is occasionally seen on chest radiograph, MRI, or CT scan (fig. 6-10) (4,27,33). The background can be focally myxoid.

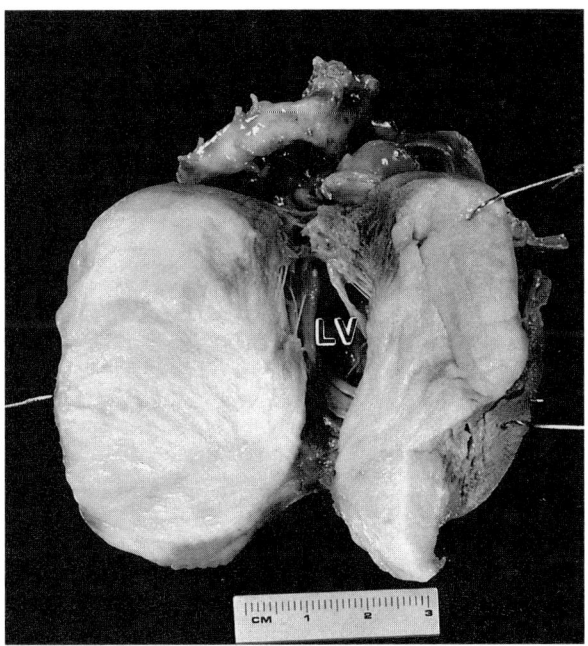

Figure 6-3
CARDIAC FIBROMA
Cut surface of the tumor shown in figure 6-2. The left
ventricular (LV) cavity is present behind the mass. The patient
was a 4-month-old child who died suddenly without a previous
medical history.

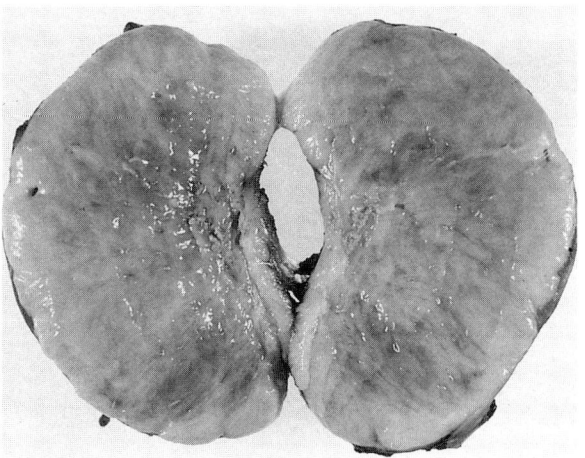

Figure 6-4
CARDIAC FIBROMA
Cut section of this surgically resected specimen shows a
homogenous mass that was easily shelled out.

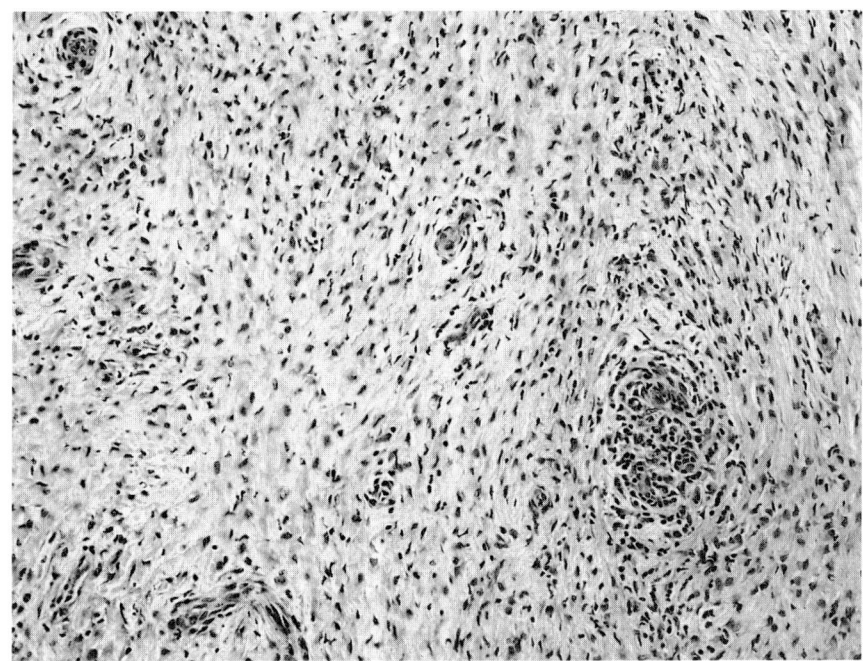

Figure 6-5
CARDIAC FIBROMA
In newborns and infants, the lesions can be quite cellular with little collagen deposition. There can be a sparse lymphocytic
perivascular infiltrate.

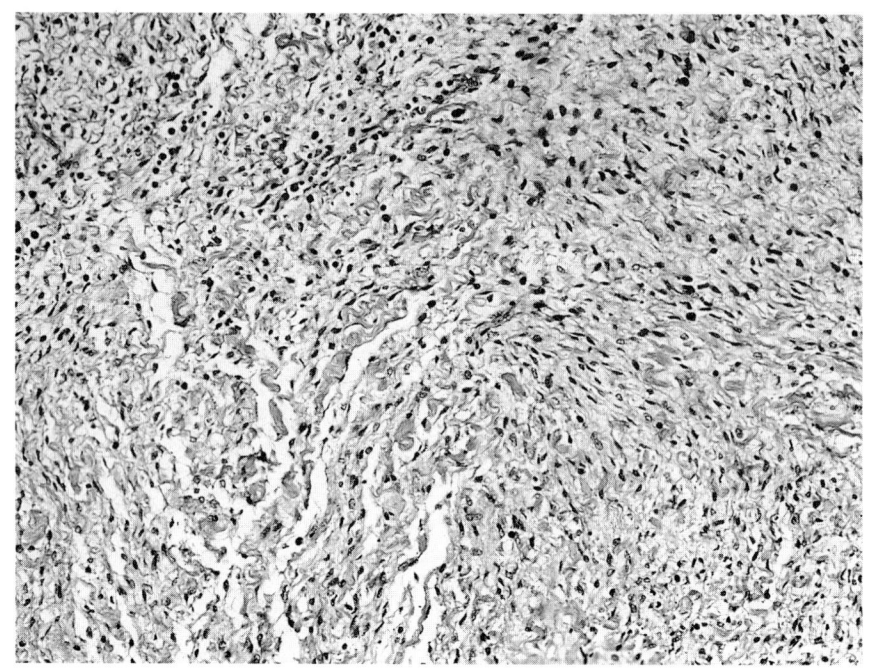

Figure 6-6
CARDIAC FIBROMA
This tumor has a mild degree of collagen deposition.

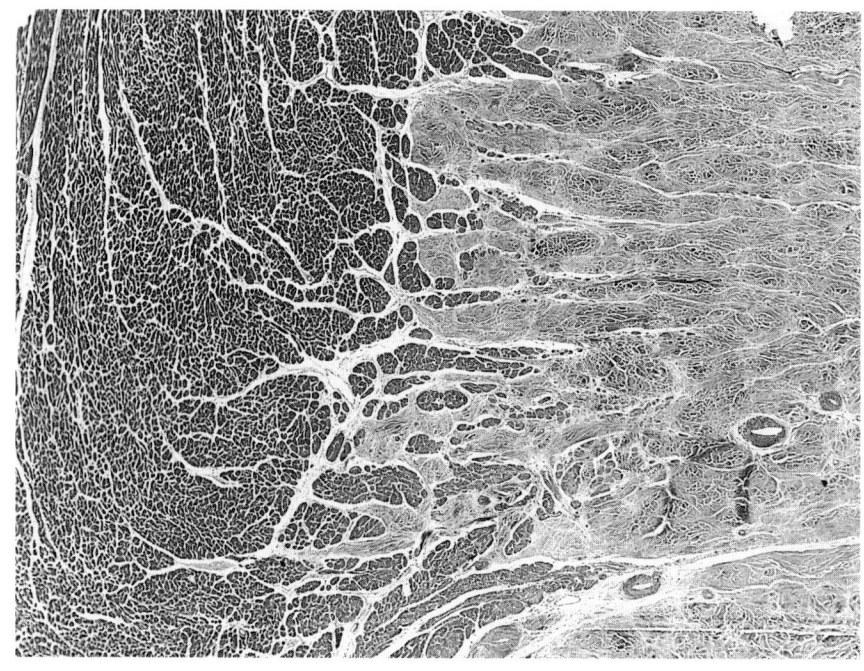

Figure 6-7
CARDIAC FIBROMA
In older children and adults, these tumors are acellular masses of collagen. (Masson trichrome stain)

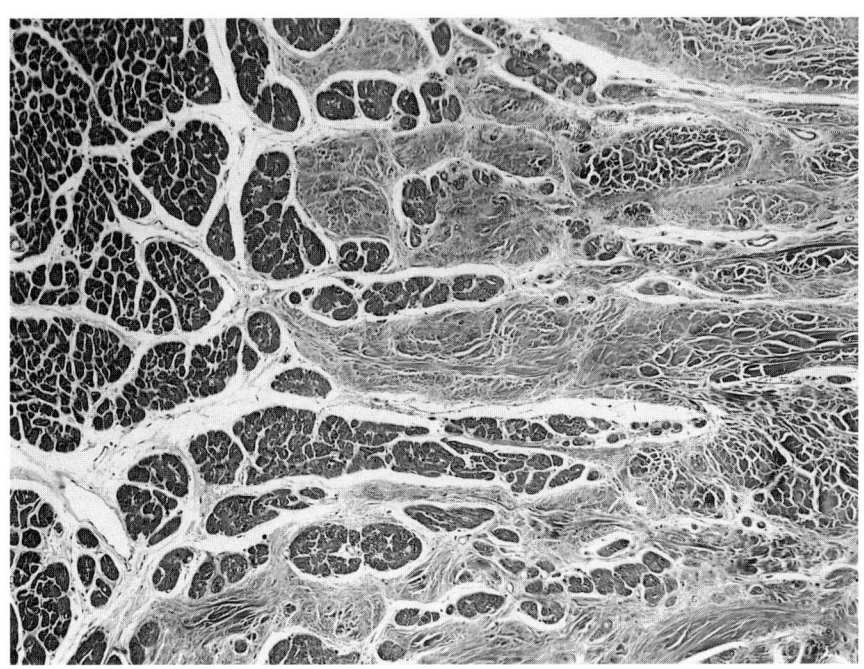

Figure 6-8
CARDIAC FIBROMA
This is a higher magnification view of figure 6-7. Although the tumors can grossly appear circumscribed, there is usually an infiltrating margin that can be appreciated histologically. (Masson trichrome stain)

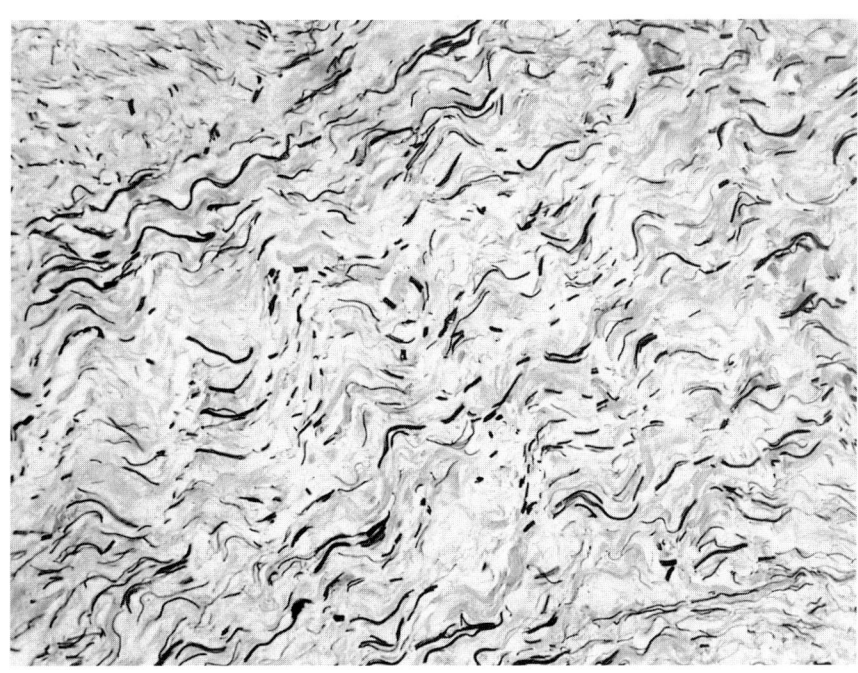

Figure 6-9
CARDIAC FIBROMA
Elastic fibers are common. (Elastin van Gieson stain)

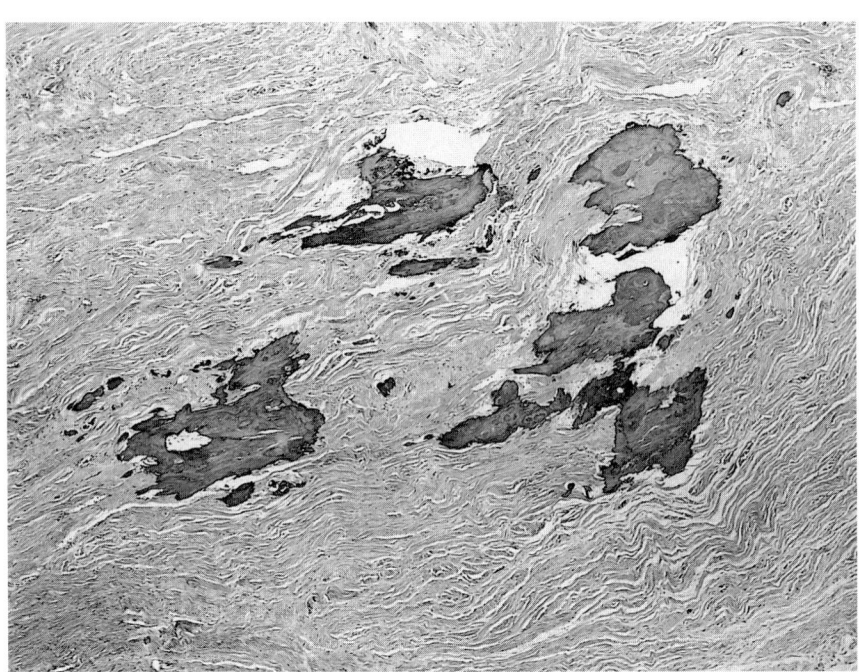

Figure 6-10
CARDIAC FIBROMA
Calcification is a common feature.

There have been several ultrastructural studies of cardiac fibroma with similar results (10,12, 17,32,34). The tumor cells resemble fibroblasts with few cellular organelles and an extensive endoplasmic reticulum, incompletely developed or absent basement membrane, ramifications of cytoplasmic processes, and a centrally placed ovoid nucleus with a distinct nucleolus (12,32). The stroma consists of proteoglycans, mast cells, collagen bundles, and elastic fibers (12,32). In addition to fibroblasts, there are cells of intermediate differentiation which contain myofilaments resembling smooth muscle myofilaments, and characteristic dense bodies against the plasma membrane and within intracellular filaments. However, these cells lack well-defined basement membranes, contain an abundant rough endoplasmic reticulum, and have extensive cytoplasmic processes, unlike smooth muscle cells (32).

Differential Diagnosis. The histologic diagnosis of cardiac fibroma is usually straightforward: there is a discrete mass of partly or completely collagenized stroma with intervening fibroblasts. However, if the tumor is unresectable, the pathologist sees only a wedge or needle biopsy (fig. 6-11). The differential diagnosis includes fibrosarcoma, which generally does not occur in the heart during the first few years of life. Histologically, the distinction between cellu-

lar fibromas of infants and fibrosarcoma is difficult, and is made on the basis of the sparse mitotic activity in fibroma. It is possible that rare examples of recurrent fibroma in infancy may in fact represent a low-grade fibrosarcoma (32). Fibromas in patients 6 months of age and older are relatively acellular, do not possess mitotic figures, and are therefore not histologically similar to fibrosarcoma. Inflammatory pseudotumors have a much more prominent inflammatory infiltrate and the tumor cells are stellate, rather than spindled, with the appearance of myofibroblasts. Also in the differential diagnosis is fibrous histiocytoma, an extremely rare cellular cardiac tumor that is composed of spindle cells and lipid-laden histiocytes. In older patients, the tumor can histologically simulate a scar, but grossly there is always a mass that results in a thickening or bulging of the ventricle not encountered in healed infarcts.

Treatment. Cardiac fibromas have been successfully removed from infants as young as 1 month of age (19). However, some attempts at resection in infants younger than 4 months have resulted in death (4,5,35). There is evidence that tumors may remain dormant for as long as 31 years (7), and spontaneous regression may occur (16). For this reason, some patients may be followed without surgery, especially if they are

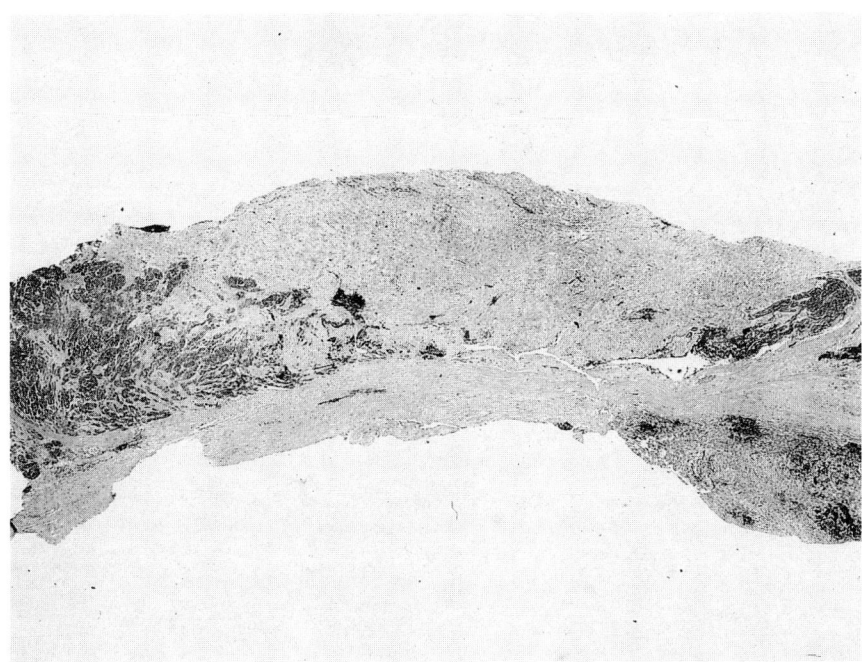

Figure 6-11
CARDIAC FIBROMA
Occasionally, the tumors are unresectable. This tumor was biopsied for diagnosis. Tumor cells are present within the light staining area in the center; darker surrounding areas are cardiac muscle. (Masson trichrome stain)

elderly (33). However, there are many arguments in favor of surgery in younger individuals. The propensity for cardiac fibroma to cause arrhythmias is increasingly evident (11), and surgery has been shown to ablate ventricular arrhythmias (30) which may be lethal (4,33,35). Successful resection with recurrence-free, long-term follow-up has been documented in over 30 patients (2,4, 5,19,22,25,31,33,35). However, complete excision is not always possible because of the infiltrative nature of these tumors, which may occasionally encase a coronary artery (26). Despite incomplete excision, with residual tumor that may be noted on echocardiography or chest radiography, patients may remain asymptomatic (6,31,33). In patients with large unresectable tumors, cardiac transplantation may be needed for refractory arrhythmias (15,32). For adequate surgical removal, patch repair of the septum or ventricular wall, valve replacement, or coronary artery grafting may be necessary (4).

SOLITARY FIBROUS TUMOR OF THE PERICARDIUM

Definition. Benign fibrous tumor is a neoplasm of fibroblasts that arises in close proximity to a mesothelial surface. Most benign fibrous tumors have been described in the pleura and

extrapericardial mediastinum (41). Other sites include the peritoneum, liver, paranasal sinuses, and thyroid gland (37). Synonyms include *pericardial fibroma* and *benign fibrous mesothelioma,* although the latter term is a misnomer.

Incidence. Solitary fibrous tumors of the pericardium are extremely rare: we know of only three cases reported in the medical literature (36,38), and there are two in the Armed Forces Institute of Pathology (AFIP) files. It is possible that seven pericardial fibromas reported by Mahaim in 1945 (39) represent the same entity.

Clinical Features. Pericardial fibrous tumors cause symptoms of pericarditis and pericardial effusion, and are found in adults of any age. Surgery is generally curative, but because of lack of knowledge of long-term behavior, close follow-up is recommended (36). Rare malignant examples of solitary fibrous tumors have been reported in the pleura and mediastinum (41), and analogous tumors of the pericardium have probably been classified as pericardial fibrosarcomas (see chapters 12 and 14).

Pathologic Findings. Grossly, the tumor is white, with a whorled appearance on cut section, and is attached to the pericardial surface either by a broad or narrow pedicle. There is no intracardiac extension. One tumor in the AFIP files measured 10 cm and was attached by a narrow pedicle to the

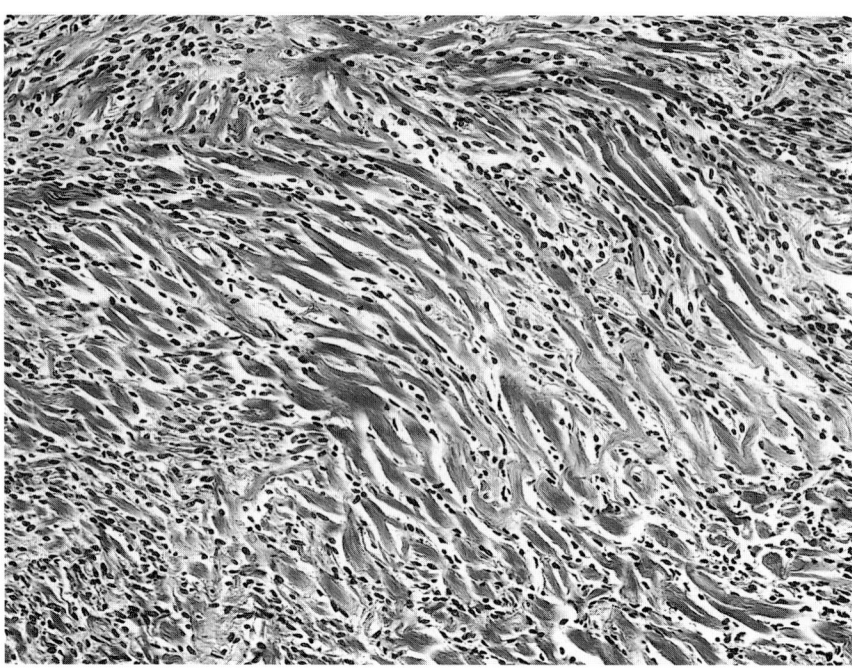

Figure 6-12
FIBROUS TUMOR:
PERICARDIUM
There is dense collagen and a proliferation of monomorphic spindle cells. Grossly, the tumor was a large, relatively circumscribed mass attached to the epicardium by a narrow pedicle (not shown).

epicardial surface. Histologically, the tumor consists of spindle cells with interspersed hyalinized collagen, focally arranged in bundles of collagen fibers (fig. 6-12). Small foci of calcification may be present, similar to cardiac fibroma. Mitotic figures, necrosis, and cellular atypia are generally absent. However, in 8 of 14 solitary fibrous tumors of the mediastinum reported by Witkin and Rosai (41), cellular areas with mitoses and necrosis were described. Myxoid areas and a vascular pattern reminiscent of hemangiopericytoma have been described in mediastinal tumors (41). Ultrastructural studies demonstrate spindle cells poor in organelles with occasional strands of rough endoplasmic reticulum (38,40). Immunohistochemically, the cells express vimentin and do not express cytokeratin (38,41), in contrast to mesothelioma.

Differential Diagnosis. There are few entities in the differential diagnosis of benign solitary fibrous tumor. Pericardial leiomyomas and neural tumors may be excluded by immunohistochemical stains for neural markers and trichrome stain for smooth muscle. Cardiac fibroma is histologically similar, if not indistinguishable, from solitary fibrous tumor. Unlike the latter, however, cardiac fibroma is an intramyocardial, not pericardial, mass. The diagnosis of malignant lesions of similar

histology is more complicated, and is discussed in chapters 12 and 14.

BENIGN FIBROUS HISTIOCYTOMA

In the differential diagnosis of fibroma and inflammatory pseudotumor is benign fibrous histiocytoma. There has been a report of an intracardiac fibrous histiocytoma (42); we have seen an intracardiac tumor in a patient who was free from recurrence more than 8 years after surgical removal of the histiocytoma (fig. 6-13). Benign fibrous histiocytomas may be true neoplasms or unusually cellular fibromas with a large number of histiocytes. In contrast to malignant fibrous histiocytoma, mitoses and pleomorphism are absent and the course is presumably benign, based on limited follow-up (42).

INFLAMMATORY PSEUDOTUMOR

Inflammatory pseudotumors are masses of chronic inflammatory and mesenchymal cells. Synonyms include *plasma cell granuloma* and *inflammatory fibrohistiocytic tumor.* The cardiac lesion is analogous to that described in the lung, thyroid, gastrointestinal tract, oral cavity, central nervous system, and genitourinary system. It is uncertain whether the lesion is a neoplasm

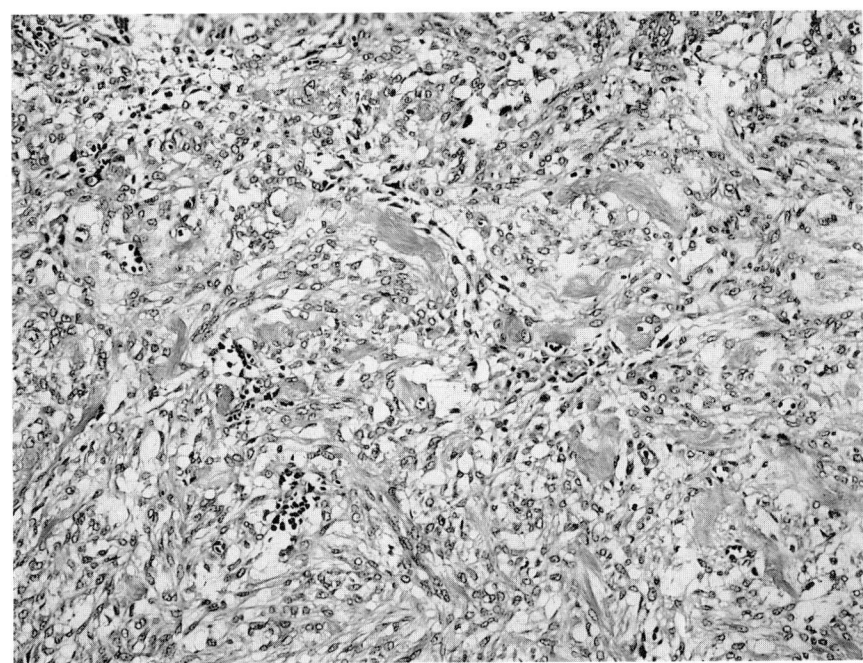

Figure 6-13
FIBROUS HISTIOCYTOMA:
HEART
This tumor was removed from a young man and was originally considered a malignant fibrous histiocytoma because of its cellularity. However, mitotic figures were absent, and the patient is alive and well 8 years postoperatively without recurrence.

(a fibrous histiocytoma with an inflammatory component) or a reactive process.

Inflammatory pseudotumors of the heart are extremely rare: only 3 cases have been reported in the medical literature (43–45). Like extracardiac inflammatory pseudotumors, reported cases that have occurred in the heart, as one case at the AFIP, have occurred in children under 11 years of age. Another lesion was removed from the left atrium of a 40-year-old man (AFIP files). Other cardiac sites include the left atrioventricular groove, right atrium, and right ventricular outflow tract. One cardiac inflammatory pseudotumor was associated with a systemic vasculitis (45) and another regressed spontaneously (44).

Inflammatory pseudotumors of the heart are large lesions, measuring up to 8 cm. Microscopically, they resemble their extracardiac counterparts, containing proliferations of fibroblasts with a dense plasmacytic and lymphocytic stromal infiltrate and a moderate vascular proliferation.

REFERENCES

Fibroma

1. Arciniegas E, Hakimi M, Farooki ZQ, Truccone NJ, Green EW. Primary cardiac tumors in children. J Thorac Cardiovasc Surg 1980;79:582–91.
2. Blondeau P. Primary cardiac tumors—French studies of 533 cases. Thorac Cardiovasc Surg 1990;38:192–5.
3. Brown IW, McGoldrick JP, Robles A, Curelly GW, Gula G, Ross DN. Left ventricular fibroma: echocardiographic diagnosis and successful surgical excision in three cases. J Cardiovasc Surg 1990;31:536–40.
4. Burke AP, Rosado-de-Christenson M, Templeton PA, Virmani R. Cardiac fibroma: clinicopathologic correlates and surgical treatment. J Thor Cardiovasc Surg 1994;108:862–70.
5. Chan HS, Sonley MJ, Moes CA, Daneman A, Smith CR, Martin DJ. Primary and secondary tumors of childhood involving the heart, pericardium, and great vessels. A report of 75 cases and review of the literature. Cancer 1985;56:825–36.
6. Ceithaml EL, Midgley FM, Perry LW, Dullum MK. Intramural ventricular fibroma in infancy: survival after partial excision in 2 patients. Ann Thorac Surg 1990;50:471–2.
7. Charuzi Y, Mills H, Buchbinder NA, Marshall LA. Primary intramural cardiac tumor: long-term follow-up. Am Heart J 1983;106:414–9.
8. Coffin CM. Congenital cardiac fibroma associated with Gorlin syndrome. Pediatr Pathol 1992;12:255–62.

9. de Leon GA, Zaeri N, Donner RM, Karmazin N. Cerebral rhinocele, hydrocephalus, and cleft lip and palate in infants with cardiac fibroma. J Neural Sci 1990;99:27–36.
10. Feldman PS, Meyer MW. Fibroelastic hamartoma (fibroma) of the heart. Cancer 1976;38:314–23.
11. Filiatrault M, Beland MJ, Neilson KA, Paquet M. Cardiac fibroma presenting with clinically significant arrhythmias in infancy. Pediatr Cardiol 1991;12:118–20.
12. Fine G, Osamura RY, Lee MW. Ultrastructure of the myocardial fibroma. Arch Pathol Lab Med 1979;103:11–7.
13. Gonzalez-Crussi F, Eberts TJ, Mirkin DC. Congenital fibrous hamartoma of the heart. Arch Pathol Lab Med 1978;102:491–3.
14. Gorlin RJ. Nevoid basal cell carcinoma syndrome. Medicine (Baltimore) 1987;66:98–113.
15. Jamieson SW, Gaudiani VA, Reitz BA, Oyer PE, Stinson EB, Shumway NE. Operative treatment of an unresectable tumor of the left ventricle. J Thorac Cardiovasc Surg 1981;81:797–9.
16. Lee YC, Singleton RT, Tang CK. Benign mesenchymal tumor of the heart. Spontaneous regression and disappearance of pulmonary artery stenosis. Chest 1982;82:503–5.
17. Marin-Garcia J, Fitch CW, Shenefelt RE. Primary right ventricular tumor (fibroma) simulating cyanotic heart disease in a newborn. J Am Coll Cardiol 1984;3:868–71.
18. McAllister HA Jr, Fenoglio JJ Jr. Tumors of the cardiovascular system. Atlas of Tumor Pathology. 2nd Series, Fascicle 15, Washington D.C.: Armed Forces Institute of Pathology, 1978:32–34.
19. Murphy MC, Sweeney MS, Putnam JB Jr, et al. Surgical treatment of cardiac tumors: a 25-year experience. Ann Thorac Surg 1990;49:612–7.
20. Nadas HS, Ellison RC. Cardiac tumors in infancy. Am J Cardiol 1968;21:363–6.
21. Oliva PB, Breckinridge JC, Johnson ML, Brantigan CO, Meara OP. Left ventricular outflow obstruction produced by a pedunculated fibroma in a newborn. Chest 1978;74:590–3.
22. Otsuka T, Asano K, Murota Y, Fukuda S, Hada Y, Fujii J. Successful removal of a cardiac fibroma in an elderly patient. J Cardiovasc Surg 1990;31:55–7.
23. Parks FR Jr, Adams F, Longmire WR Jr. Successful excision of a left ventricular hamartoma: report of a case. Circulation 1962;26:1316–20.
24. Parmley LF, Salley RK, Williams JP, Head GB III. The clinical spectrum of cardiac fibroma with diagnostic and surgical considerations: noninvasive imaging enhances management. Ann Thorac Surg 1988;45:455–65.
25. Reece IJ, Cooley DA, Frazier OH, Hallman GL, Powers PL, Montero CG. Cardiac tumors. Clinical spectrum and prognosis of lesions other than classical benign myxoma in 20 patients. J Thorac Cardiovasc Surg 1984;88:439–46.
26. Reece IJ, Houston AB, Pollock JC. Interventricular fibroma. Echocardiographic diagnosis and successful surgical removal in infancy. Br Heart J 1983;50:590–1.
27. Reul GJ, Howell JF, Rubio PA, Peterson PK. Successful partial excision of an intramural fibroma of the left ventricle. Am J Cardiol 1975;36:262–5.
28. Shnitka TK, Asp DM, Horner RH. Congenital generalized fibromatosis. Cancer 1958;11:627–39.
29. Tahernia AX, Bricker JT, Ott DA. Intracardiac fibroma in an asymptomatic infant. Clin Cardiol 1990;13:506–12.
30. Takahashi I, Kamata E, Takuro M, Ishida K. Successful surgical ablation of reentrant ventricular tachycardia caused by myocardial fibroma. J Thorac Cardiovasc Surg 1984;87:469–73.
31. Tazelaar HD, Locke TJ, McGregor CG. Pathology of surgically excised primary cardiac tumors. Mayo Clin Proc 1992;67:957–65.
32. Turi GK, Albala A, Fenoglio JJ. Cardiac fibromatosis: an ultrastructural study. Hum Pathol 1980;11:577–80.
33. Williams DB, Danielson GK, McGoon DC, Feldt RH, Edwards WD. Cardiac fibroma: long-term survival after excision. J Thorac Cardiovasc Surg 1982;84:230–6.
34. Valente M, Cocco P, Thiene G, et al. Cardiac fibroma and heart transplantation. J Thorac Cardiovasc Surg 1993;106:1208–12.
35. Yamaguchi M, Hosokawa Y, Ohashi H, Imai M, Oshima Y, Minamiji K. Cardiac fibroma. Long-term fate after excision. J Thorac Cardiovasc Surg 1992;103:140–5.

Fibrous Tumor of the Pericardium

36. Bortolotti U, Calabro F, Loy M, Fasoli G, Altavilla G, Marchese D. Giant intrapericardial solitary fibrous tumor. Ann Thorac Surg 1992;54:1219–20.
37. Cameselle-Teijeiro J, Varela-Duran J, Fonseca E, Villanueva JP, Sobrinho-Simoes M. Solitary fibrous tumor of the thyroid. Am J Clin Pathol 1993;101:535–8.
38. El-Naggar AK, Ro JY, Ayala AG, Ward R, Ordonez NG. Localized fibrous tumor of the serosal cavities. Immunohistochemical, electron microscopic, and flow cytometric DNA study. Am J Clin Pathol 1989;92:561–5.
39. Mahaim K. Les tumeurs et les polypes de coeur: etude anatomo-clinique. Paris: Masson, 1945.
40. Weidner N. Solitary fibrous tumor of the mediastinum. Ultrastruct Pathol 1991;15:489–92.
41. Witkin G, Rosai J. Solitary fibrous tumor of the mediastinum. A report of 41 cases. Am J Surg Pathol 1989;13:547–57.

Benign Fibrous Histiocytoma

42. Rose AG. Fibrous histiocytoma of the heart [Letter]. Arch Pathol Lab Med 1978;102:389.

Inflammatory Pseudotumor

43. Chou P, Gonzalez-Crussi F, Cole R, Reddy VB. Plasma cell granuloma of the heart. Cancer 1988;62:1409–13.
44. Pearson PJ, Smithson WA, Driscoll DJ, Banks PM, Ehman RL. Inoperable plasma cell granuloma of the heart: spontaneous decrease in size during an 11-month period. Mayo Clin Proc 1988;63:1022–25.
45. Stark P, Sandbank JC, Rudnicki C, Zahavi I. Inflammatory pseudotumor of the heart with vasculitis and venous thrombosis. Chest 1992;102:1884–5.

7
VASCULAR TUMORS AND TUMOR-LIKE CONDITIONS

BLOOD CYST

Definition. Blood cysts are congenital cysts found on the endocardium, particularly along the lines of closure of heart valves. The cysts are lined by flattened endothelium and filled with nonorganized blood.

Histogenesis. Blood cysts are a result of microscopic invaginations of atrial endothelium into atrioventricular valves, and ventricular endothelium into semilunar valves. The cyst lumen is connected to the ventricular lumen or to the aortic or pulmonary arterial lumen, depending on the location; they are, therefore, strictly considered diverticula (3).

Clinical Features. Blood cysts are incidental autopsy findings on cardiac valves in approximately 50 percent of infants under 2 months of age (3). Although they were once believed to be associated with asphyxia, this theory has been refuted (3). Rarely, they may be large and result in ventricular or valvular obstruction (1,2).

Blood cysts are rare after 2 years of age; the reason for their disappearance is not clear. It has been suggested that collapse of the cyst with adhesion and fibrosis of opposite surfaces of the endothelium leads to its disappearance. Small deposits of hemosiderin, fibrosis, and lymphocytes have been observed adjacent to blood cysts (3), indicating a tissue reaction possibly related to resolution of the cyst.

Pathologic Findings. Blood cysts are multiple in over 50 percent of cases, and up to 20 cysts may coexist. They usually affect the mitral and tricuspid valves, with infrequent pulmonary or aortic valvular involvement (3). They range from microscopic to 3 mm in diameter, although they may occasionally grow much larger (fig. 7-1). Microscopically, the cysts are thin walled and lined by cobblestone-shaped endothelial cells.

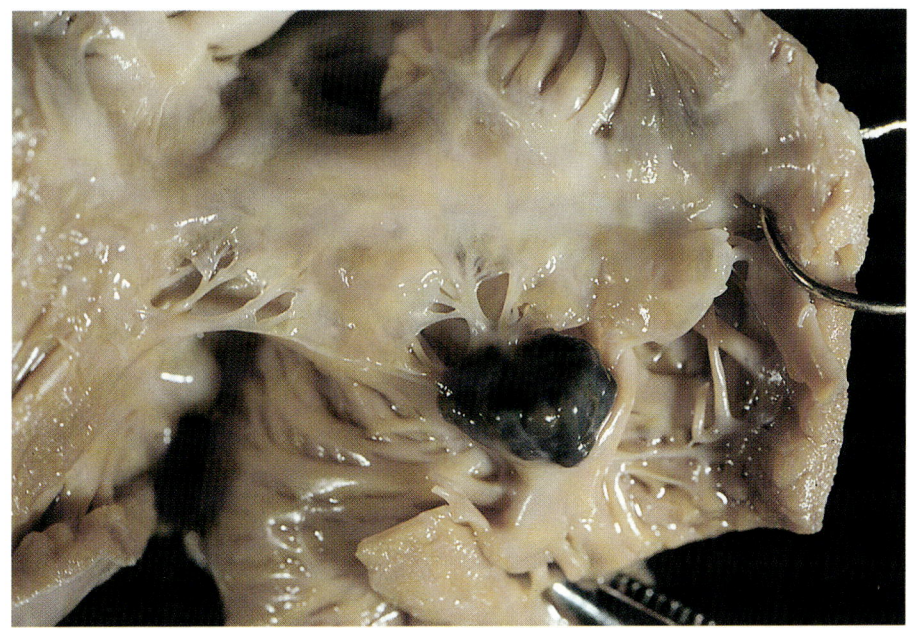

Figure 7-1
BLOOD CYST
The lesion was an incidental finding on the tricuspid valve of a 4-month-old infant who died of unrelated causes. The large size of the cyst (4 mm) and the age of the patient are unusual for congenital blood cysts, which are usually less than 2 mm in diameter and regress by 2 months of age.

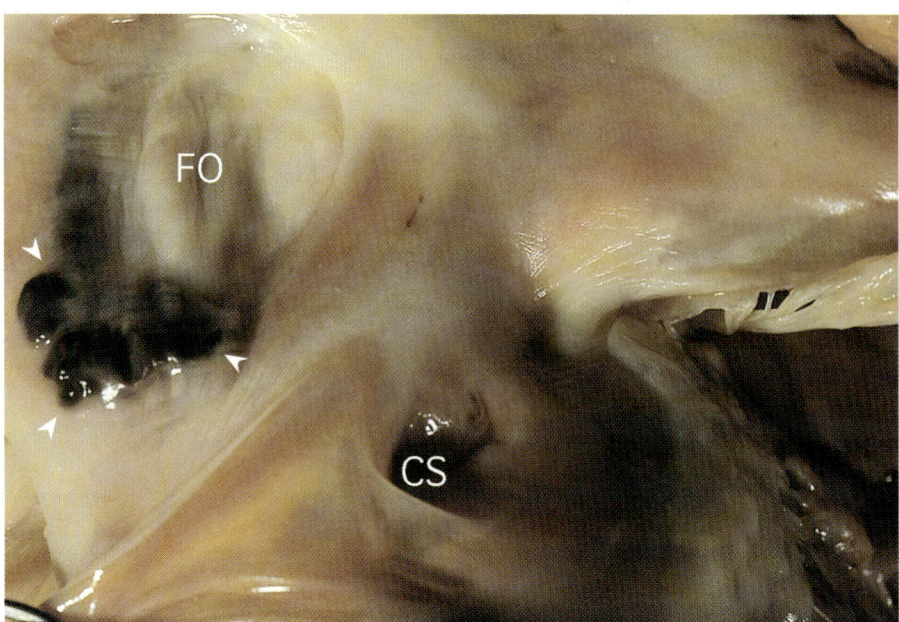

Figure 7-2
VARIX
There is a bluish discoloration of the endocardium (arrowheads) just above the coronary sinus (CS) posterior to the rim of the fossa ovalis (FO).

VARIX

Definition. Varices are endocardial, unilocular, blood-filled cysts lined by endothelial cells and filled with organizing thrombi. They are usually found in the right atrium and are dilated thrombosed veins. The term *venous malformation* is preferred by Rose (7), because it implies a congenital, rather than acquired, defect. However, venous malformation may be confused with arteriovenous malformation, which is generally considered a form of hemangioma (see below). For this reason, the more descriptive term, varix, is preferred.

Histogenesis. The inferior rim of the fossa ovalis, which is the site of virtually all cardiac varices, is the location of small veins (7). The cause for their dilatation and formation into varices may be the embryonic incorporation of remnants of the left valve of the sinus venosus into the right side of the interatrial septum (5,7). This explanation, however, does not account for the rare cardiac varices that occur in the ventricles (6).

Incidence. The incidence of atrial varices has been estimated to be as high as 2.5 percent at autopsy (5). We agree with Rose (7) that the incidence is probably far lower; he estimates an incidence of approximately 0.07 percent.

Clinical Features. Atrial varices do not cause symptoms. Theoretically, they may be de-

tected by imaging studies and result in diagnostic confusion with atrial tumors (7). An incidental atrial varix was detected by coronary angiography in a patient with atrial myxoma (4). A tumor described as a varix was successfully removed from the right ventricular outflow tract after a loud murmur was detected in an essentially asymptomatic patient (6).

Pathologic Findings. Grossly, varices are raised, bluish areas inferior to the fossa ovalis (fig. 7-2). Histologically, they are endothelial-lined cysts containing blood which may be organizing (fig. 7-3).

HEMANGIOMA

Definition. Hemangiomas (angiomas) are benign tumors composed predominantly of blood vessels. Histologically, benign vascular tumors are classified as those composed of multiple, dilated, thin-walled vessels (cavernous type); smaller vessels resembling capillaries (capillary type); and dysplastic malformed arteries and veins (arteriovenous hemangioma, cirsoid aneurysm).

Histogenesis. Hemangiomas are generally considered benign neoplasms, although the distinction between vascular malformations, vascular hamartomas, and true benign neoplasms of blood vessels is vague (15). Cardiac hemangiomas often have combined features of cavernous,

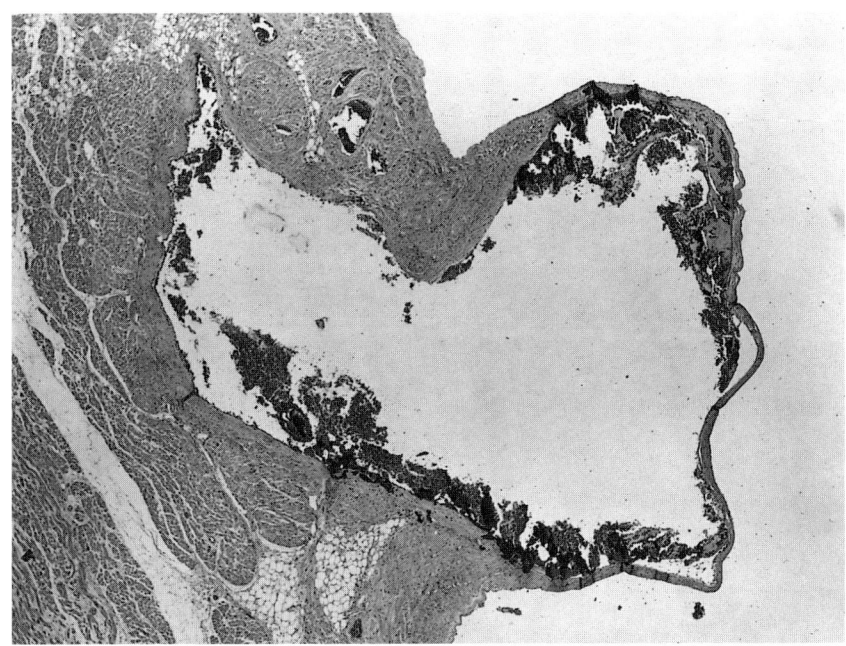

Figure 7-3
VARIX
Microscopic section demonstrates a dilated vein with a focally attenuated wall.

capillary, and arteriovenous hemangiomas, and many contain fibrous tissue and fat. These features are reminiscent of intramuscular hemangiomas of skeletal muscle, and it is possible that some cardiac hemangiomas and intramuscular hemangiomas are related lesions.

Incidence. Hemangiomas of the heart and pericardium are quite rare: fewer than 75 cases have been reported (8–10,14,19,23,24,26). In surgical series, they represent 5 to 10 percent of benign cardiac tumors (9,16,17,24,26). Approximately 15 percent of cardiac hemangiomas involve the epicardium or pericardium (10,23,33).

Clinical Features. Cardiac hemangiomas occur in patients of all ages, from 4 months (12) to the seventh decade (8,10,23). The mean age at presentation of 45 patients from three series was 43 years (8,10,23); there were 29 males and 16 females, suggesting a male predominance. Most cardiac hemangiomas are asymptomatic and discovered incidentally at autopsy or cardiac surgery. Increasingly, asymptomatic cardiac hemangiomas are discovered by an increased cardiothoracic ratio on routine chest radiograph or after evaluation for incidental murmurs. In symptomatic patients, cardiac hemangiomas cause arrhythmias (10,32), pericardial effusions (10,12), congestive heart failure (8,23), outflow tract obstruction (27,28), and coronary insuffi-

ciency (20). Occasionally, the presenting symptom is sudden cardiac death, and the forensic pathologist is the first to diagnose the tumor (8). Hemangiomas causing sudden cardiac death generally cause conduction disturbances in the heart, and may be located in the region of the atrioventricular node or in the ventricles. A rare mechanism of sudden death in individuals with cardiac hemangioma is rupture of the tumor and pericardial tamponade (22).

Echocardiography is a sensitive, noninvasive method for detecting cardiac masses, including hemangiomas (10,13). A specific diagnosis of hemangioma was made preoperatively by cardiac catheterization (29).

There is an occasional association of cardiac hemangioma with extracardiac hemangiomas of the gastrointestinal tract (10) and port-wine stain of the face (32). Giant cardiac hemangiomas can result in thrombosis and coagulopathies (Kasabach-Merritt syndrome) (14,18).

Pathologic Findings. Hemangiomas may occur in any location of the heart. Of 45 cases (8,10, 23), 15 were located in the atria, 12 in the left ventricle or ventricular septum, 11 in the right ventricle, 6 in the pericardium or on the epicardium, and 1 on the mitral valve. Cardiac hemangiomas can be well-demarcated, lobulated tumors (fig. 7-4), or have grossly and microscopically

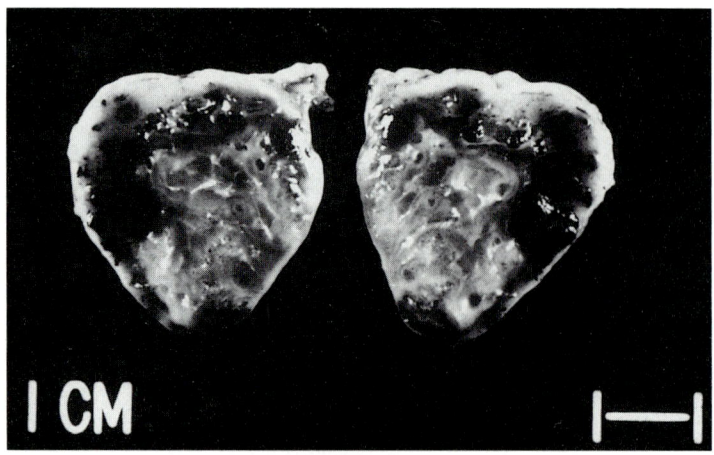

Figure 7-4
CARDIAC HEMANGIOMA
This tumor was resected from the right atrium of a 1-year-old boy with pericardial effusions. Note areas of hemorrhage and dilated vessels. The patient was well 49 months postoperatively.

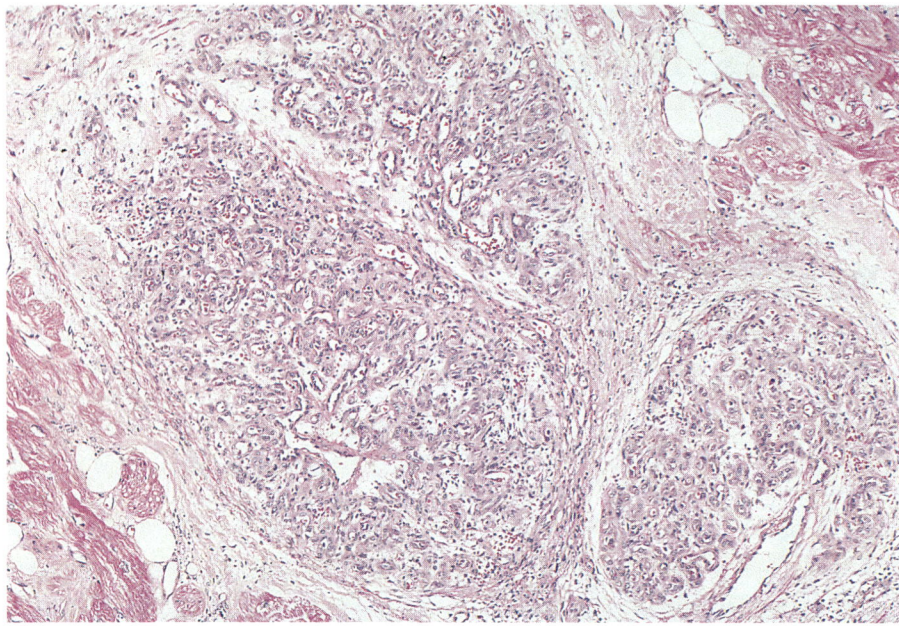

Figure 7-5
CARDIAC HEMANGIOMA, CAPILLARY TYPE
Note the small capillary channels.

infiltrating margins, making them difficult to completely resect. They range in size from less than 1 cm to 8 cm or larger (8). Approximately 75 percent are mural lesions and the remainder are endocardial tumors that project into the atrial or ventricular cavity.

The histologic appearance of cardiac hemangioma is similar to that of extracardiac hemangioma. A variety of histologic patterns may be seen. Capillary hemangioma (figs. 7-5, 7-6) is composed of lobules of endothelial cells, with scattered pericytes and fibroblasts. There may be open capillary lumens, especially at the periphery of the tumor, and cavernous and capillary channels may coexist (figs. 7-7, 7-8). Over

half of capillary hemangiomas of the heart are endocardial lesions that project into the cavity, often by a narrow pedicle; these tumors typically have a myxoid background. In contrast, cavernous hemangiomas (fig. 7-9) are composed of thin- or thick-walled capillary or venous structures filled with blood, and are usually mural tumors.

Approximately half of cardiac hemangiomas have areas of dysplastic, irregularly thickened arterial and venous structures which are typical of arteriovenous malformations. These hemangiomas are mural tumors that are likely to be poorly circumscribed. Histologically, they may contain fibrous tissue and fat and have areas indistinguishable from capillary hemangioma;

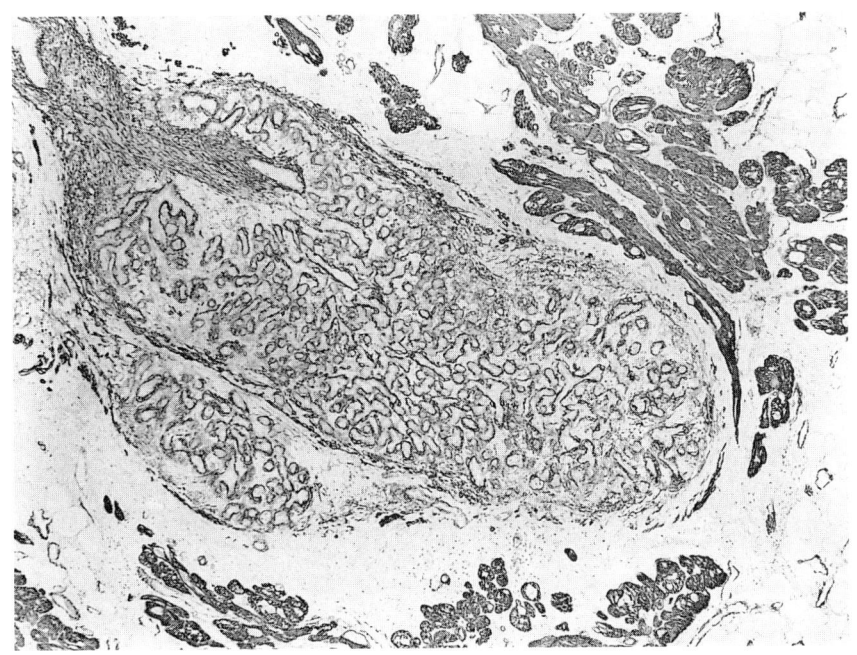

Figure 7-6
CARDIAC HEMANGIOMA,
CAPILLARY TYPE
The vascular channels are outlined by immunohistochemical staining with antimuscle-specific actin. Same tumor as that shown in figure 7-5.

Figure 7-7
CARDIAC HEMANGIOMA,
CAVERNOUS-CAPILLARY TYPE
This tumor, resected postpartum from a young woman, protruded into the ventricular cavity.

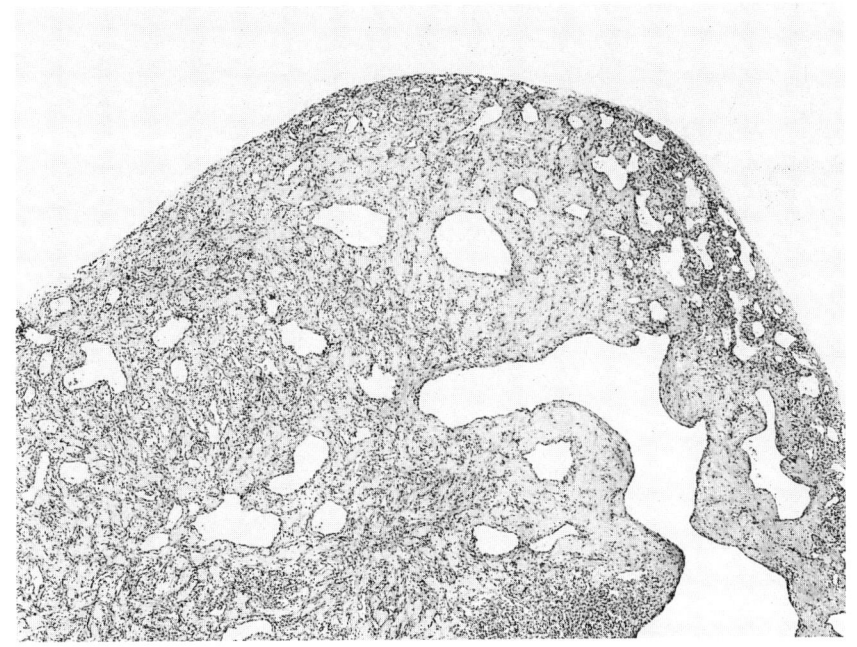

they are similar in appearance to intramuscular hemangiomas of skeletal muscle (15).

Three cardiac hemangiomas with epithelioid cells have been reported (fig. 7-10) (10,11,21). These cells, which are of endothelial origin, have been distinguished from true histiocytes by immunohistochemical or ultrastructural methods (21). Another unusual histologic feature of car-

diac hemangioma is papillary endothelial hyperplasia (fig. 7-11) (8,10), a reactive, unusually exuberant form of endothelial proliferation that may be a component of an organizing thrombus. Papillary endothelial hyperplasia has no clinical significance, but may be histologically confused with angiosarcoma. Unlike angiosarcoma, necrosis and marked nuclear atypia are absent,

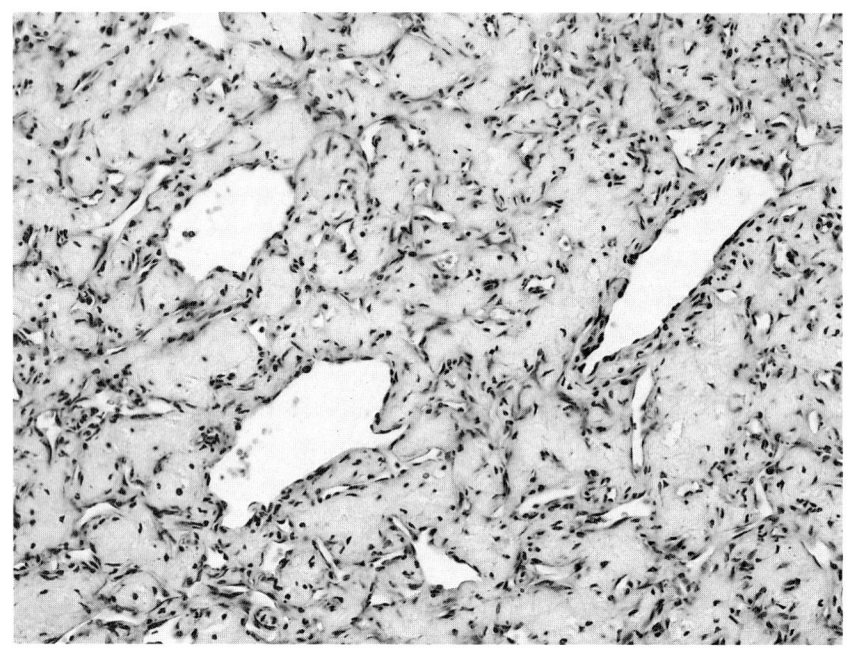

Figure 7-8
CARDIAC HEMANGIOMA, CAVERNOUS-CAPILLARY TYPE
There are both dilated, cavernous vessels and smaller capillary channels.

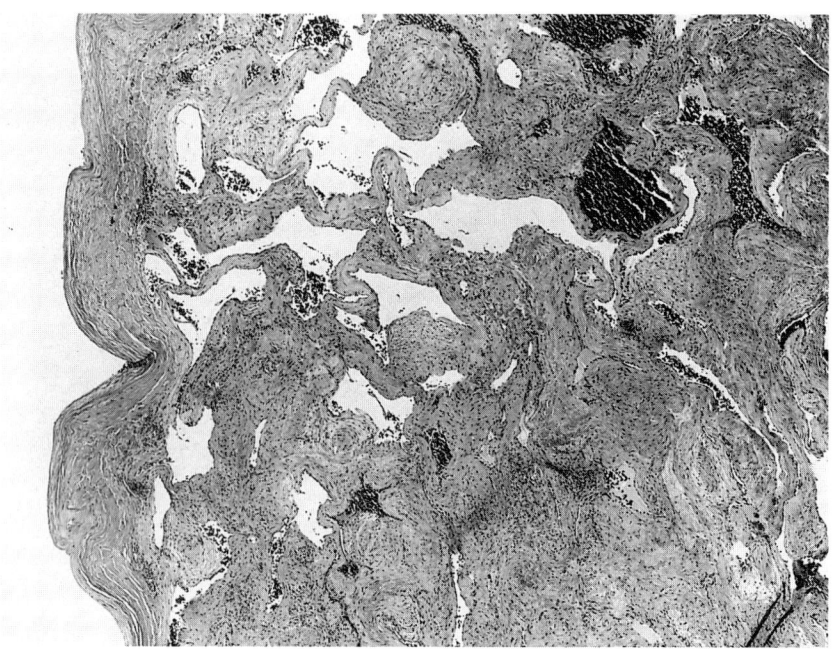

Figure 7-9
CARDIAC HEMANGIOMA, CAVERNOUS TYPE

The tumor was resected from an asymptomatic 56-year-old man. The tumor involved the right atrium and ventricle. The patient is well 12 months postoperatively. (Fig. 2 from Burke AP, Johns JP, Virmani R. Hemangiomas of the heart, a clinicopathologic study of ten cases. Am J Cardiovasc Pathol 1990;3:283-90.)

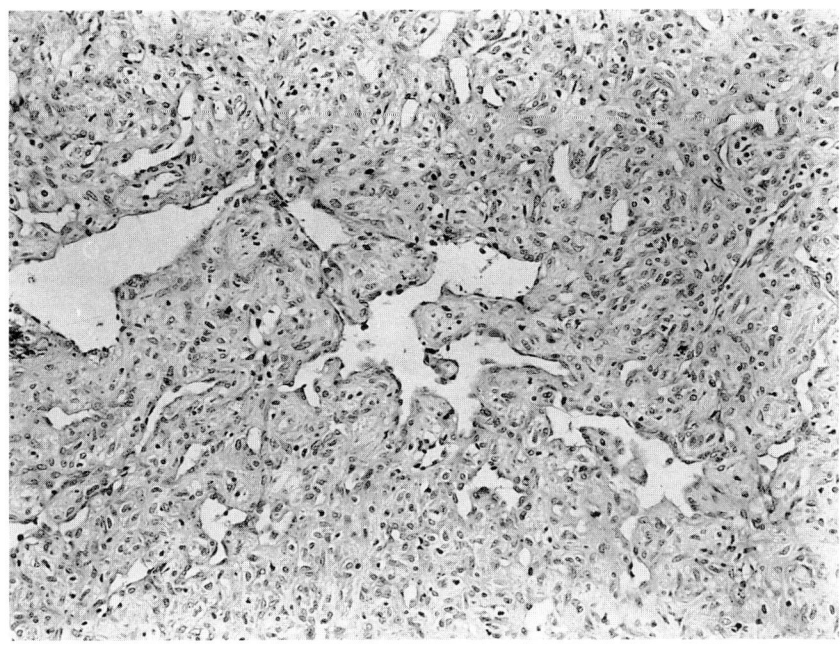

Figure 7-10
CARDIAC HEMANGIOMA

Irregular vascular channels with a pronounced pericytic component. Some of the cells between the open channels have a histiocytoid appearance. Histologic section from tumor shown in figure 7-4. (Fig. 3 from Burke AP, Johns JP, Virmani R. Hemangiomas of the heart, a clinicopathologic study of ten cases. Am J Cardiovasc Pathol 1990;3:283-90.)

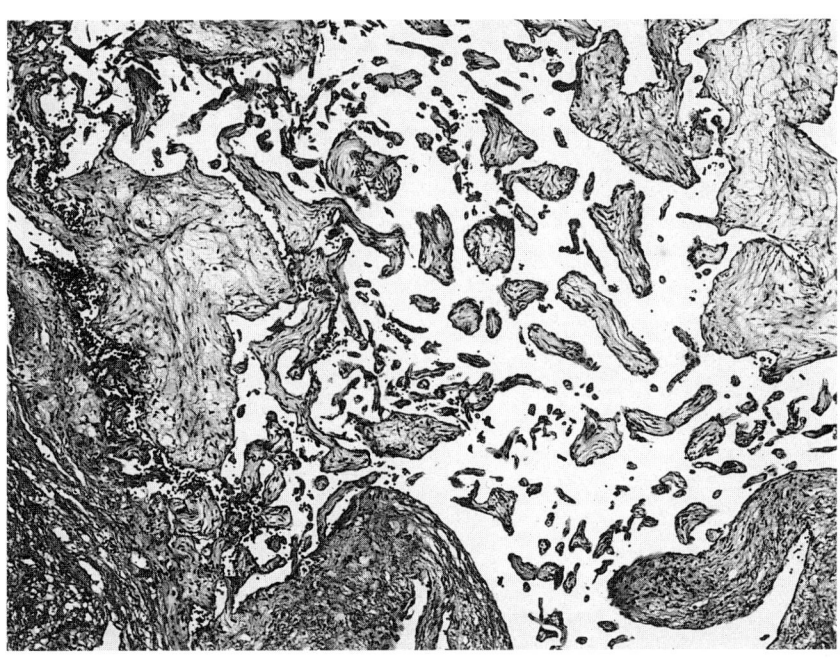

Figure 7-11
CARDIAC HEMANGIOMA, PAPILLARY ENDOTHELIAL HYPERPLASIA

Fibrin deposition and endothelial atypia characterizes these structures. Other areas of the tumor were typical of cavernous hemangioma. The patient was a 27-year-old woman who died suddenly; at autopsy an infiltrating hemangioma was present in the left ventricle.

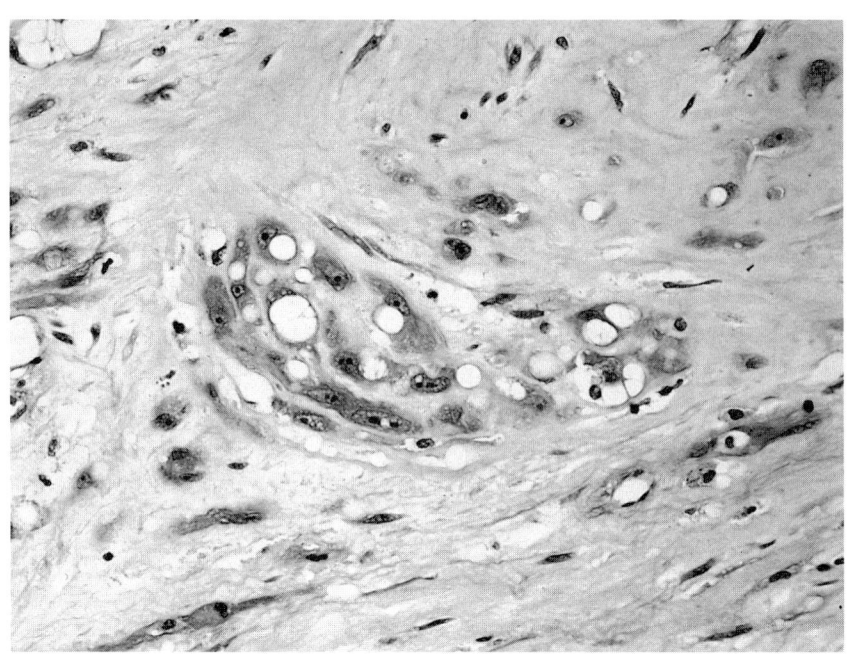

Figure 7-12
EPITHELIOID
HEMANGIOENDOTHELIOMA
Tumor cells have abundant cytoplasm with characteristic large, intracytoplasmic vacuoles. Left atrial mass in a 71-year-old woman with palpitations.

and there is usually an organizing fibrin thrombus within the papillae.

Differential Diagnosis. Cardiac hemangioma is rarely misdiagnosed histologically. There are two entities in the differential diagnosis. Intracavity cardiac hemangiomas typically possess a myxoid background and may be erroneously diagnosed as myxoma. However, there are no myxoma cells or ring structures in cardiac hemangioma, and cellular areas with numerous capillaries are usually present. In addition, cardiac hemangiomas are rarely, if ever, attached to the fossa ovalis of the left atrium; those that are pedunculated are often ventricular lesions. Papillary endothelial hyperplasia, as discussed above, may mimic angiosarcoma. However, with complete tumor sampling, angiosarcoma is readily excluded because most of the cardiac hemangioma is composed of bland vascular structures lacking endothelial atypia; such areas are absent in angiosarcoma.

Treatment. There have been at least 37 reports of surgically resected cardiac hemangiomas (8–10,16,19,24,26,30,31). In approximately 30 of these cases, complete excision was possible; in the remainder, biopsy or partial excision was performed. Reconstruction of ventricular outflow with Dacron grafts may be necessary (10). In rare instances, massive, unresectable cardiac hemangiomas are found in relatively asymptomatic individuals (19), and they can occasionally regress (25). In one case of infantile hemangioma of the heart, steroids were successfully used for treatment (12). There is a single reported case of angiosarcoma developing 7 years after surgical excision of a cardiac hemangioma (11); however, in most cases, excision is considered curative.

HEMANGIOENDOTHELIOMA

Hemangioendothelioma is a term generally used for vascular neoplasms of intermediate malignancy (15). The term has occasionally been used to describe childhood hemangiomas (12). It is best reserved, however, for specific histopathologic entities, including epithelioid hemangioendothelioma, that may occasionally occur within the heart. In this tumor, epithelioid cells form short strands or solid nests of round or oval endothelial cells; these strands or nests form small intracellular lumina and infiltrate muscular walls of vessels (fig. 7-12). The lumens may mimic the vacuoles of adenocarcinoma, which may be initially considered in the microscopic differential diagnosis. Immunohistochemical stains for factor VIII–related antigen or CD34 identify the cells as endothelial in origin (fig. 7-13).

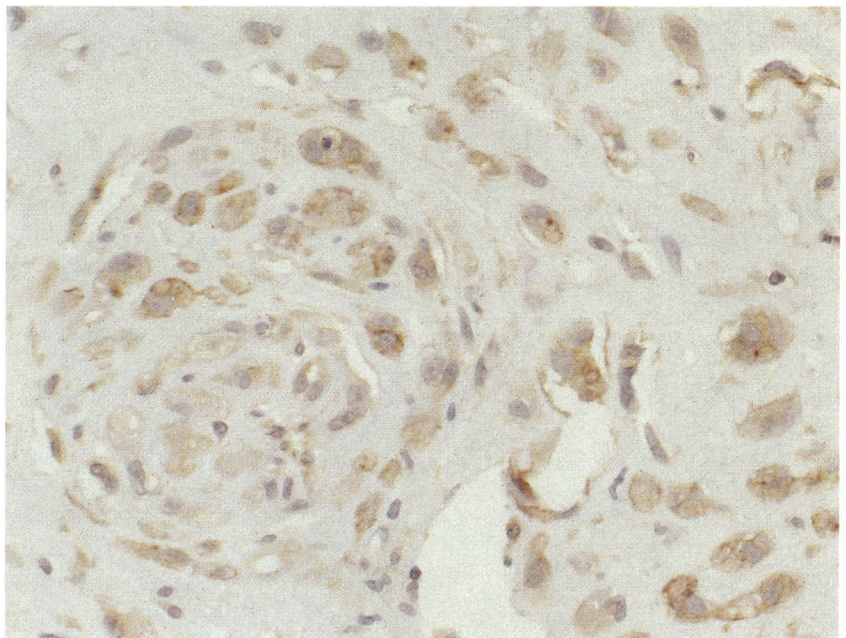

Figure 7-13
EPITHELIOID
HEMANGIOENDOTHELIOMA
Characteristic vacuolated cells demonstrate endothelial differentiation in this immunohistologic preparation using anti-CD34. (Avidin-biotin stain)

Approximately 10 percent of extracardiac hemangioendotheliomas result in metastases, and up to one third recur (15). Epithelioid hemangioendotheliomas of the heart are quite rare, and their biologic behavior is thus unknown. They should be considered potentially malignant based on available data on histologically similar extracardiac tumors.

HEMANGIOPERICYTOMA

Hemangiopericytomas are neoplasms of pericytes and may be benign or malignant. There have been rare reports of primary pericardial or myocardial hemangiopericytoma, although few with histologic documentation (35–39). Histologically, hemangiopericytomas are highly vascular tumors composed of tightly packed cells with round to oval nuclei and indistinct cytoplasm. These pericytic cells surround endothelial-lined vascular channels, are cuboidal or spindled, and do not generally form fascicles or long bundles. The vascular spaces form characteristic anastomosing vascular channels that have been compared to "staghorns." The diagnosis is made after careful exclusion of other soft tissue neoplasms, such as synovial sarcoma and fibrous histiocytoma, that may possess a similar vascular architecture. Electron microscopy is helpful in confirming the pericytic nature of these tumors (34): elongated cytoplasmic processes, pi-

nocytotic vesicles, poorly developed desmosomes, a paucity of organelles, and a well-developed basal lamina (34).

The first reported case of cardiac hemangiopericytoma (37) described multiple masses in the pericardium of a 33-year-old man, who remained asymptomatic 10 months postoperatively. Subsequent reports have demonstrated cardiac rupture due to hemangiopericytoma (35), cardiac hemangiopericytoma after radiation (39), presentation with dysphagia, and resulting pseudoaneurysms of the pulmonary artery (38). Several reported cases of cardiac hemangiopericytoma were considered malignant (36,38).

LYMPHANGIOMA

Occasionally designated as *hygromas*, lymphangiomas are composed of dilated lymphatic channels arising from sequestered lymphatic tissue that fails to communicate normally with the lymphatic tree (41). The formation of a mass is secondary to accumulation of fluid, which results in cystic dilatation and cellular proliferation. Intrapericardial lymphangiomas are extremely rare (40,43), and occur in infants, children, and young adults. Only two cases were reported in the previous Fascicle on cardiac tumors (42). Lymphangiomas of the heart are generally located

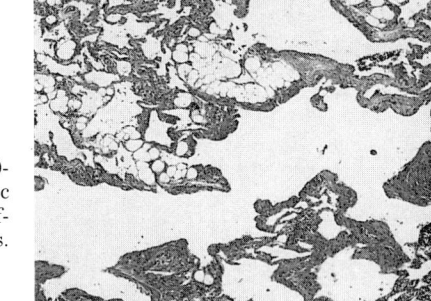

Figure 7-14
LYMPHANGIOMA
This tumor was excised from a 10-year-old girl with an enlarged cardiac silhouette and chylous pericardial effusion. Note the lymphoid aggregates.

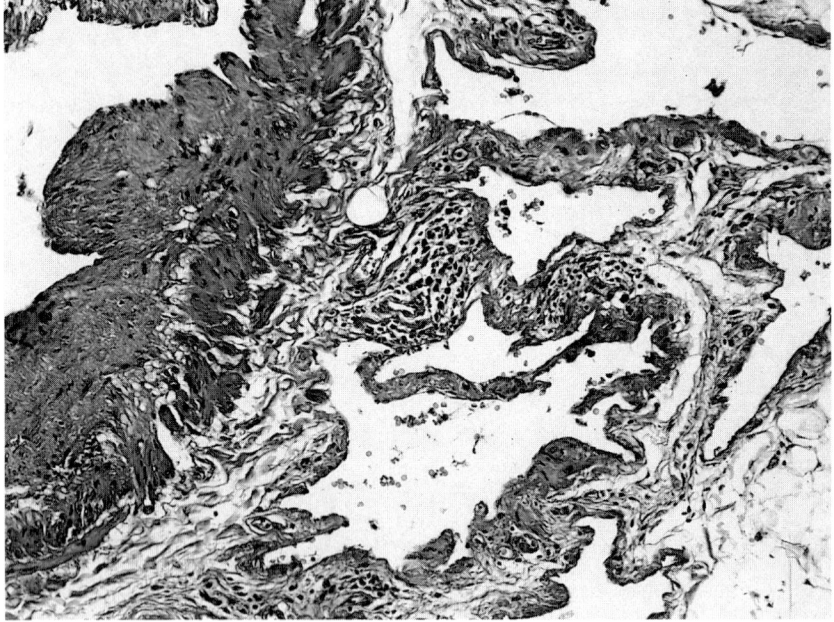

Figure 7-15
LYMPHANGIOMA
A higher magnification of figure 7-14 demonstrates smooth muscle bundles. Smooth muscle and lymphoid aggregates are not prominent in mesothelial cysts.

within the pericardial sac and exhibit no myocardial infiltration. The histologic appearance of intrapericardial lymphangioma is identical to lymphangiomas of the mesentery. In contrast to mesothelial pericardial cysts, lymphangiomas are multilocular, lined by flattened endothelial cells, contain proteinaceous fluid and lymphocytes, and often have smooth muscle cells and lymphoid aggregates within the cyst wall (figs. 7-14, 7-15). Immunohistochemical staining for factor VIII–related antigen and cytokeratin is helpful in distinguishing these tumors from mesothelial cysts. The cells lining the lymphangioma express endothelial markers, whereas the mesothelial lining cells of mesothelial cysts strongly express cytokeratins.

REFERENCES

Blood Cyst

1. Arnold IR, Hubner PJ, Firmin RK. Blood filled cyst of the papillary muscle of the mitral valve producing severe left ventricular outflow tract obstruction. Br Heart J 1990;63:132–3.

2. Pasaoglu I, Dogan R, Demircin M, Bozer AY. Blood cyst of the pulmonary valve causing pulmonic valve stenosis. Am J Cardiol 1993;72:493–4.
3. Zimmerman KG, Paplanus SH, Dong S, Nagle RB. Congenital blood cysts of the heart valves. Hum Pathol 1983;14:699–703.

Atrial Varix

4. Fueredi GA, Knechtges TE, Czarnecki DJ. Coronary angiography in atrial myxoma: findings in nine cases. Am J Roentgenol 1989;152:737–8.
5. Heggtveit HA. Thrombosed varices of the heart [Abstract]. Am J Pathol 1966;48:50.

6. Murphy MC, Sweeney MS, Putnam JB, et al. Surgical treatment of cardiac tumors: a 25-year experience. Ann Thorac Surg 1990;49:612–7.
7. Rose AG. Venous malformations of the heart. Arch Pathol Lab Med 1979;103:18–20.

Hemangioma

8. Abad C, Campo E, Estruch R, et al. Cardiac hemangioma with papillary endothelial hyperplasia: report of a resected case and review of the literature. Ann Thorac Surg 1990;49:305–8.
9. Blondeau P. Primary cardiac tumors—French studies of 533 cases. Thorac Cardiovasc Surg 1990;38:192–5.
10. Burke AP, Johns J, Virmani R. Hemangiomas of the heart: a clinicopathologic study of 10 cases. Am J Cardiovasc Pathol 1991;13:283–90.
11. Chalet Y, Mace L, Frac B, Neveux JY, Lancelin B. Angiosarcoma 7 years after surgical excision of histiocytoid haemangioma in the left atrium [Letter]. Lancet 1993;341:1217.
12. Chang JS, Young ML, Chiu WM, Lue HC. Infantile cardiac hemangioendothelioma. Pediatr Cardiol 1992;13:52–5.
13. Cunningham T, Lawrie GM, Stavinoha J Jr, Quinones MA, Zoghbi WA. Cavernous hemangioma of the right ventricle: echocardiographic-pathologic correlates. J Am Soc Echocardiogr 1993;6:335–40.
14. Dein JR, Frist WH, Stinson EB, et al. Primary cardiac neoplasms. Early and late results of surgical treatment in 42 patients. J Thorac Cardiovasc Surg 1987;93:502–11.
15. Enzinger FM, Weiss SW. Benign tumors and tumorlike lesions of blood vessels. In: Enzinger FM, Weiss SW, eds. Soft tissue tumors. St Louis: CV Mosby, 1988:489–532.
16. Fabian JT, Rose AG. Tumours of the heart. A study of 89 cases. S Afr Med J 1982;16:71–7.
17. Fine G. Primary tumors of the pericardium and heart. Cardiovasc Clin 1973;5:207–38.
18. Gengenbach S, Ridker PM. Left ventricular hemangioma in Kasabach-Merritt syndrome. Am Heart J 1991;121:202–3.
19. Grenadier E, Margulis T, Palant A, Safadi T, Merin G. Huge cavernous hemangioma of the heart: a completely evaluated case report and review of the literature. Am Heart J 1989;117:479–81.
20. Kemme DJ, Rainer WG. Subendocardial arteriovenous malformation in a patient with unstable angina. Clin Cardiol 1991;14:82–4.
21. Kuo TT, Hsueh S, Su IJ, Gonzalez-Crussi F, Chen JS. Histiocytoid hemangioma of the heart with peripheral eosinophilia. Cancer 1985;55:2854–61.

22. Lefas JP. Mort subite par rupture d'angiome péricardique. Bull Soc Anat (Paris) 1989;73:464–9.
23. McAllister HA, Fenoglio JJ Jr. Tumors of the cardiovascular system. Atlas of Tumor Pathology. 2nd Series, Fascicle 15. Washington, D.C.: Armed Forces Institute of Pathology, 1978:46–52.
24. Murphy MC, Sweeney MS, Putnam JB, et al. Surgical treatment of cardiac tumors: a 25-year experience. Ann Thorac Surg 1990;49:612–7.
25. Palmer TE, Tresch DD, Bonchek LI. Spontaneous resolution of a large, cavernous hemangioma of the heart. Am J Cardiol 1986;58:184–5.
26. Reece IJ, Cooley DA, Frazier OH, et al. Cardiac tumors. Clinical spectrum and prognosis of lesions other than classical benign myxoma in 20 patients. J Thorac Cardiovasc Surg 1984;88:439–46.
27. Reiss N, Theissen P, Feaux de Lacroix W. Right-ventricular hemangioma causing serious outflow-tract obstruction. Thorac Cardiovasc Surg 1991;39:234–6.
28. Soberman MS, Plauth WH, Winn KJ, Forest GC, Hatcher CR Jr, Sink JD. Hemangioma of the right ventricle causing outflow tract obstruction. J Thorac Cardiovasc Surg 1988;96:307–9.
29. Sulayman R, Cassels DE. Myocardial coronary hemangiomatous tumors in children. Chest 1975;68:113–5.
30. Tabry IF, Nassar VH, Rizk G, Touma A, Dagher IK. Cavernous hemangioma of the heart: case report and review of the literature. J Thorac Cardiovasc Surg 1975;69:415–20.
31. Tadros NB, Akl BF, Avasthi P, Crotta P. Arteriovenous and capillary hemangiomas of the interventricular septum. Ann Thorac Surg 1988;46:236–8.
32. Weston CF, Hayward MW, Seymour RM, Stephens MR. Cardiac hemangioma associated with a facial port-wine stain and recurrent atrial tachycardia. Eur Heart J 1988;9:668–71.
33. Yoshikawa M, Hayashi T, Sato T, Akiba T, Watarai J, Nakamura C. A case of pericardial hemangioma with consumption coagulopathy cured by radiotherapy. Pediatr Radiol 1987;17:149–50.

Hemangiopericytoma

34. Enzinger FM, Weiss SW. Benign tumors and tumorlike lesions of blood vessels. In: Enzinger FM, Weiss SW, eds. Soft tissue tumors. St Louis: CV Mosby, 1988:489–532.
35. Fujii B, Matsuzaki M, Takashiba K, et al. Primary cardiac hemangiopericytoma causing rupture of the right atrium and chronic atrial tamponade. Jpn Circ J 1991;55:1206–10.
36. Galvin IF, Bowe P, Mellon K, Gibbons JR, Maghout M, Bharucha H. Pericardial hemangiopericytoma as a cause of dysphagia. Ann Thorac Surg 1988;45:94–6.
37. Ishikawa K, Tsuya T, Shirato C, et al. Primary hemangiopericytoma of the heart. A case report. Jpn Circ J 1981;45:62–8.
38. Nakamura Y, Nishiya Y, Kawada M, et al. Primary hemangiopericytoma of the heart associated with psuedoaneurysm of the pulmonary artery—a case report. Angiology 1987;38:788–92.
39. Schmid KW, Thurner J Jr, Gruenwald K. Hemangiopericytoma of the heart following treatment of Hodgkin's disease. A case report. Virchows Arch [A] 1987;411:485–8.

Lymphangioma

40. Anbe DT, Fine G. Cardiac lymphangioma and lipoma. Report of a case of simultaneous occurrence in association with lipomatous infiltration of the myocardium and cardiac arrhythmia. Am Heart J 1973;86:227–35.
41. Enzinger FM, Weiss SW. Tumors of lymph vessels In: Enzinger FM, Weiss SW, eds. Soft tissue tumors. St. Louis: CV Mosby 1988;614–37.
42. McAllister HA, Fenoglio JJ Jr. Tumors of the cardiovascular system. Atlas of Tumor Pathology. 2nd Series, Fascicle 15. Washington, D.C.: Armed Forces Institute of Pathology, 1978:46–52.
43. Moore TC, Cobo JC. Massive symptomatic cystic hygroma confined to the thorax in early childhood. J Thorac Cardiovasc Surg 1985;89:459–62.

8
BENIGN TUMORS OF FATTY TISSUE

LIPOMATOUS HYPERTROPHY OF THE INTERATRIAL SEPTUM

Definition. Lipomatous hypertrophy of the atrial septum is a nonencapsulated accumulation of mature fat, adipose cells resembling brown fat cells, and enlarged cardiac myocytes. Any deposit of fat in the atrial septum at the level of the fossa ovalis which exceeds 2 cm in transverse dimension is considered lipomatous hypertrophy (20). The upper limit of normal fat deposit has also been defined as 1.5 cm in young adults, with increasing limits as age progresses (14). Synonyms are *lipomatous hamartoma of the atrial septum* (1,9) and *massive fatty deposits of the atrial septum* (20). The increase in mass in the atrial septum is likely secondary to an increased number of fat cells, as opposed to hypertrophied myocytes. Therefore, the word "hypertrophy" in lipomatous hypertrophy of interatrial septum (1,18) is a misnomer.

Histogenesis. The precise nature of lipomatous hypertrophy of the atrial septum is unknown. Because there is an association between this lesion and obesity, advanced age, and cardiomegaly (5,20) it is, most likely, an acquired process and may be a metabolic disturbance. In support of the theory that lipomatous hypertrophy is a metabolic disturbance, it has recently been described as a complication of parenteral nutrition (2). However, not all patients with lipomatous hypertrophy are obese, and in some cases a massive tumor results in cardiac symptoms, suggesting a hamartoma (4,9).

Incidence. Lipomatous hypertrophy is a rare lesion: approximately 200 cases have been reported (3–5,13–17,19,20). The true incidence is probably higher since most reported cases are incidental findings and may be overlooked at autopsy. In one series, the estimated incidence was 1.1 percent in over 7,000 autopsies, but these were cases with cardiovascular disease (20).

Clinical Features. The mean age of 190 patients from six combined series of cases of lipomatous hypertrophy of the atrial septum was 69 years (4,5,13,14,17,20); there were 122 males and 68 females, with an age range of 22 to 91 years. There is no race predilection (20). Over one third

of patients are obese (17) and there is an association between increased body weight and increased thickness of the atrial septum (4). However, mean body weight of patients with fatty accumulations in the atrial septum of greater than 3 cm are not significantly greater than those with fatty accumulations of greater than 2 cm but less than 3 cm (20). An association with starvation or anemia has not been reported, which is significant because of the known association between brown fat deposition and cachexia.

The association between atrial arrhythmias and fatty infiltrates of the atrium was initially made in 1969 (12) and has been corroborated by other investigators (8,10). The incidence of atrial arrhythmias in autopsy cases of lipomatous hypertrophy of the atrial septum ranges from 40 to 70 percent (14,17,20). Although both advancing age and coronary artery disease contribute to atrial arrhythmias in many patients, Shirani et al. (20) provide convincing statistical evidence that lipomatous hypertrophy is in itself causatory. The arrhythmias are atrial fibrillation, atrial premature complexes, junctional rhythms, and ectopic atrial rhythms.

Although it is impossible to prove that these tumors cause sudden death, lipomatous hypertrophy is generally accepted as a presumptive cause of fatal arrhythmias. Lipomatous hypertrophy was the only finding to explain sudden death in three cases in a series published by McAllister and Fenoglio (13). In addition to arrhythmias or sudden death, lipomatous hypertrophy can cause compression of the superior vena cava (19) and massive tumors may cause congestive heart failure, requiring surgical removal (3,4,7,22). There is a single report, without histologic documentation, of an atrial "lipoma," which may actually represent lipomatous hypertrophy. The tumor resulted in recurrent embolization necessitating amputation of the left arm (23).

The first antemortem diagnosis of lipomatous hypertrophy occurred in 1982 (10); recently, magnetic resonance imaging (MRI) and transesophageal echocardiography have been used for presurgical diagnosis (11,15).

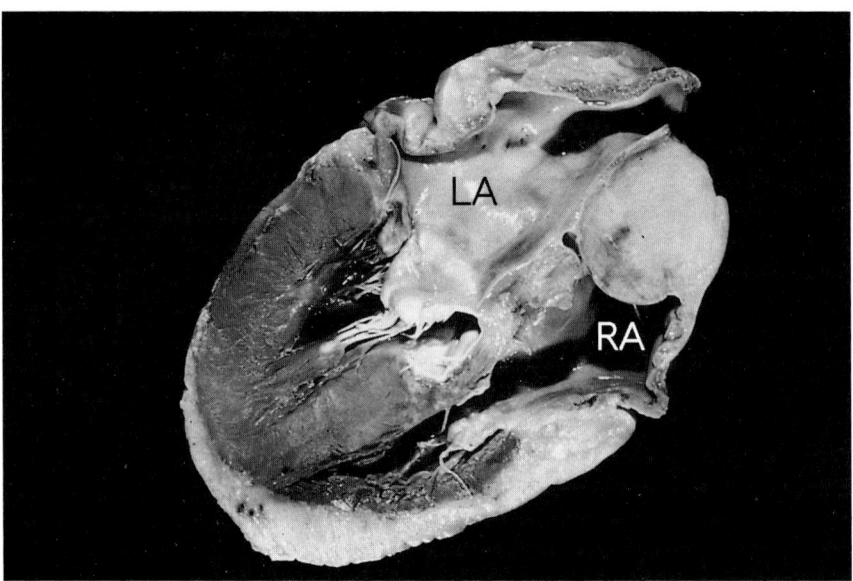

Figure 8-1
LIPOMATOUS HYPERTROPHY:
ATRIAL SEPTUM

There is a nearly spherical fatty mass projecting into the right atrium limited inferiorly by the fossa ovalis. RA = right atrium, LA = left atrium. (Figure 9A from Shirani J, Roberts WC. Clinical, electrocardiographic and morphologic features of massive fatty deposits ("lipomatous hypertrophy") in the atrial septum. J Am Coll Cardiol 1993;22:226–38.)

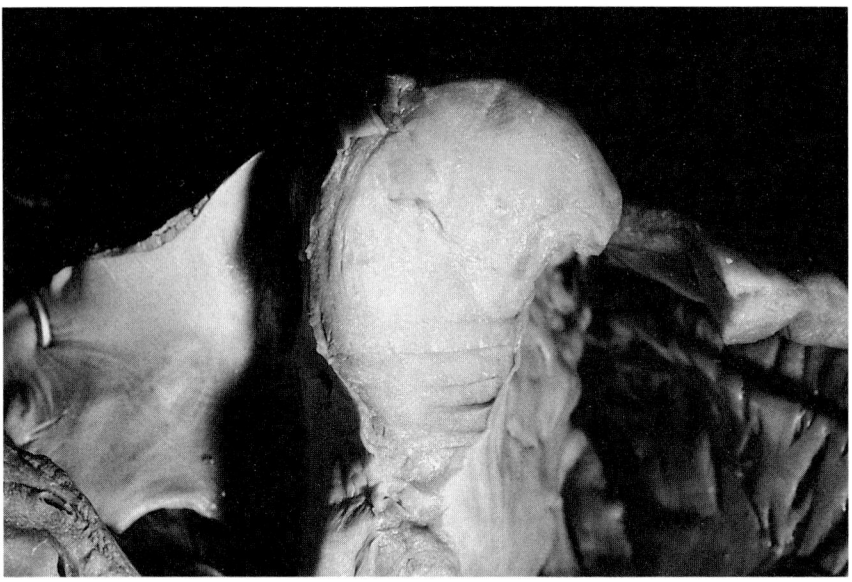

Figure 8-2
LIPOMATOUS HYPERTROPHY:
ATRIAL SEPTUM

A higher magnification of a different example demonstrating the fatty deposit superior to the fossa ovalis.

Pathologic Findings. Grossly, the atrial septum is thickened up to several centimeters (figs. 8-1, 8-2), and the fatty mass generally extends into the right atrium (5). The thickness of the atrial septum cephalad to the fossa ovalis is always greater than that caudal to the fossa ovalis (20). These tumors can be very large, occasionally attaining a size of 15 cm (19). There can be involvement of the entire septum or, occasionally, the bulk of the tumor may be attached to the atrial surface. Although histologically the lesions are infiltrating, they can appear circum-scribed grossly (fig. 8-1) because of the bulging of the endocardial surfaces. Usually, the fossa ovalis is spared, although there can be mild fatty infiltration at this site.

Microscopically, the characteristic feature is a mixture of fat and cardiac myocytes. At least some of the fat is vacuolated, with centrally placed nuclei (figs. 8-3, 8-4); these cells resemble brown fat and fat cells in malnourished or starving patients. In most cases, the interspersed cardiac myocytes are bizarre and greatly enlarged. However, mitoses are absent, distinguishing this

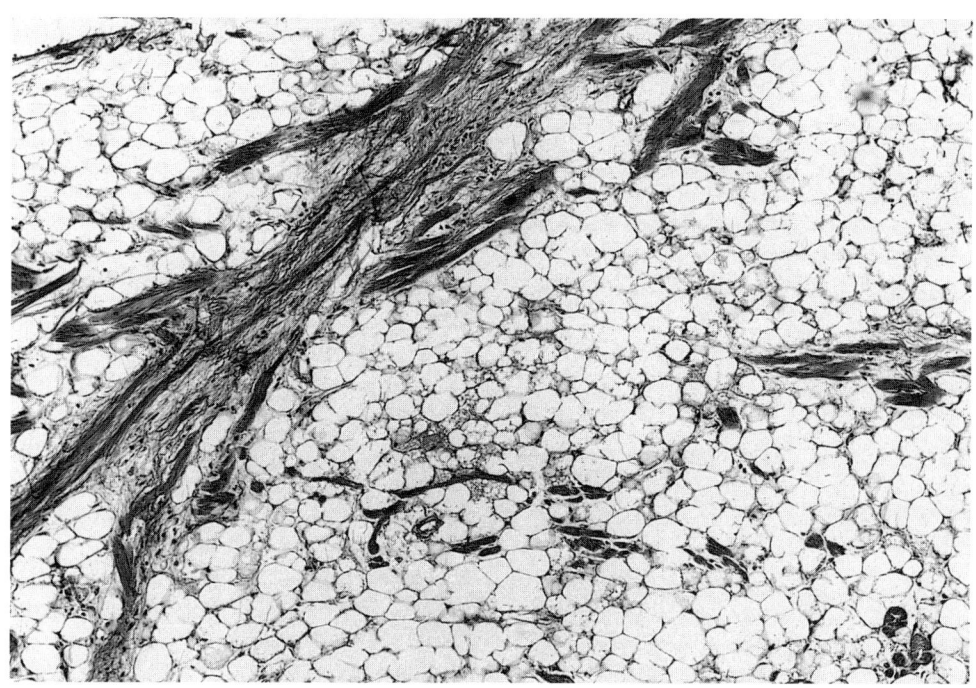

Figure 8-3
LIPOMATOUS HYPERTROPHY: ATRIAL SEPTUM
There is a mixture of normal-appearing fat, vesicular fat, and hypertrophied cardiac myocytes.

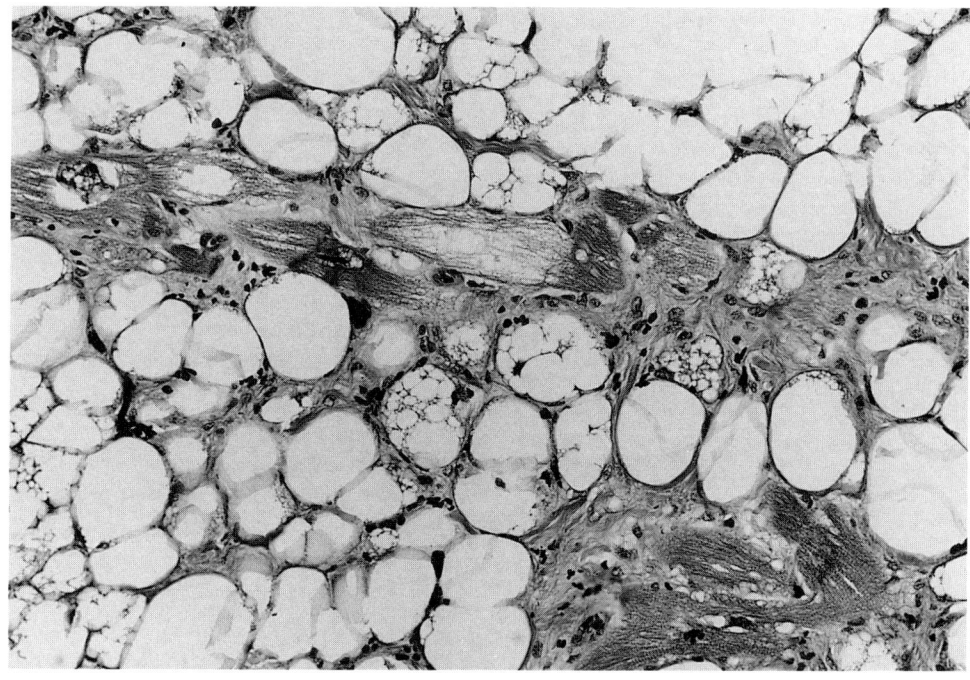

Figure 8-4
LIPOMATOUS HYPERTROPHY: ATRIAL SEPTUM
A higher magnification of the same case illustrated in figure 8-3. Note the vesicular and normal-appearing fat cells and interspersed myocytes.

lesion from a malignancy. Abundant vacuolated fat cells and atypical myocytes with a nuclear length exceeding 40 μm are significantly more prevalent in cases of lipomatous hypertrophy than in controls, independent of age (4). There is an association between interatrial thickness and cardiomegaly and obesity (4,20). We did not find an association between lipomatous hypertrophy of the atrial septum and coronary atherosclerosis (4), as has been suggested by Shirani and Roberts (20). Ultrastructurally, the vesiculated fat cells contain abundant mitochondria, characteristic of brown fat (4).

The differential diagnosis includes liposarcoma and other sarcomas, especially if a large mass is resected surgically. The brown fat cells in lipomatous hypertrophy are sometimes mistaken for lipoblasts. Unlike lipoblasts, fat cells in lipomatous hypertrophy do not form signet ring structures and do not have enlarged, hyperchromatic, indented nuclei. The hyperchromatic enlarged myocytes are also sometimes mistaken for malignant cells, but the lack of mitotic figures and the other features of lipomatous hypertrophy point to the correct diagnosis. Rarely, the diagnosis is made on the basis of transvenous biopsy (21). In such instances, clinical correlation is recommended due to small sample size, and the mere presence of benign fat is compatible with the diagnosis.

Treatment. Although once only diagnosed at autopsy, lipomatous hypertrophy of the atrial septum is now a recognized surgical entity. Seven of 12 recent cases on file at the Armed Forces Institute of Pathology (AFIP) were surgical specimens. There are at least 7 additional cases of successful surgical removal of this tumor in the medical literature (7,18,19,22). In many cases, there was postoperative resolution of atrial arrhythmias or improvement of cardiac function.

LIPOMA

Definition. Like lipomas of extracardiac soft tissue, lipomas of the heart are benign neoplasms of adipose tissue.

Incidence. Lipomas of the heart are quite rare: there were 17 examples in Mahaim's monograph on cardiac tumors (28). Thirty cases had been reported by 1968 (26). It is difficult to determine how many of these cases were actually lipomatous hypertrophy of the atrial septum. Eight cardiac and five pericardial lipomas were reported in the previous Fascicle on cardiac tumors (29). In several recent series of surgically excised cardiac tumors, there were 22 cases of lipomas (24,25,30,31,33,35), but at least 5 of these were lipomatous hypertrophy of the atrial septum and not true lipomas (25,33,35).

Clinical Features. In contrast to lipomatous hypertrophy, lipomas are usually found on the epicardial surfaces and do not generally cause symptoms. Several large epicardial lipomas, however, caused preoperative left ventricular dysfunction (32,35), and one tumor infiltrated soft tissue surrounding an epicardial coronary artery, necessitating complex surgery (31). These reports indicate that cardiac lipomas are not always completely innocent lesions. One case of multiple lipomas of the posterior wall in the right ventricle of a patient with a partial atrioventricular canal has been reported (33), as well as multiple tumors in patients with tuberous sclerosis (29).

Reports of surgical excision were all without complication (24,30,31,33,35). Preoperative diagnosis can be made with MRI (34).

Pathologic Findings. Nearly all cardiac lipomas are epicardial (figs. 8-5, 8-6): they may occur at any site on the atrial or ventricular surface. We have recently encountered a lipoma of the right ventricle that was predominantly intracavitary. Most are single lesions, except for the case mentioned in association with congenital heart defect (33), three cases in the previous Fascicle associated with tuberous sclerosis (29), and a patient with multiple tumors that resulted in cardiac compression (32). Histologically, cardiac lipomas are composed essentially of mature adipocytes (29,33), although there may be entrapped myocytes at the base of the tumor. A capsule is usually present (29), although it may be focally absent or attenuated. There is a report of an incidental mural angiolipoma infiltrating the posterior wall of the left ventricle (27); its location, infiltration, nonencapsulated appearance, and large number of vessels, described as veins, capillaries, and arterioles within the tumor, suggest to us that the lesion is best classified as a hemangioma. Cardiac hemangiomas are typically mural, rather than epicardial lesions and may contain significant accumulations of fat (see chapter 7).

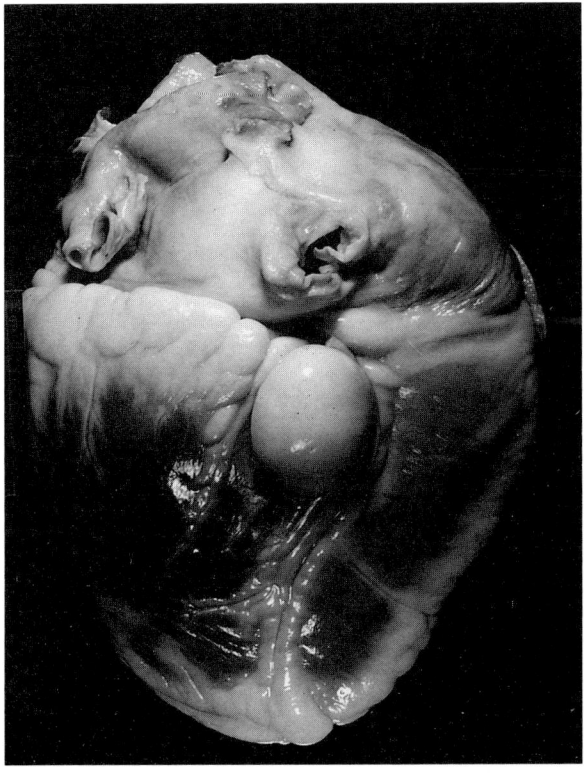

Figure 8-5
CARDIAC LIPOMA
There is a circumscribed mass on the inferior aspect of the heart at the base.

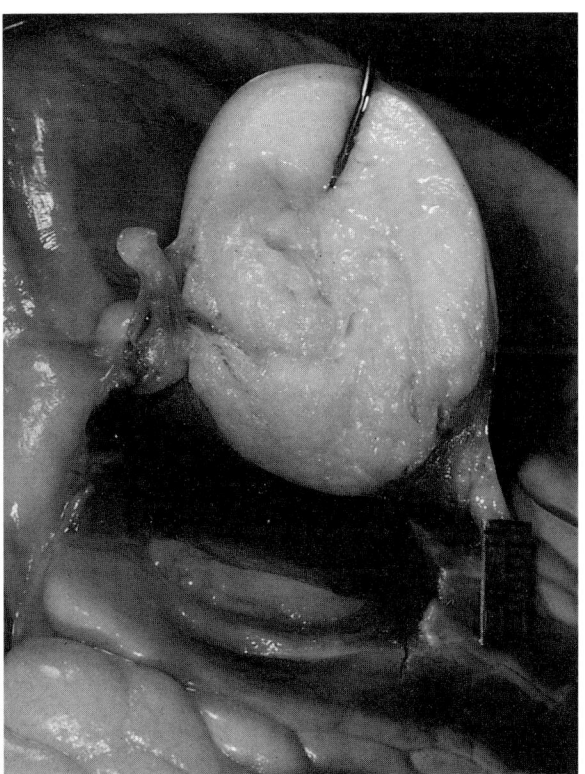

Figure 8-6
CARDIAC LIPOMA
A higher magnification of the lipoma illustrated in figure 8-5 reveals homogeneous fat. Histologically the lesion consisted entirely of mature fat (not shown).

LIPOMATOUS HAMARTOMA OF CARDIAC VALVES

There have been at least six reports of lipomatous tumors involving the mitral or tricuspid valves (36–41). The patients have ranged from 2 to 76 years at presentation (38,40), and no sex predilection is apparent. One patient was obese (41). Patients present with symptoms of valve incompetence, and preoperative diagnosis is facilitated by echocardiography and computed tomography (CT) (36). The tumors may be multiple, and valve replacement may be necessary because of involvement of the papillary muscle or adjacent atrial tissue (36,38,41). Histologically, the lesions are composed of varying proportions of mature fat and fibrous tissue. They are considered to be hamartomas because there is often an admixture of fibrous tissue and a lack of encapsulation (40).

THE FATTY HEART

Diffuse lipomatous infiltration of the epicardial surfaces of the heart, with areas of infiltration of the myocardium, has been termed *the fatty heart* and *lipomatous infiltration of the heart*. In contrast to lipomas and lipomatous hamartomas, the fatty infiltrates are not discrete. There is a severe increase in fat in the atrioventricular sulci, over both ventricles, and occasionally within the ventricular walls.

There is no clear definition of an abnormal accumulation of epicardial fat. Five percent of hearts in a large autopsy series had extensive fat deposits resulting in "floating" hearts when immersed in water (43). In all cases the fatty infiltration was an incidental finding, associated with obesity and lipomatous infiltration of the atrial septum (43). Rarely, lipomatous infiltration that is not limited to the atrial septum may

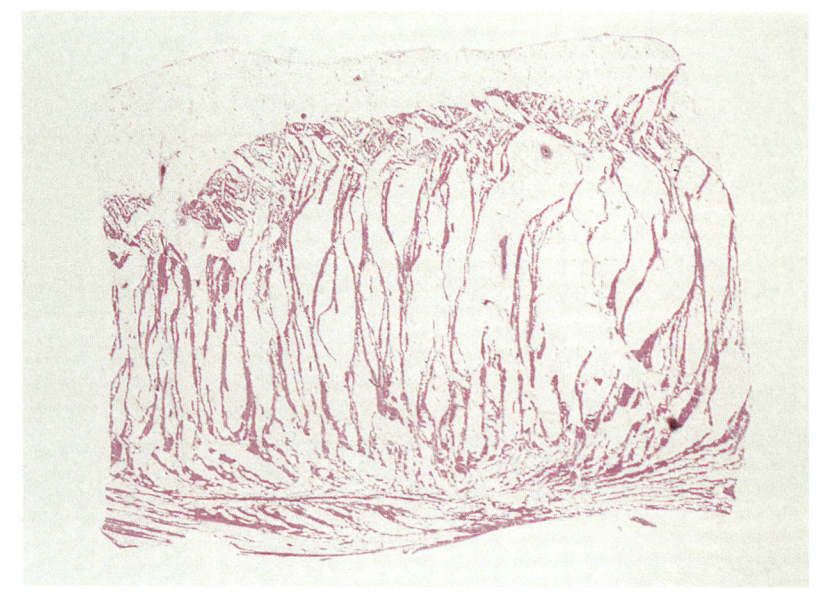

Figure 8-7
MASSIVE FATTY INFILTRATION:
RIGHT VENTRICLE
The patient was a 50-year-old obese woman who died suddenly. At autopsy, there was severe coronary atherosclerosis, as well as marked thickening of the right ventricular wall of up to 2 cm.

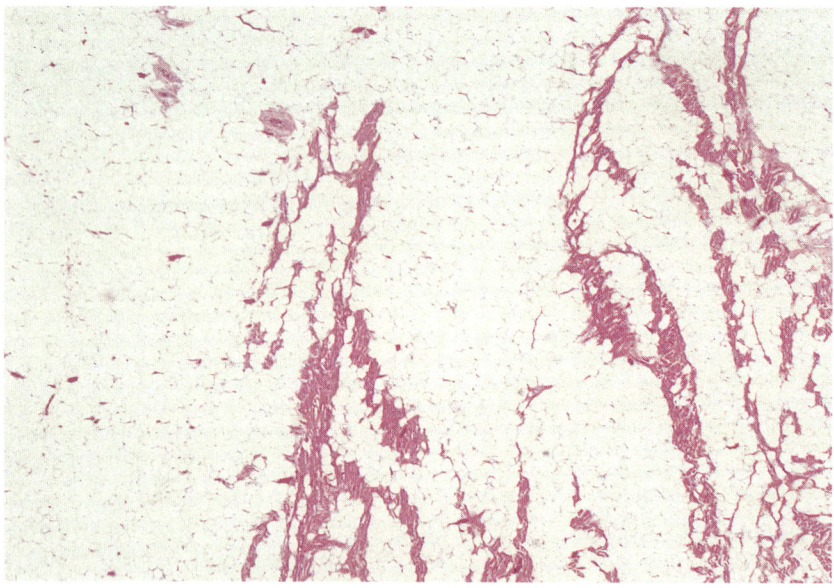

Figure 8-8
MASSIVE FATTY INFILTRATION:
RIGHT VENTRICLE
A higher magnification of figure 8-7 shows fat cells dispersed among muscle cells.

cause sudden death (44). Histologically, the fatty deposits are composed of mature fat that may diffusely infiltrate the ventricles (figs. 8-7, 8-8).

Right ventricular dysplasia (right ventricular cardiomyopathy) is a related condition that may result in focal fatty infiltrates in the right ventricle (42). It is a rare familial cardiomyopathy that causes symptomatic ventricular dysrhyth-mias and sudden death. There is infiltration of fat and fibrous tissue in the right ventricle, especially in the posterior and anterior walls, with loss of myocytes. Unlike the other entities discussed in this chapter, right ventricular dysplasia does not cause a tumor-like infiltrate, but, rather, thinning of the ventricular wall.

REFERENCES

Lipomatous Hypertrophy of the Interatrial Septum

1. Agbamu DA, McMahon RF. Lipomatous hamartoma of the interatrial septum. Am J Cardiovasc Pathol 1993;4:371–3.
2. Beau P, Michel P, Coisne D, Morichau-Beauchant M. Lipomatous hypertrophy of the cardiac interatrial septum: an unusual complication in long-term home parenteral nutrition in adult patients. JPEN 1991;15:659–62.
3. Bhattacharjee M, Neligan MC, Dervan P. Lipomatous hypertrophy of the interatrial septum: an unusual intraoperative finding. Br Heart J 1991;65:49–50.
4. Burke AP, Litovsky S, Virmani R. Lipomatous hypertrophy of the interatrial septum presentating as a right atrial mass. Am J Surg Pathol (in press).
5. Crocker D. Lipomatous infiltrates of the heart. Arch Pathol Lab Med 1978;102:69–72.
6. Dein JR, Frist WH, Stinson EB, et al. Primary cardiac neoplasms. Early and late results of surgical treatment in 42 patients. J Thorac Cardiovasc Surg 1987;93:502–11.
7. Fisher MS, Edmonds P. Lipomatous hypertrophy of interatrial septum. Diagnosis by magnetic resonance imaging. J Comput Tomogr 1988;12:267–9.
8. Hutter AM Jr, Page DL. Atrial arrhythmias and lipomatous hypertrophy of the cardiac interatrial septum. Am Heart J 1971;82:16–21.
9. Inoue T, Mohri N, Nagahara T, Takanashi R. A case report of lipomatous hypertrophy of the cardiac interatrial septum with a proposal for a new term, lipomatous hamartoma of the cardiac atrial septum. Acta Pathol Jpn 1988;38:1583–9.
10. Isner JM, Swan CS, Mikus JP, Carter BL. Lipomatous hypertrophy of the interatrial septum: in vivo diagnosis. Circulation 66:1982;470–3.
11. Levine RA, Weyman AE, Dinsmore RE, et al. Noninvasive tissue characterization: diagnosis of lipomatous hypertrophy of the atrial septum by nuclear magnetic resonance imaging. J Am Coll Cardiol 1986;7:688–92.
12. Kluge WF. Lipomatous hypertrophy of the interatrial septum. Northwest Med 1969;68:25–30.
13. McAllister HA, Fenoglio JJ Jr. Tumors of the cardiovascular system, Atlas of Tumor Patholgy. 2nd Series, Fascicle 15. Washington, D.C.: Armed Forces Institute of Pathology 1978:40–6.
14. Page DL. Lipomatous hypertrophy of the cardiac interatrial septum: its development and probable clinical significance. Hum Pathol 1970;1:151–63.
15. Pochis WT, Saeian K, Sagar KB. Usefulness of transesophageal echocardiography in diagnosing lipomatous hypertrophy of the atrial septum with comparison to transthoracic echocardiography. Am J Cardiol 1992;70:396–8.
16. Prior JT. Lipomatous hypertrophy of cardiac interatrial septum. Arch Pathol 1964;78:11–5.
17. Reyes CV, Jablokow VR. Lipomatous hypertrophy of the cardiac interatrial septum. A report of 38 cases and review of the literature. Am J Clin Pathol 1979;72:785–8.
18. Rokey R, Mulvagh SL, Cheirif J, Mattox KL, Johnston DL. Lipomatous encasement and compression of the heart: antemortem diagnosis by cardiac nuclear magnetic resonance imaging and catheterization. Am Heart J 1989;117:952–3.
19. Scully RE, Mark EJ, McNeely WF, McNeely BU. Case records of the Massachusetts General Hospital. Weekly clinicopathological exercises. Case 10. N Engl J Med 1989;320:652–60.
20. Shirani J, Roberts WC. Clinical, electrocardiographic and morphologic features of massive fatty deposits (lipomatous hypertrophy) in the atrial septum. J Am Coll Cardiol 1993;22:226–38.
21. Stone GW, O'Kell RT, Good TH, Hartzler GO. Lipomatous hypertrophy of the interatrial septum: diagnosis by percutaneous transvenous biopsy. Am Heart J 1990;119:406–8.
22. Tschirkov A, Stegaru B. Lipomatous hypertrophy of interatrial septum presenting as recurring pericardial effusion and mistaken for constrictive pericarditis. Thorac Cardiovasc Surg 1979;27:400–3.
23. Verkkala K, Kupari M, Maamies T, et al. Primary cardiac tumours—operative treatment of 20 patients. Thorac Cardiovasc Surg 1989;37:361–4.

Cardiac Lipoma

24. Blondeau P. Primary cardiac tumors—French studies of 533 cases. Thorac Cardiovasc Surg 1990;38:192–5.
25. Dein JR, Frist WH, Stinson EB, et al. Primary cardiac neoplasms. Early and late results of surgical treatment in 42 patients. J Thorac Cardiovasc Surg 1987;93:502–11.
26. Heath D. Pathology of cardiac tumors. Am J Cardiol 1968;21:315–27.
27. Kiaer HW. Myocardial angiolipoma. Acta Pathol Microbiol Immunol Scand [A] 1984;92:291–2.
28. Mahaim K. Les tumeurs et les polypes de coeur: etude anatomo-clinique. Paris: Masson, 1945.
29. McAllister HA, Fenoglio JJ Jr. Tumors of the cardiovascular system, Atlas of Tumor Patholgy. 2nd Series, Fascicle 15. Washington, D.C.: Armed Forces Institute of Pathology 1978,40–46.
30. Murphy MC, Sweeney MS, Putnam JB, et al. Surgical treatment of cardiac tumors: a 25-year experience. 1990;49:612–7.
31. Reece IJ, Cooley DA, Frazier OH, Hallman GL, Powers PL, Montero CG. Cardiac tumors. J Thorac Cardiovasc Surg 1984;88:439–46.
32. Rokey R, Mulvagh SL, Cheirif J, Mattox KL, Johnston DL. Lipomatous encasement and compression of the heart: antemortem diagnosis by cardiac nuclear magnetic resonance imaging and catheterization. Am Heart J 1989;117:952–3.
33. Tazelaar HD, Locke TJ, McGregor CG. Pathology of surgically excised primary cardiac tumors. Mayo Clin Proc 1992;67:957–65.
34. Tuna IC, Julsrud PR, Click RL, Tazelaar HD, Bresnahan DR, Danielson GK. Tissue characterization of an unusual right atrial mass by magnetic resonance imaging. Mayo Clin Proc 1991;66:498–501.
35. Verkkala K, Kupari M, Maamies T, et al. Primary cardiac tumours—operative treatment of 20 patients. Thorac Cardiovasc Surg 1989;37:361–4.

Lipomatous Hamartoma of Cardiac Valves

36. Anderson DR, Gray MR. Mitral incompetence associated with lipoma infiltrating the mitral valve. Br Heart J 1988;60:169–71.
37. Barberger-Gateau P, Paquet M, Desaulniers D, Chenard J. Fibrolipoma of the mitral valve in a child. Clinical and echocardiographic features. Circulation 1978;58:955–8.
38. Behnam R, Williams G, Gerlis L, Walker D, Scott O. Lipoma of the mitral valve and papillary muscle. Am J Cardiol 1983;51:1459–60.

39. Crocker D. Lipomatous infiltrates of the heart. Arch Pathol Lab Med 1978;102:69–72.
40. Crotty TB, Edwards WD, Oh JK, Rodeheffer RJ. Lipomatous hamartoma of the tricuspid valve: echocardiogaphic- pathologic correlations. Clin Cardiol 1991;14:262–6.
41. Dollar AL, Wallace RB, Kent KM, Burkhart MW, Roberts WC. Mitral valve replacement for mitral lipoma associated with severe obesity. Am J Cardiol 1989;64:1405–7.

Lipomatous Infiltration of the Heart

42. Goodin J, Farb A, Field F, Smialek J, Virmani R. Right ventricular dysplasia associated with sudden death in young adults. Mod Pathol 1991;4:702–6.
43. Roberts WC, Roberts JD. The floating heart or the heart too fat to sink: analysis of 55 necropsy patients. Am J Cardiol 1983;52:1286–9.

44. Voigt J, Agdal N. Lipomatous infiltration of the heart. An uncommon cause of sudden unexpected death in a young man. Arch Pathol Lab Med 1982;106:497–8.

9
BENIGN MESOTHELIAL PROLIFERATIONS

MESOTHELIAL CYSTS

Definition. Mesothelial cysts are non-neoplastic cysts lined by mesothelial cells. Synonyms and related terms include *pericardial coelomic cyst, pericardial cyst, hydrocele of the mediastinum,* and *pericardial diverticulum.* We prefer the more precise term mesothelial cyst to pericardial cyst, which fails to specify the cyst's cell of origin.

Histogenesis. Mesothelial cysts are considered to be pericardial diverticula, in which the site of communication with the pericardium is no longer intact (3). They are developmental anomalies, probably caused by the persistence of the ventral parietal recess of the pericardium.

Incidence. The true incidence of mesothelial cysts of the pericardium is unknown because most are incidental findings on chest radiographs (1). At the Armed Forces Institute of Pathology (AFIP) they are the most common cystic lesion of the heart and pericardium, and are approximately one third as common as cardiac myxoma.

Clinical Features. Since 1976, 32 cases of mesothelial cyst were accessioned to the AFIP files. Most patients are adults: the age at the time of presentation ranges from 16 to 68 years. There is no sex predilection. Sixty percent of these patients had no symptoms referable to their cyst. For the remaining 40 percent, manifestations included precordial or substernal chest pain, dyspnea, cough, hemoptysis, pneumothorax, fever, and, rarely, palpitations. Odynophagia secondary to mesothelial cyst has been reported once, in a 39-year-old woman (4).

The most common location for mesothelial cyst of the pericardium is the right cardiophrenic angle (fig. 9-1), followed by the left costophrenic angle. Rarely, mesothelial cysts are located in the anterior, superior, or posterior mediastinum.

The gold standards for the radiologic diagnosis of mediastinal cysts are magnetic resonance imaging (MRI) and computed tomography (CT) (4). Transesophageal echocardiography is an excellent alternative if rapid diagnosis is necessary (4).

Pathologic Findings. Mesothelial cysts are morphologically similar to the normal pericardium. Grossly, they are usually unilocular, thin-walled, and translucent; 20 percent are multiloculated (fig. 9-2) and a few are continuous with the pericardial sac (pericardial diverticulum). Mesothelial cysts range in diameter from 2 to 16 cm. They contain clear fluid and are lined by a flattened, single layer of mesothelial cells and, occasionally, by hyperplastic mesothelial cells (fig. 9-3). The cyst wall is made up of connective tissue rich in collagen with scattered elastic fibers. Rarely, lymphocytes and plasma cells are present in aggregates, and calcification of the cyst wall may occur.

Differential Diagnosis. The differential diagnosis of mesothelial cyst includes mediastinal pseudocysts, which usually result from trauma; healed infections; and lymphangioma. Lymphangiomas are more likely to be multilocular than mesothelial cysts, and occur in infants and children. Histologically, lymphangiomas contain lymphoid aggregates and smooth muscle within

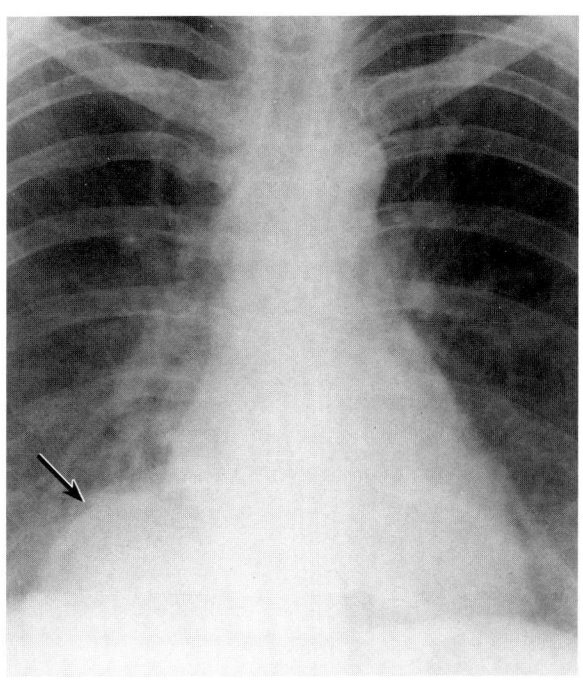

Figure 9-1
MESOTHELIAL CYST OF THE PERICARDIUM
Note the rounded mass in the right costophrenic angle (arrow).

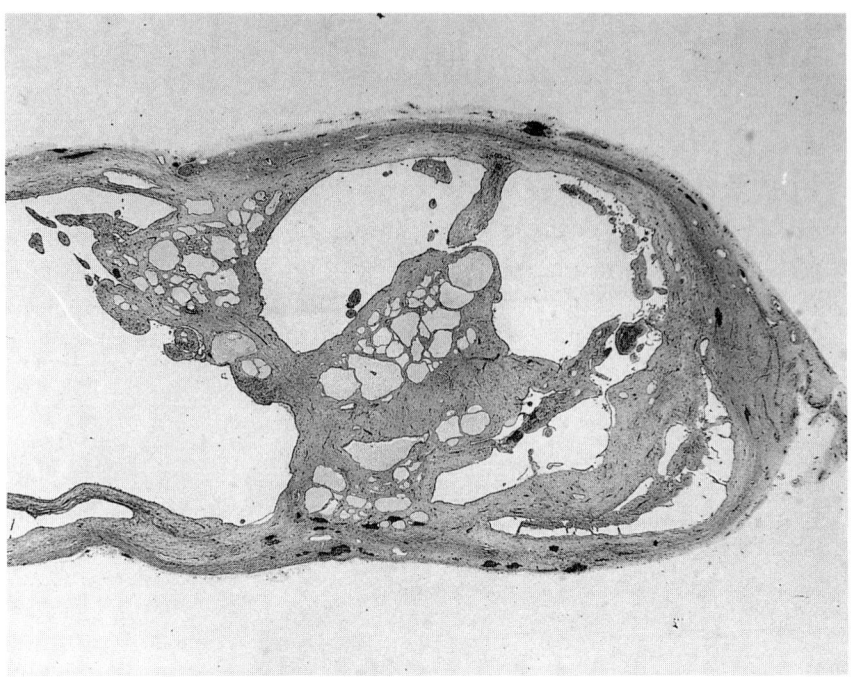

Figure 9-2
MESOTHELIAL CYST
Although usually unilocular, this example has many cysts of varying sizes.

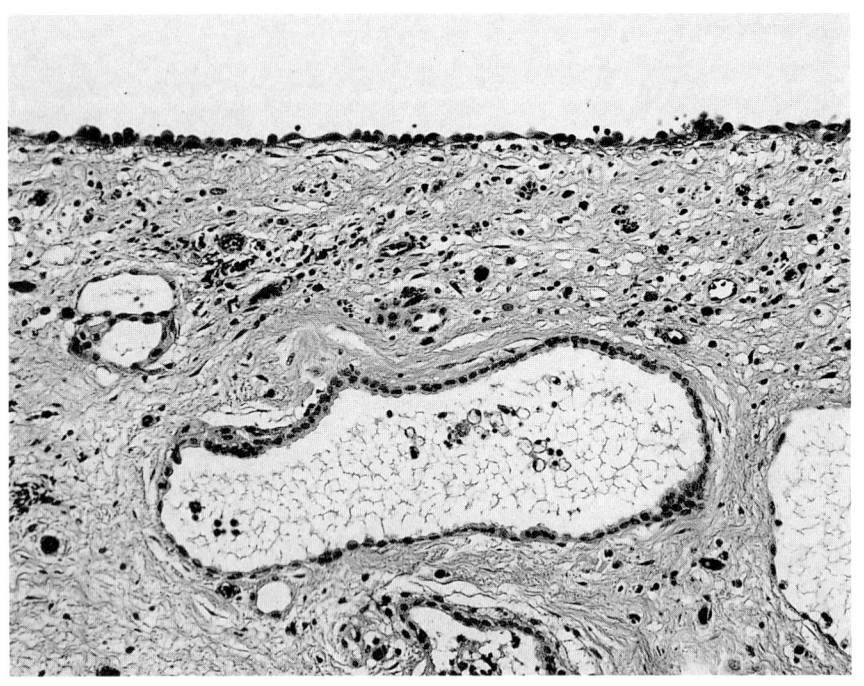

Figure 9-3
MESOTHELIAL CYST
Note the typical cuboidal mesothelial lining cells.

the cyst wall, unlike the majority of mesothelial cysts. Immunohistochemical stains differentiate between these two entities by demonstrating positivity for endothelial markers in lymphangioma and positivity for cytokeratin in lining cells of mesothelial cysts (fig. 9-4). Pseudocysts, by definition, lack a cellular lining, and are instead composed of collagen, with variable amounts of granulation tissue and inflammation. Usually, a history of trauma or infectious pericarditis is elicited.

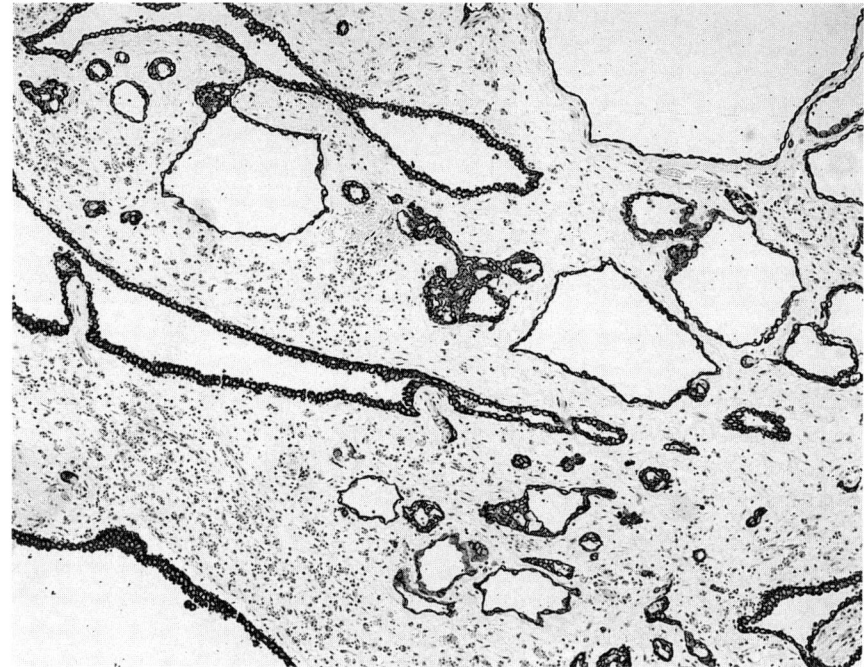

Figure 9-4
MESOTHELIAL CYST
The mesothelial lining cells stain strongly with anticytokeratin. (Avidin-biotin stain)

Treatment. Patients with mesothelial cysts generally require no treatment. Surgical management has been recommended for patients with symptoms of chest pain, dyspnea, or airway obstruction, or if the mass is increasing in size (2). Reports of spontaneous rupture of pericardial cysts and subsequent resolution (2) underscore the prudence of conservative management.

MESOTHELIAL/MACROPHAGE INCIDENTAL CARDIAC EXCRESCENCES

Definition. Mesothelial/macrophage incidental cardiac excrescences (MICE) are fragmented collections of benign mesothelial cells, fat cells, and macrophages that lack intervening stroma. They are found exclusively within the heart, aorta, or pericardium, generally during surgical procedures.

Histogenesis. Although originally considered a form of tumor possibly related to histiocytoid hemangioma (6), MICE are now considered artifacts of cardiovascular surgery, having been discovered in cardiotomy suction devices (5). This theory does not, however, explain rare similar collections of cells found during transvenous right ventricular biopsy (6).

Incidence. The true incidence of cardiac MICE is unknown. If they are indeed artifacts of surgery, as we currently believe, they may be quite common. There were 14 cases when originally reported (6) and two recently published series have added 6 new cases (5,7). Of 110 cardiac myxomas reviewed at the AFIP, 3 had MICE attachments, indicating that they are probably not rare (fig. 9-5). Courtice et al. (5) processed, for light microscopy, the contents of extracorporeal bypass pump filters and material adherent to mediastinal and pericardial drains in cardiac surgery cases. They demonstrated cardiac MICE in 82 percent of pump filters and 13 percent of drains, further suggesting their common occurrence as surgical artifacts.

Clinical Features. Cardiac MICE are considered to be incidental artifacts and therefore without clinical relevance. In a series of 14 cases, 7 were in women; 6 were found within atria, 2 on the mitral valve, 1 on the aortic valve, 3 in the pericardium, and 1 in a dissecting aortic aneurysm. The fourteenth case was not found at cardiac surgery but at endomyocardial biopsy (6).

Histologic Findings. Histologically, there are compact clusters of histiocytes, fat globules, and mesothelial cells, without intervening stroma. The mesothelial components of these "tumors" stain strongly with anticytokeratin antibodies (fig. 9-6).

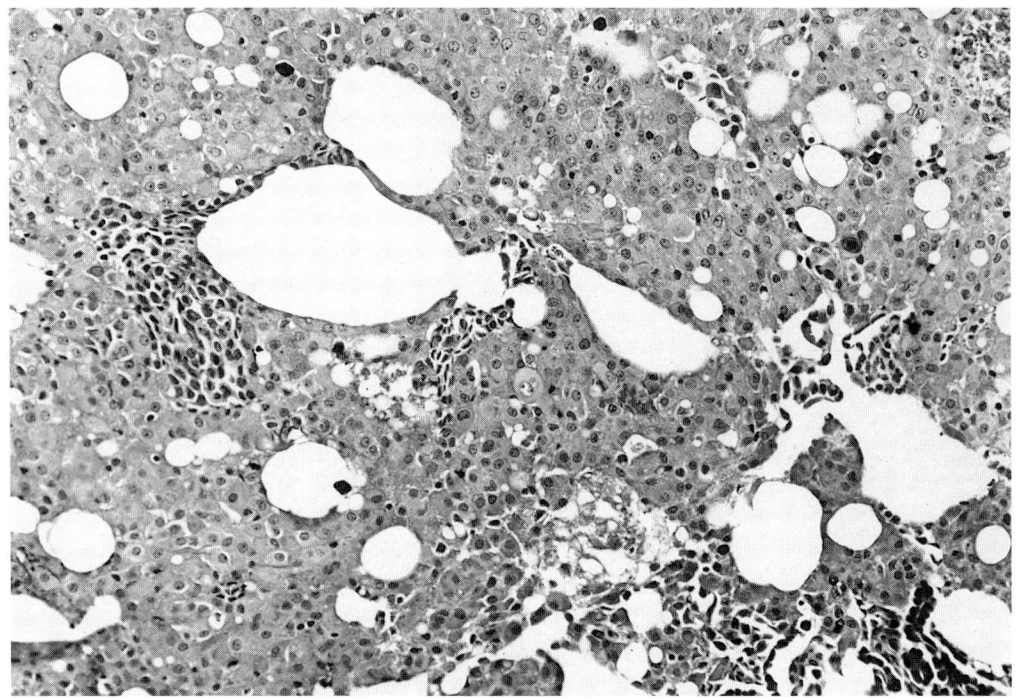

Figure 9-5
MACROPHAGE/MESOTHELIAL INCIDENTAL CARDIAC EXCRESCENCE
There are fat globules, mesothelial cells, and histiocytes. There is no stroma.

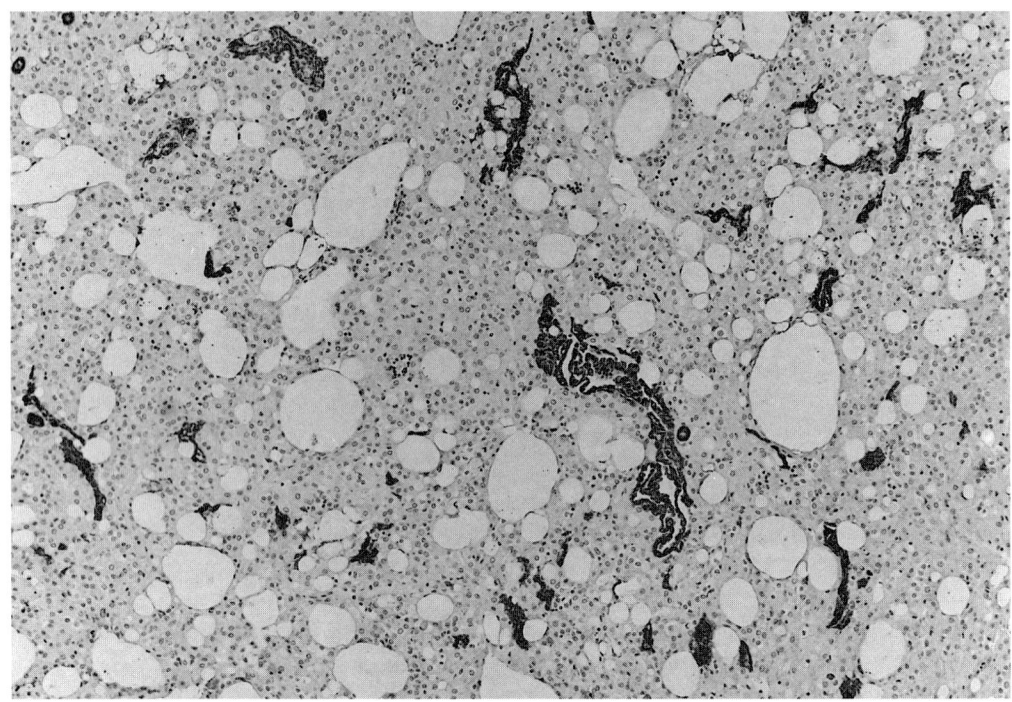

Figure 9-6
MACROPHAGE/MESOTHELIAL INCIDENTAL CARDIAC EXCRESCENCE
Mesothelial cells are highlighted by stain for anticytokeratin. (Avidin-biotin stain)

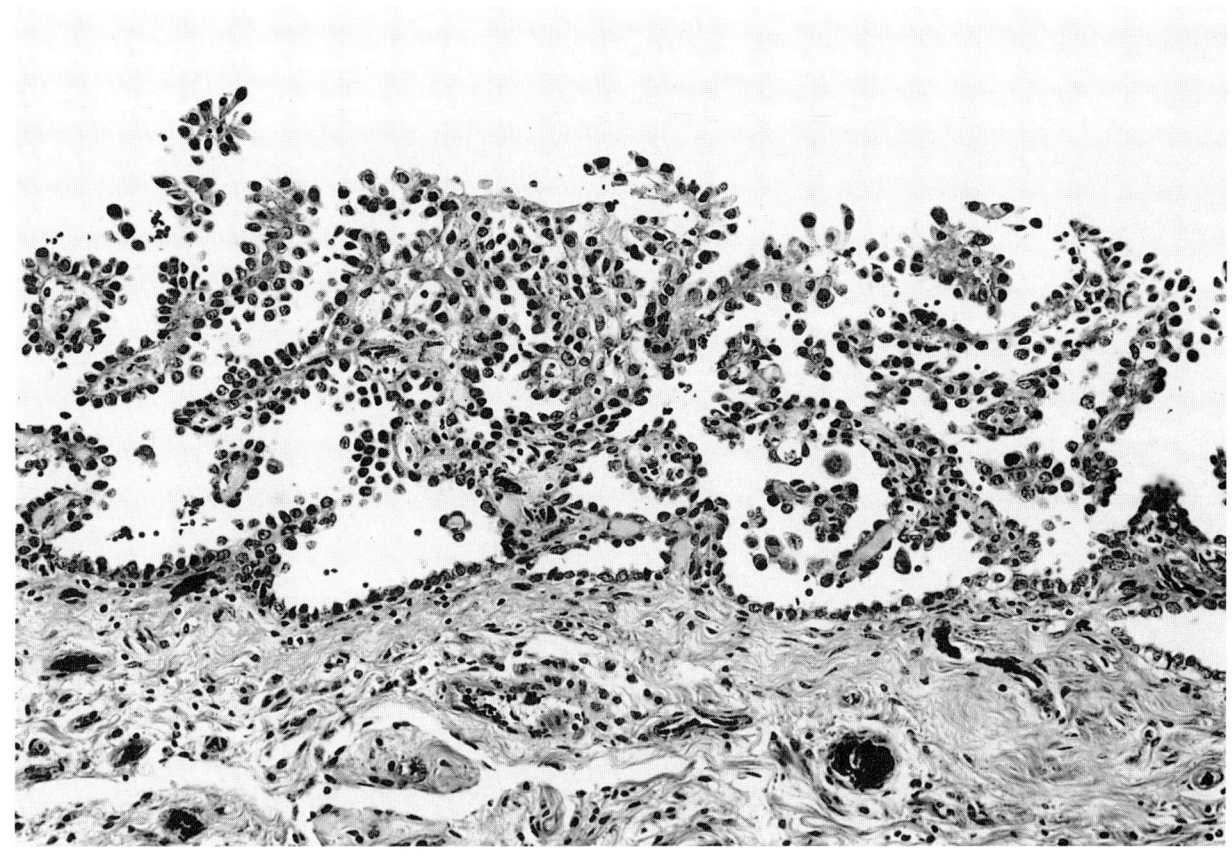

Figure 9-7
MESOTHELIAL PAPILLOMA
Note the papillary structure lined by mesothelial cells identical to those of the pericardial lining. There is little cytologic pleomorphism, and no infiltration of underlying structures. This "tumor" was an incidental finding at autopsy. Although there was no apparent stimulus for a reactive process, the term "reactive mesothelial hyperplasia" may also be used here.

MESOTHELIAL PAPILLOMA OF THE PERICARDIUM

Definition. Benign mesotheliomas of cuboidal or epithelioid cells are found in the peritoneum, pleural surfaces, and pericardial surfaces. These lesions have been called *benign papillary mesothelioma, adenomatoid tumors of the omentum, papillomatosis peritonei, serosal papillomas, mesothelial papillomas, papilloma of the epicardium* (11), and *localized pleural mesothelioma of the epithelial type* (9). Whether these lesions are reactive proliferations, benign neoplasms, or a heterogeneous group of entities is unknown, largely because too few have been described for precise classification. They are composed of epithelioid mesothelial cells, in contrast to benign fibrous tumors of the serosal surfaces, which are composed entirely of spindle cells that ultrastructurally and immunohistochemically resemble fibroblasts.

Incidence. Mesothelial papillomas of the pericardium are extremely rare (8-10).

Clinical Features. They may be incidental findings at autopsy (10) or result in pericardial effusions (8,9). Cytologic examination may suggest a malignant diagnosis (8,9).

Pathologic Findings. Mesothelial papillomas are discrete papillary tumors that arise from the epicardial surface via a narrow pedicle (10). In contrast to reactive mesothelial hyperplasia, there is little inflammation in cytologic specimens or biopsies of the pericardium. Unlike malignant mesothelioma, there are no mitotic figures and significant cellular atypia and pleomorphism are absent (fig. 9-7).

REFERENCES

Mesothelial Pericardial Cysts

1. Feigin DS, Fenoglio JJ, McAllister HA, Madewell JE. Pericardial cysts. A radiologic-pathologic correlation and review. Radiology 1977;125:15–20.
2. Kruger SR, Michaud J, Cannon DS. Spontaneous resolution of a pericardial cyst. Am Heart J 1985; 109:1390–1.
3. Lillie WI, McDonald JR, Clagett OT. Pericardial celomic cysts and pericardial diverticula. A concept of etiology and report of cases. J Thoracic Cardiovasc Surg 1950; 20:494–504.
4. Santoro MJ, Ford LJ, Chen YK, Solinger MR. Odynophagia caused by a pericardial diverticulum. Am J Gastroenterol 1993;88:943–4.

Cardiac MICE

5. Courtice RW, Stinson WA, Walley VM. Tissue fragments recovered at cardiac surgery masquerading as tumoural proliferations. Evidence suggesting iatrogenic or artefactual origin and common occurrence. Am J Surg Pathol 1994;18:167–74.
6. Luthringer DJ, Virmani R, Weiss SW, Rosai J. A distinctive cardiovascular lesion resembling histiocytoid (epithelioid) hemangioma. Evidence suggesting mesothelial participation. Am J Surg Pathol 1990;14:993–1000.
7. Veinot JP, Tazelaar HD, Edwards WD, Colloy TV, Davy C. Mesothelial/monocytic incidental cardiac excrescences: cardiac MICE. Mod Pathol 1994;7:9–16.

Benign Pericardial Mesothelioma

8. Becker SN, Pepin DW, Rosenthal DL. Mesothelial papilloma: a case of mistaken identity in a pericardial effusion. Acta Cytol 1986;20:266–8.
9. Hansen RM, Caya JG, Clowry LJ Jr, Anderson T. Benign mesothelial proliferation with effusion. Clinicopathologic entity that may mimic malignancy. Am J Med 1984;77:887–92.
10. Larsen TE. Serosal papilloma of the epicardium. Report of a case. Arch Pathol 1974;97:271–2.
11. McAllister HA, Fenoglio JJ, Jr. Tumors of the cardiovascular system. Atlas of Tumor Pathology. 2nd Series, Fascicle 15. Washington, D.C.: Armed Forces Institute of Pathology, 1978:25.

BENIGN TUMORS OF NEURAL OR SMOOTH MUSCLE ORIGIN

GRANULAR CELL TUMOR

Definition. Granular cell tumors of the heart are benign epicardial neoplasms composed of cells with a characteristic granular cytoplasm. They are histologically identical to granular cell tumors at extracardiac sites.

Histogenesis. Although originally considered of smooth muscle origin, most evidence suggests that granular cell tumors are proliferations of modified nerve sheath cells. They are often found in proximity to nerves, are diffusely positive for S-100 protein, and ultrastructurally demonstrate, in some cases, myelinated and nonmyelinated axon-like structures.

Granular cell epulis, or *congenital granular cell tumor,* is a related tumor found in the gingiva of infants. Despite its histologic similarity to granular cell tumor of adults, it is unlikely that congenital granular cell tumors are of nerve sheath derivation (4). It is mentioned here because, in rare instances, it may involve the heart in cases of disseminated tumor (4).

Incidence. There are very few reported granular cell tumors of the heart: to date, approximately five cases have been reported in the English language literature (1,5,6). Many cases are not diagnosed because they are generally incidental epicardial nodules that are easily overlooked. Since the publication of the previous Fascicle on cardiac tumors (3), which described three cases, four additional cases are on file at the Armed Forces Institute of Pathology (AFIP).

Clinical Features. Patients are adults aged 24 to 55 years. Granular cell tumors are always incidental autopsy findings and are located on the ventricular or atrial epicardial surface close to the base of the heart where nervous tissue is abundant. In two patients, extracardiac granular cell tumors were present in the oropharynx, esophagus, stomach, intestine, and subcutaneous tissue.

Pathologic Findings. Grossly, cardiac granular cell tumors are circumscribed, gray or tan, and firm (figs. 10-1, 10-2). Microscopically, the tumor cells merge with the surrounding cardiac tissue and scattered normal myocytes are en-

trapped within the tumor mass. The tumor is histologically identical to extracardiac granular cell tumor (figs. 10-3–10-5). Tumor cells are round to elongated, and are filled with granular cytoplasm that is weakly positive with periodic acid–Schiff (PAS) reagent after diastase pretreatment. Glycogen is absent. Tumor cells express S-100 protein, neuron-specific enolase, and various myelin proteins; they are negative for neurofilaments and glial fibrillary acidic protein. The intracellular granules, by electron microscopy, consist of membrane-bound, autophagic vacuoles containing cellular debris of mitochondria, rough endoplasmic reticulum, and myelinated and nonmyelinated structures resembling axons.

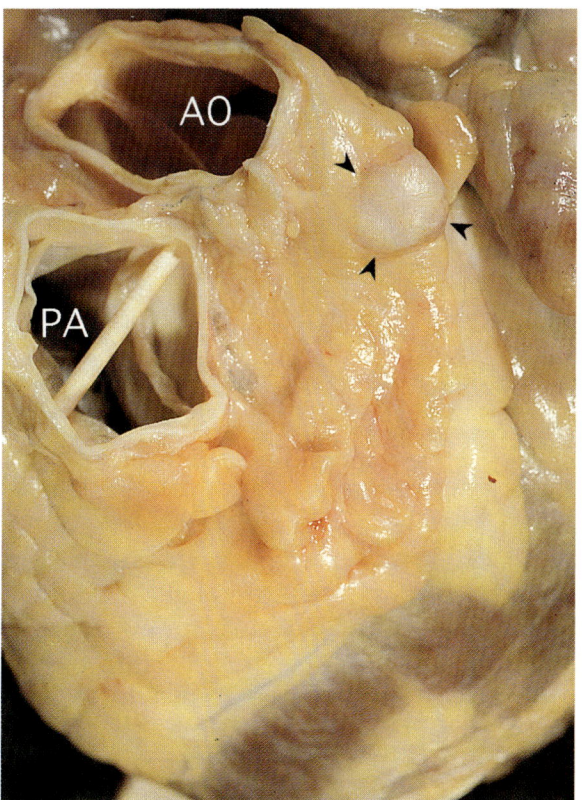

Figure 10-1
GRANULAR CELL TUMOR
Localized epicardial tumor (arrowheads) overlying the left main coronary artery close to its takeoff. Note aorta (AO) posterior to the pulmonary artery (PA).

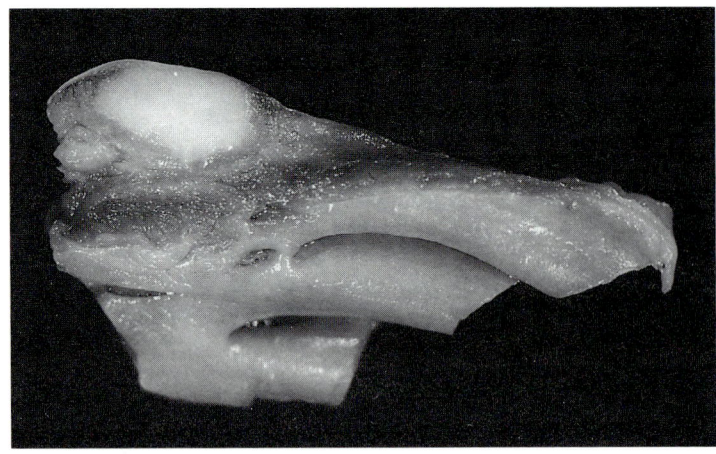

Figure 10-2
GRANULAR CELL TUMOR
Note the cut surface of circumscribed white tumor on the epicardial surface and the underlying right ventricular trabeculations.

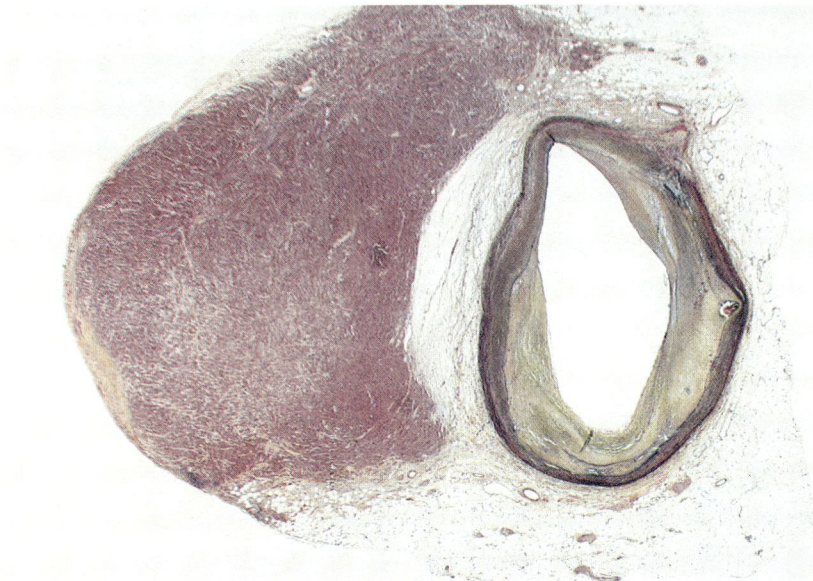

Figure 10-3
GRANULAR CELL TUMOR
Movat stain shows well-demarcated tumor adjacent to a coronary artery. This is the same tumor as seen in figure 10-1.

Despite their presumed neural origin, only one granular cell tumor of the heart has been shown to be continuous with nervous tissue (4): this tumor was in direct contact with the sinus node and perinodal tissue. Malignant granular cell tumors constitute fewer than 2 percent of all granular cell tumors, and have not been reported in the myocardium except as metastatic deposits (2) or as part of disseminated congenital granular cell tumor (4).

PARAGANGLIOMA

Definition. Cardiac paraganglioma is a neoplasm of paraganglial cells, which are generally located within the atria. There are a variety of synonyms for paraganglioma. Extra-adrenal paragangliomas that secrete catecholamines are generally chromaffin positive and have been termed *chromaffin paragangliomas* or *pheochromocytoma* (12). Tumors of similar morphology that occur in the region of the carotid body and aortic body are generally called *chemodectomas*. These latter tumors are generally chromaffin negative or weakly positive, and rarely secrete significant amounts of catecholamines (12). The terms pheochromocytoma (11, 17,20,21) and chemodectoma (13) have been used for cardiac paragangliomas that are functional or nonfunctional, respectively. There are no consistent histologic differences between functioning and nonfunctioning paragangliomas

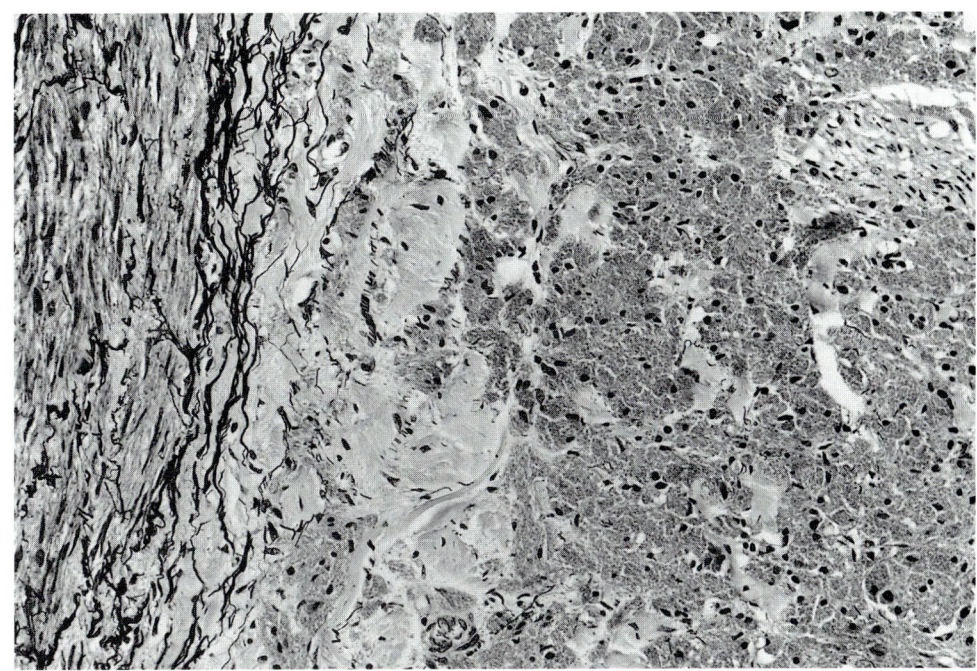

Figure 10-4
GRANULAR CELL TUMOR
This example was adjacent to the left anterior descending coronary artery. Elastic lamellae of the media of the coronary artery are seen at the left. (Movat pentachrome stain)

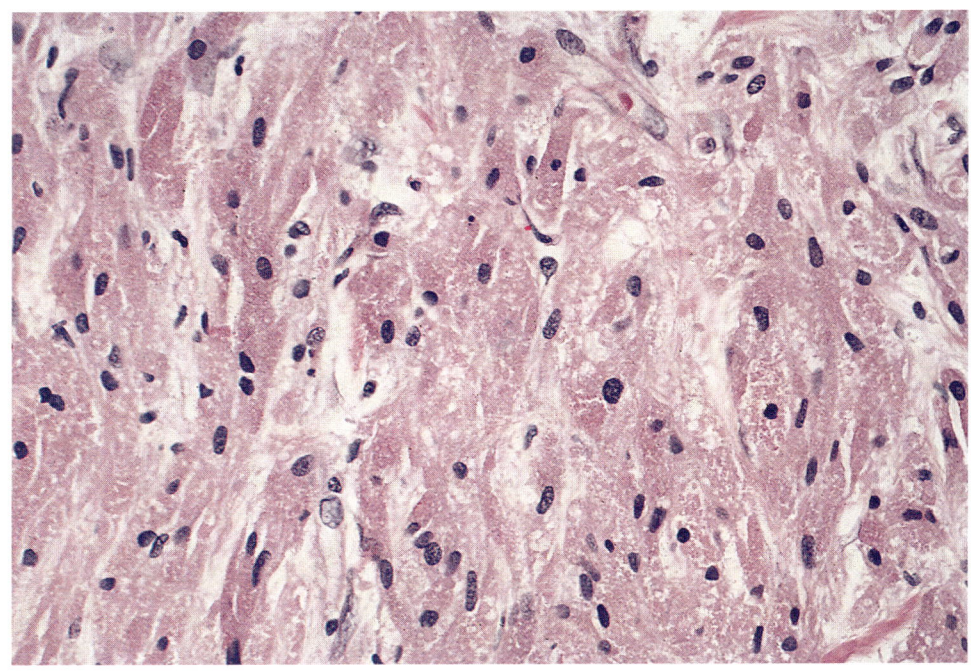

Figure 10-5
GRANULAR CELL TUMOR
Higher magnification of figure 10-3 demonstrating pyknotic nuclei, granular cytoplasm, and ill-defined cell margins.

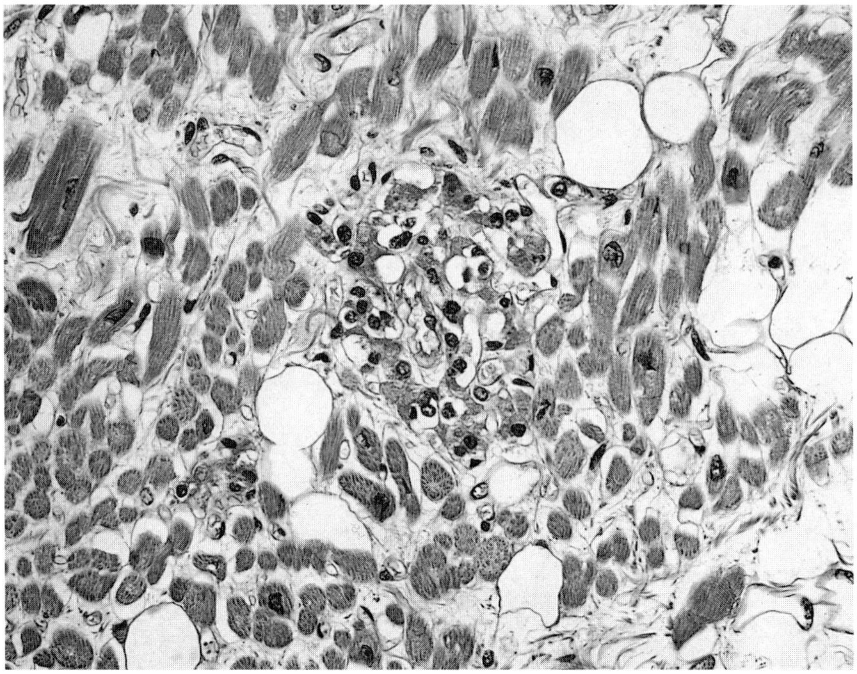

Figure 10-6
PARAGANGLIAL CELLS:
NORMAL RIGHT ATRIUM
This aggregate of paraganglial cells within the atrial muscle was an incidental finding at autopsy.

(12), and the chromaffin reaction does not reliably separate these tumors. Therefore, we prefer the use of the terms *nonfunctional* and *functional paraganglioma* for cardiac tumors, as has been recommended for extra-adrenal paragangliomas of soft tissue (12).

Histogenesis. The cells of origin of cardiac paraganglioma are most likely the intrinsic cardiac ganglia, which are located in the atria (fig. 10-6) along the atrioventricular sulcus and near the roots of the great vessels. Ganglia are rare in the ventricles, accounting for the rarity of ventricular paragangliomas. The atria and atrial septum are enervated by visceral autonomic paraganglia, as opposed to aorticopulmonary paragangliomas, which are derived from branchial arch structures (21).

Incidence. Cardiac paragangliomas are rare: approximately 25 cases have been reported in the English language literature (7–11,13–19).

Clinical Features. Most patients are young adults, with an age range at diagnosis from 15 to 60 years. Slightly more than 50 percent of patients present with hypertension and symptoms of pheochromocytoma (8), indicating that these tumors are functional. Other signs and symptoms include palpitations, murmurs, angina, and mitral regurgitation (8,15). Imaging studies, such as

magnetic resonance imaging (MRI), have proven useful in preoperative management (9). ^{131}I-metaiodobenzylguanidine scintigraphy is useful for localizing mediastinal paragangliomas (21). Rare malignant cardiac paragangliomas, with recurrences, have been reported (10).

Pathologic Findings. Cardiac paragangliomas are large, poorly circumscribed masses that are 5 to 15 cm in greatest dimension (8). Most are located on the epicardial surface of the base of the heart or atria; five have been intracavitary atrial lesions (8), two of which occurred within the atrial septum (15,17). Left ventricular paragangliomas are quite rare (13). Histologically, cardiac paragangliomas are unencapsulated and formed of typical nests or zellballen surrounded by sustentacular cells. Their histologic appearance (fig. 10-7) and immunohistochemical profile are identical to extracardiac paragangliomas (16). Immunohistochemically, they are positive for chromogranin, neuron-specific enolase, and often met-enkephalin; the sustentacular cells are positive for S-100 protein (16). Endocrine polypeptides have not been demonstrated within tumor cells (16). Ultrastructurally, both epinephrine- and norepinephrine-type granules have been demonstrated, although the latter predominate (16).

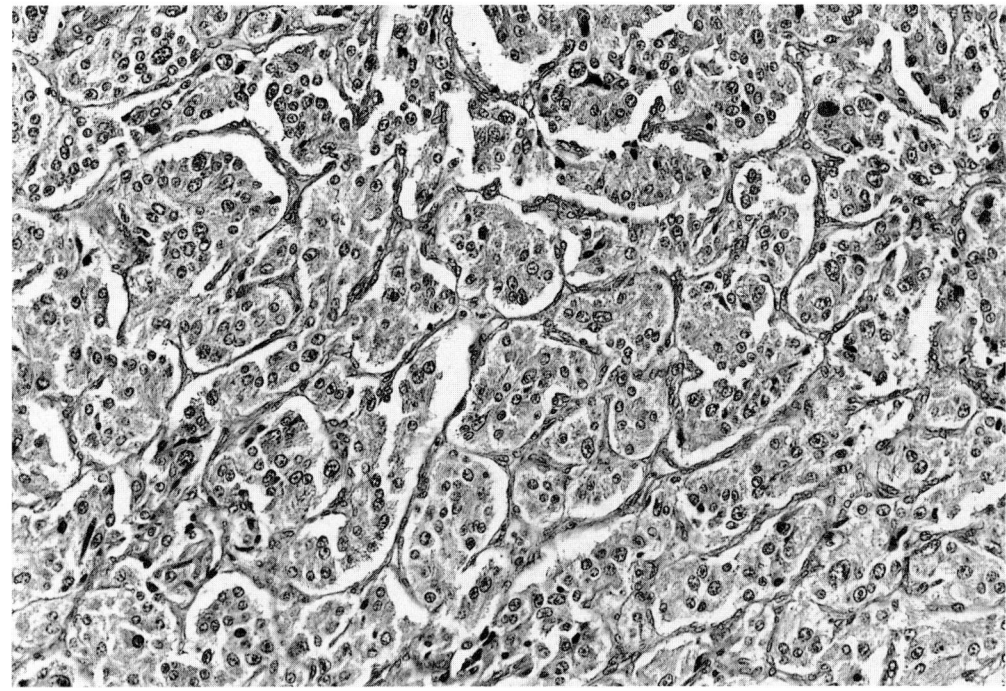

Figure 10-7
PARAGANGLIOMA: ATRIUM

The tumor was excised from a middle-aged woman with hypertension and elevated serum catecholamines. The histologic appearance of nested cells in an "organoid" pattern is typical of paraganglioma.

Treatment. Cardiac paragangliomas are generally benign, and patients may survive for long periods with partial excision (7). There have been at least 16 reports of surgical excision, with 3 postoperative deaths (8). Normalization of blood pressure is usual in patients with preoperative hypertension (14).

NEUROFIBROMA/NEURILEMOMA

Neurofibromas and neurilemomas are benign tumors of nerve sheath origin. Although there is a spectrum of histologic features shared by these two entities, they are easily separated by clinical, histologic, and immunohistochemical findings.

Like other neural tumors, nerve sheath tumors of the heart are quite rare (22–26). There appears to be a predilection for location in the atria (23,24). There have been reports of a cardiac neurofibroma occurring in patients with von Recklinghausen's disease (26), and in a patient who had received prior radiation therapy (23); in addition, a neural tumor with features of a neuroma and neurofibroma has been described in the

atrioventricular nodal area of a 3-month-old infant (23). Occasionally, primary cardiac neurilemoma may be an incidental finding discovered at autopsy (23). There are reports of surgically resected neurilemomas, one obstructing the right ventricular outflow tract (22,24). There is no evidence that the microscopic features of cardiac nerve sheath tumors differ from those of extracardiac neurofibromas and neurilemomas (23).

LEIOMYOMA AND LEIOMYOMATOSIS

Primary leiomyomas of the pericardium are extremely rare (27). Benign smooth muscle tumors of extracardiac sites may extend into the right atrium, generally via the inferior vena cava. Such tumors may initially present with cardiac symptoms and are termed intracardiac leiomyomatosis (30,31). Most arise within the uterus (29). However, not all uterine leiomyomas with intravascular extension (intravascular leiomyomatosis) reach the right atrium. Rarely, intracardiac leiomyomatosis may result from hepatic vein (28) or iliac vein (31) leiomyomas.

REFERENCES

Cardiac Granular Cell Tumor

1. Fenoglio JJ Jr, McAllister HA Jr. Granular cell tumors of the heart. Arch Pathol Lab Med 1976;100:276–8.
2. Kubac G, Doris I, Ondro M, Davey PW. Malignant granular cell myoblastoma with metastatic cardiac involvement: case report and echocardiogram. Am Heart J 1980;100:227–9.
3. McAllister HA, Fenoglio JJ Jr. Tumors of the cardiovascular system. Atlas of Tumor Pathology, 2nd Series, Fascicle 15. Washington D.C.: Armed Forces Institute of Pathology, 1978:70–1.
4. Park SH, Kim TJ, Chi JG. Congenital granular cell tumor with systemic involvement. Immunohistochemical and ultrastructural study. Arch Pathol Lab Med 1991;115:934–8.
5. Roth D, Spain DM. Granular cell myoblastoma of the myocardium. Cancer 1952;5:302–6.
6. Wang J, Kragel AH, Friedlander ER, Cheng JT. Granular cell tumor of the sinus node. Am J Cardiol 1993;71:490–2.

Cardiac Paraganglioma

7. Abad C, Jimenez P, Santana C, et al. Primary cardiac paraganglioma. Case report and review of surgically treated cases. J Cardiovasc Surg 1992;33:758–72.
8. Aravot DJ, Banner NR, Cantor AM, Theodoropoulos S, Yacoub MH. Location, localization and surgical treatment of cardiac pheochromocytoma. Am J Cardiol 1992;69:283–5.
9. Conti VR, Saydjari R, Ampara EG. Paraganglioma of the heart. The value of magnetic resonance imaging in the preoperative evaluation. Chest 1986;90:604–6.
10. Cruz PA, Mahidhara S, Ticzon A, Tobon H. Malignant cardiac paraganglioma: follow-up of a case [Letter]. J Thorac Cardiovasc Surg 1984;87:942–4.
11. David TE, Lenkei SC, Marquez-Julio A. Pheochromocytoma of the heart. Ann Thorac Surg 1986;41:98–100.
12. Enzinger F, Weiss SW. Paraganglioma. In: Enzinger F, Weiss SW, eds. Soft tissue tumors. St. Louis: C.V. Mosby, 1988:836–60.
13. Gopalakrishnan R, Ticzon AR, Cruz PA, et al. Cardiac paraganglioma (chemodectoma). A case report and review of the literature. J Thorac Cardiovasc Surg 1978;76:183–9.
14. Hodgson SF, Sheps SG, Subramanian R, Lie JT, Carney JA. Catecholamine-secreting paraganglioma of the interatrial septum. Am J Med 1984;77:157–61.
15. Hui G, McAllister HA, Angelini P. Left atrial paraganglioma: report of a case and review of the literature. Am Heart J 1987;113:1230–4.
16. Johnson TL, Shapiro B, Beierwalters WH, et al. Cardiac paragangliomas. A clinicopathologic and immunohistochemical study of four cases. Am J Surg Pathol 1985;11:827–34.
17. Kawasuji M, Matsunaga Y, Iwa T. Cardiac phaeochromocytoma of the interatrial septum. Eur J Cardiothorac Surg 1989;3:175–7.
18. Levi B, Cain AS, Dorzab WE. Coronary paraganglioma. Clin Cardiol 1982;5:505–10.
19. Orringer MB, Sisson JC, Glazer G, et al. Surgical treatment of cardiac pheochromocytomas. J Thorac Cardiovasc Surg 1985;89:753–7.
20. Renoult E, Danchin N, Mathieu P, et al. Intrapericardial phaeochromocytoma associated with two intercarotid paragangliomas: diagnostic considerations [Letter]. Postgrad Med J 1992;68:842–3.
21. Shapiro B, Sisson J, Kalff V, et al. The location of middle mediastinal pheochromocytomas. J Thorac Cardiovasc Surg 1984;87:814–20.

Cardiac Neurofibroma and Neurilemoma

22. Betancourt B, Defendini EA, Johnson C, et al. Severe right ventricular outflow tract obstruction caused by an intracavitary cardiac neurilemoma: successful surgical removal and postoperative diagnosis. Chest 1979;75:522–4.
23. Factor S, Turi G, Biempica L. Primary cardiac neurilemoma. Cancer 1976;37:883–90.
24. Forbes AD, Schmidt RA, Wood DE, Cochran RP, Munkenbeck F, Verrier ED. Schwannoma of the left atrium: diagnostic evaluation and surgical resection. Ann Thorac Surg 1994;57:743–6.
25. Jaffe R. Neuroma in the region of the atrioventricular node. Hum Pathol 1981;12:375–6.
26. McAllister HA, Fenoglio JJ Jr. Tumors of the cardiovascular system. Atlas of Tumor Pathology, 2nd Series, Fascicle 15. Washington D.C.: Armed Forces Institute of Pathology, 1978:70–1.

Cardiac Leiomyoma and Leiomyomatosis

27. Brandes WW, Gray JA, Macleod NW. Leiomyoma of the pericardium. Report of a case. Am Heart J 1942;23:426–32.
28. Cleveland DC, Westaby S, Karp RB. Treatment of intraatrial cardiac tumors. J Am Med Assoc 1983;249:2799–802.
29. Dunlap HJ, Udjus K. Atypical leiomyoma arising in an hepatic vein with extension into the inferior vena cava and right atrium. Report of a case in a child. Pediatr Radiol 1990;20:202–3.
30. Norris HJ, Parmley T. Mesenchymal tumors of the uterus. V. Intravenous leiomyomatosis. A clinical and pathologic study of 14 cases. Cancer 1975;36:2164–78.
31. Politzer F, Kronzon I, Wieczorek R, et al. Intracardiac leiomyomatosis: diagnosis and treatment. J Am Coll Cardiol 1984;4:629–34.

11
HETEROTOPIAS AND TUMORS
ORIGINATING FROM ECTOPIC TISSUES

BRONCHOGENIC CYST

Definition. Bronchogenic cysts are congenital endodermal rests lined by columnar or cuboidal epithelium, usually with a muscular wall. They are located in the mediastinum, neck, lung, and rarely, heart. They contain elements derived from only two germ layers, mesoderm and endoderm. Synonyms and related terms include *inclusion cyst, epithelial cyst, entodermal cyst, heterotopic cyst, gastroenterogenous cyst,* and *enteric cyst.*

Histogenesis. During embryogenesis, bronchogenic cysts arise from abnormal budding in the distal tracheobronchial tree. Resulting structures may migrate to subpleural, pericardial, myocardial, paravertebral, and cervical locations when embryologic connections with the parent bronchus are lost. The cysts are either formed from the migration of sequestered cells, or are preformed and subsequently migrate (2).

In a minority of cases, the cysts more closely resemble primitive gut than bronchus because of a lack of cartilage in the wall and a lack of mucin-producing cells. These cysts are designated *gastroenterogenous* or *enteric cysts.* In fact, it is often impossible to determine the embryologic derivation of these structures and either term is acceptable.

Incidence. Bronchogenic or enteric cysts located within the pericardium are extremely rare, and are less common than intrapericardial teratoma (1). A recent review of 26 thoracic bronchogenic cysts showed that the majority were in the mediastinum near the pericardium and none were intrapericardial; 15 patients were girls and 11 were boys, whose ages ranged from 2 months to 14 years (2). There were four cases of intracardiac cyst, which were likely bronchogenic or enteric cysts, compiled from the literature by Gould et al. in 1960 (4); three of these were located on papillary muscles and one was intramural in the left ventricle. The term epithelial cyst was used for these lesions; two other cases in this review are better classified as cystic tumors of the atrioventricular (AV) node

(see below) because of their location in the atrial septum. In 1976, a literature review found 21 cases of intrapericardial bronchogenic cyst (1). There were seven intrapericardial bronchogenic cysts reported by McAllister and Fenoglio in 1976 (6). Since then, three more have been seen at the AFIP, and there have been a few recent case reports (3,5,7,8).

Clinical Features. There is an approximate 2 to 1 female predominance for bronchogenic cysts that occur within the pericardium (1). There may be an association between intrapericardial cysts and multiple gestation (1), and between bronchogenic cysts and complex congenital heart disease (5,8). Approximately one third of patients are infants and half are over the age of 15 years at the time of presentation (1). Generally, bronchogenic cysts are located on the epicardial surface over the right side of the heart, with blood supply derived from the root of the ascending aorta (1,6). A report of a surgically excised inclusion cyst overlying the septal leaflet of the tricuspid valve in a 5 1/2-year-old boy has recently been described (5), but this may represent a cystic tumor of the AV node (see below). Bronchogenic cysts in infants often cause symptoms, whereas those in adults are generally incidental findings. The three cases in the AFIP files are from asymptomatic adults, aged 21 to 40 years.

Pathologic Findings. Intrapericardial bronchogenic cysts may be located within the myocardium projecting into one of the cardiac ventricles, or on the epicardial surface. The cysts are usually 1 to 3 cm in diameter (fig. 11-1). Microscopically, the cyst lining is ciliated columnar or cuboidal epithelium (fig. 11-2), often resembling ciliated respiratory epithelium. Occasionally, pulmonary parenchyma reminiscent of extralobar sequestration can accompany the cyst (3). Both goblet cells and squamous epithelium may be present, especially if the cyst wall is inflamed. The wall of the cyst generally contains smooth muscle that is often concentric, cartilage, and lymphoid cells; lymphoid nodules, seromucinous glands, gastric mucosa, and pancreatic

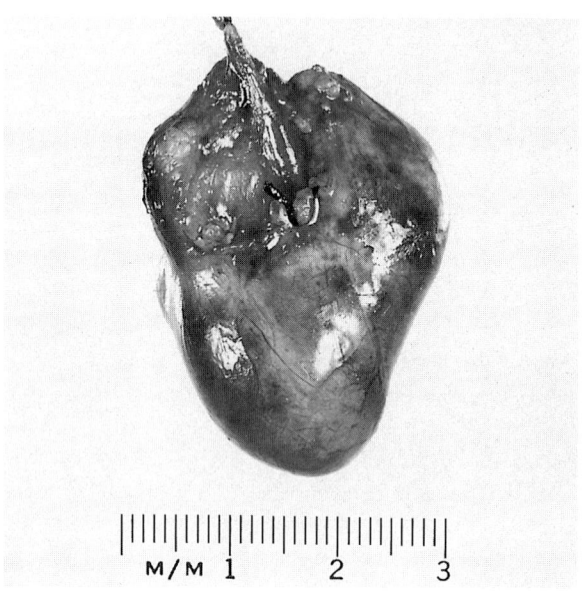

Figure 11-1
BRONCHOGENIC CYST
This example was removed from the epicardial surface of a 13-year-old.

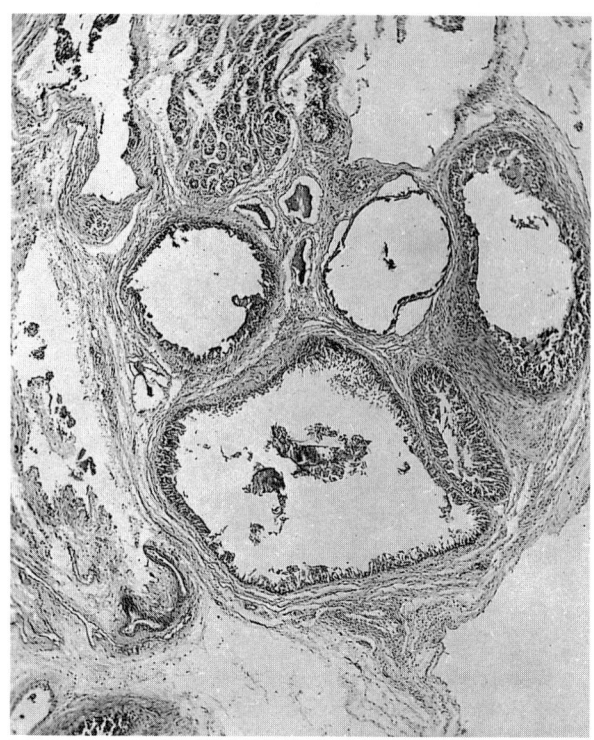

Figure 11-2
BRONCHOGENIC CYST
The lining cells are cuboidal, and the cysts are surrounded by muscle and may contain underlying seromucous glands.

tissue are variably present (1). Unlike teratomas, bronchogenic cysts lack ectodermal elements such as hair, teeth, or neural tissue.

Treatment. With current surgical techniques, bronchogenic cysts are successfully excised with little morbidity. Twenty of 25 patients whose cysts were surgically excised in the late 1960s and early 1970s survived the procedure (1).

CYSTIC TUMOR OF THE ATRIOVENTRICULAR NODE

Definition. Cystic tumor of the AV node is a benign, congenital, cystic mass located at the base of the atrial septum in the region of the AV node. Synonyms include *lymphangioma/endothelioma, mesothelioma,* and *inclusion cyst.* Unlike bronchogenic cysts, these are usually microscopic and multiple, and a muscular wall is absent.

Histogenesis. The existence and clinical significance of cystic tumors of the AV node have been known since early in this century (9). However, divergent opinions regarding the histogenesis have resulted in numerous terms for these rare tumors. The epithelial nature of the tumor is now beyond doubt, and the term "angioendothelioma" is a historic curiosity. However, there

is still disagreement as to whether these tumors are of mesothelial or endodermal origin. Strong immunohistochemical evidence suggests that they are endodermal remnants and not mesothelial rests (11,13,15,20,21); the evidence for a mesothelial origin was based on ultrastructural data that was not entirely specific (14). For these reasons, we, as well as most recent authors, have abandoned the term "mesothelioma of the AV node" and prefer the term "cystic tumor of the AV node."

Six of 66 reported cases of AV nodal tumors (11) were seen in patients with other midline defects, suggesting that these lesions represent misplaced embryologic tissue. The lesions are located in the AV nodal region because this is an area of embryologic fusion (15,17) and therefore prone to accidental incorporation of developing embryologic structures. However, the precise embryologic pathway from the primitive foregut to the atrial septum that allows for the existence of these interatrial inclusions is unknown. Travers (27) has reviewed the embryologic data

Table 11-1

REPORTED CASES OF AV NODAL TUMORS*

Years	No. Cases	Male:Female	Mean Age	Terms Used (no. cases)
1911–1970	20	4:16	38	Mesothelioma or coelothelioma (5) Foregut or endodermal inclusion (5) Squamous or epithelial cyst (4) Inclusion or heterotopia (3) Lymphangioma (3)
1970–1980	28	10:18	41	Mesothelioma (21) Heterotopia or inclusion (4) Lymphangioma (2) Endodermal rest (1)
1980–1992	19	6:13	35	Endodermal rest (15) Mesothelioma (3) Heterotopia (1)
Total	67	20:47	38	

*The data from this table are derived from reference 11, with the addition of one case (26). Another case was not included (16); we believe that tumor represents a myxoma with glandular structures.

that may explain the origin of tumors of the AV nodal region. It was argued 50 years ago that such cysts arise from sequestration or heterotopia during the period when the heart and foregut are in close approximation (24). Other authorities argue that the separation of the heart and foregut is too complete in man to allow for such a migration (23) and that a form of metaplasia of mesodermal elements results in cystic tumors of the AV node and intrapericardial bronchogenic rests.

Incidence. Cystic tumors of the AV node are rare: there have been fewer than 70 reports in the literature to date (Table 11-1), approximately twice the number of intrapericardial bronchogenic cysts. The true incidence may be greater than the literature suggests because cases may be overlooked at autopsy.

Clinical Features. The mean age at presentation is 38 years (11), and there is a female to male ratio of approximately 3 to 1. The majority of patients present with complete heart block. In the remainder, patients die suddenly without a history of heart problems, presumably as a result of ventricular arrhythmias. We recently saw an AV nodal tumor in an elderly man who died of atherosclerotic heart disease but had a recent electrocardiogram demonstrating normal sinus rhythm. We are unaware of other incidental cases of cystic AV nodal tumor.

The diagnosis of heart block in patients with AV nodal tumors may be made at birth or as late as the ninth decade of life. Because of a female predominance, it has been suggested that the diagnosis of AV nodal tumor be considered in teenage girls with complete heart block (16,25). Rarely, patients become symptomatic during pregnancy (19). The clinical differential diagnosis of congenital heart block includes maternal lupus erythematosus, which can result in intrauterine destruction of nodal pathways, presumably by an autoimmune mechanism (26).

Most cystic tumors of the AV node are first diagnosed at autopsy. There has been a report of a successfully resected tumor of the AV node (10) which was visualized initially by coronary angiography, and we recently diagnosed a surgically resectable tumor in a patient with complete heart block. With increased use of transesophageal echocardiography and new high-resolution imaging techniques, including MRI, we anticipate further reports of antemortem diagnosis of AV nodal tumors in individuals with congenital heart block.

The majority of tumors of the AV node are sporadic. However, they can occur in patients with coexisting cysts in the ovaries and breasts (18), ventricular septal defect (11,18), nasal septal defect (12), encephalocele (12), thinning of the corpus

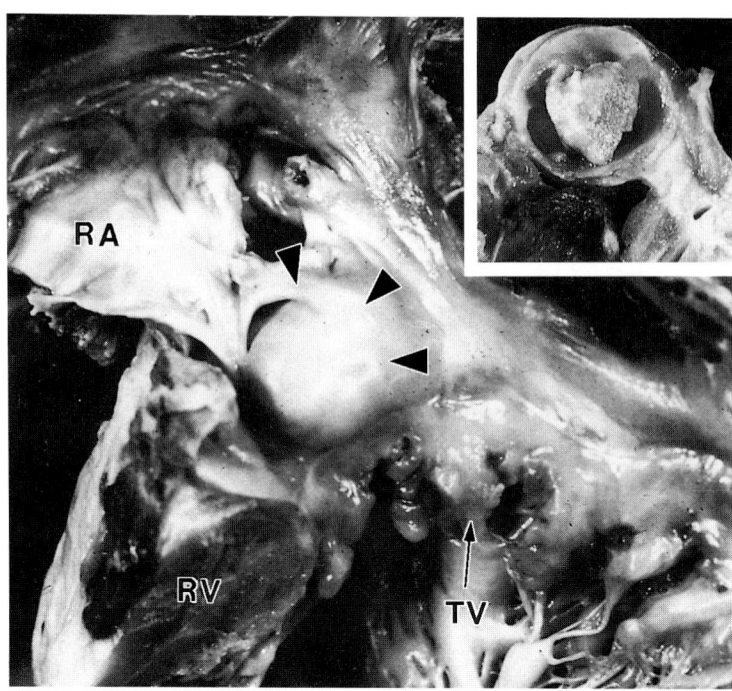

Figure 11-3
CYSTIC TUMOR OF
ATRIOVENTRICULAR NODE
The tumor is outlined by arrows. RA = right atrium; RV = right ventricle; TV = tricuspid valve. (Courtesy of Dr. Peter Anderson, Birmingham, AL.)

callosum (22), and absent septum pellucidum (22). In addition, we have seen an example in a patient with a thyroglossal duct cyst. There was a familial history of sudden unexplained death in one case in our series, as well as two reports in the literature (27), but no relative had a histologically documented AV tumor.

Pathologic Findings. These tumors are located, by definition, in the region of the AV node. Grossly, they appear as a cyst-like structure (fig. 11-3) or as an area of thickening with small, fluid-filled cysts that are barely perceptible to the naked eye. They range in size from 2 to 20 mm. Often the cysts are first recognized at the time of microscopic examination of the conduction system. In the most recent 10 cases from the AFIP files, the heart was grossly normal in 6 cases, irregular cysts were seen in the area of the AV node in 2 cases, a 3-cm cyst was noted in 1 case, and slight thickening was noted in the AV nodal area in 1 case. Microscopically, the tumor is located in the inferior interatrial septum in the region of the AV node, and respects the boundary of the central fibrous body without extending into ventricular myocardium or into valvular tissues (fig. 11-4). Nests of cells often form cysts of various sizes (figs. 11-5, 11-6): these nests can replace

myofibers within the inferior interatrial septum (fig. 11-7), and are composed of cuboidal, transitional (fig. 11-8), or squamous cells (fig. 11-9). Sebaceous cells may be interspersed among cuboidal cells, forming a two-cell population (fig. 11-10). The cysts often form two cell layers: a luminal, cuboidal, single cell layer overlying transitional cells (fig. 11-11). The epithelium can flatten and cysts can assume tortuous shapes (fig. 11-12), which may explain why early observers mistook them for endothelial cells. The lumens of the cysts contain PAS-positive, diastase-resistant material which occasionally calcifies. Often, there is dense fibrosis surrounding the cysts or cell nests, with a lymphocytic reaction. Cilia are sometimes visible on light microscopy. Endocrine granules have been reported in the epithelial cells of tumors of the AV nodal region, but we have not been able to detect these by silver stains or immunohistochemical techniques.

Immunohistochemical and Ultrastructural Findings. The immunohistochemical profile of the lining cells indicate an epithelial origin because they strongly express cytokeratin and epithelial membrane antigen. Immunohistochemical markers to distinguish mesothelial from endodermal tissues favor an endodermal

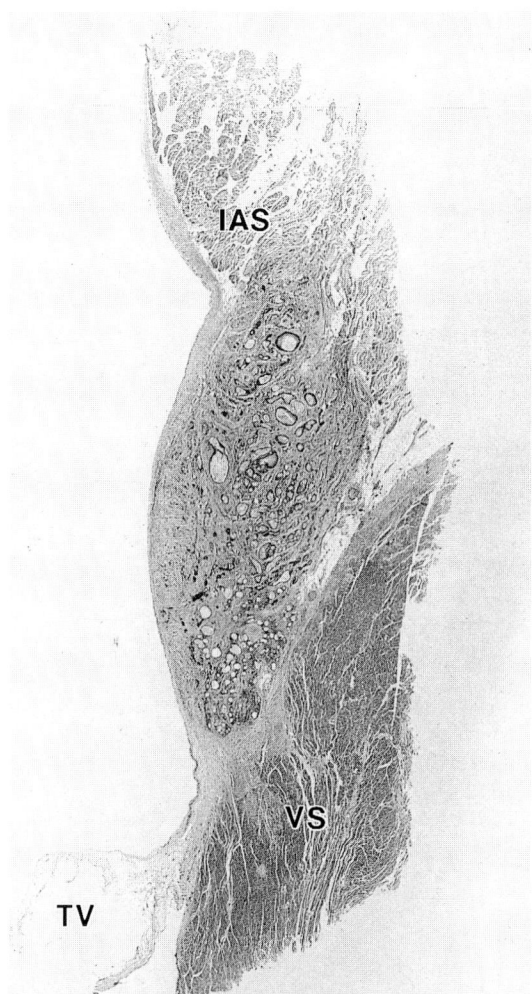

Figure 11-4
CYSTIC TUMOR OF ATRIOVENTRICULAR NODE

The cysts are located in the inferior portion of the interatrial septum and do not extend into the interventricular septum or tricuspid valve. IAS = interatrial septum; TV = tricuspid valve; VS = ventricular septum. (Courtesy of Dr. Peter Anderson, Birmingham, AL.)

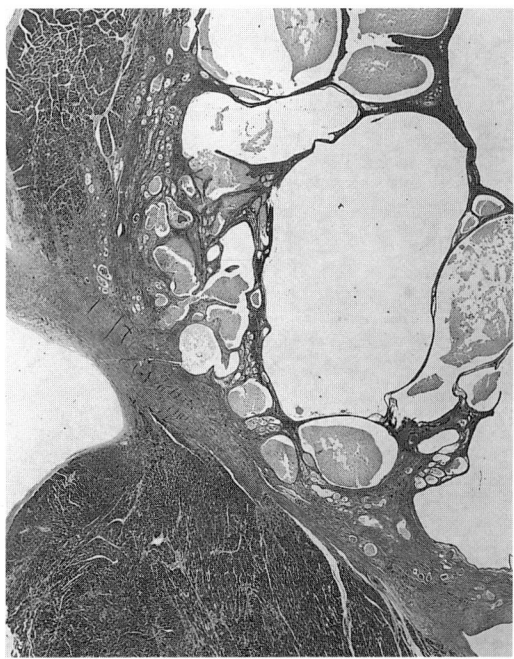

Figure 11-5
CYSTIC TUMOR OF THE ATRIOVENTRICULAR NODE

Some of the cysts become large and are filled with proteinaceous debris.

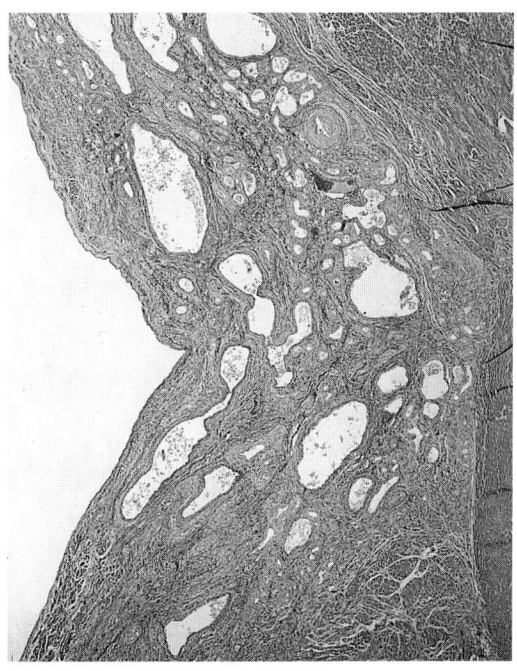

Figure 11-6
CYSTIC TUMOR OF THE ATRIOVENTRICULAR NODE

Cysts are not always visible to the naked eye. Many tumors are first discovered on microscopic examination of the conduction system.

derivation for these cells. Most cases are strongly positive for carcinoembryonic antigen (fig. 11-13) as well as B72.3 antigen (fig. 11-14) (11,13, 19,21). Both of these antigens are commonly found in embryonic or neoplastic glandular epithelium, and are generally absent in mesothelial cells. As indicated above, there has been a report of endocrine cells interspersed among the lining cells of tumors of the AV node (15). These cells stain for calcitonin and serotonin. The presence of endocrine cells in these lesions further supports an endodermal, rather than mesothelial, origin.

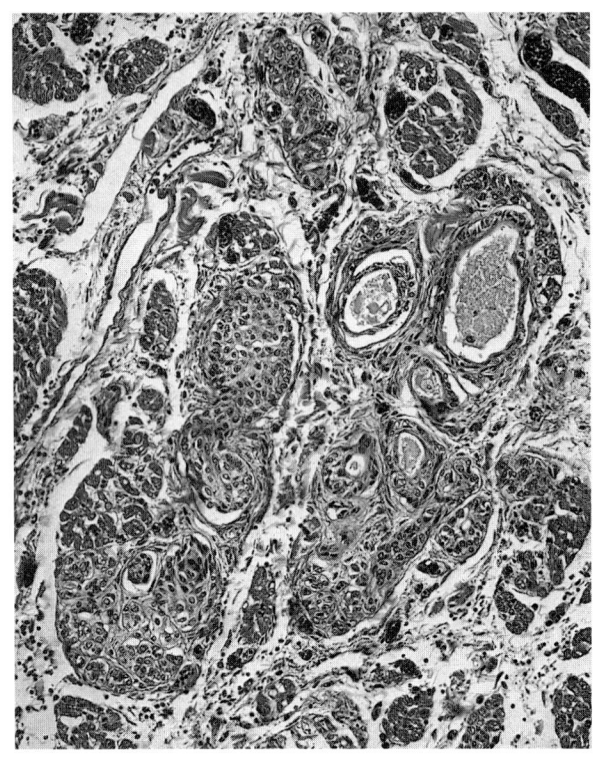

Figure 11-7
CYSTIC TUMOR OF THE
ATRIOVENTRICULAR NODE

Tumor nests and cysts often replace muscle bundles in the inferior portion of the interatrial septum.

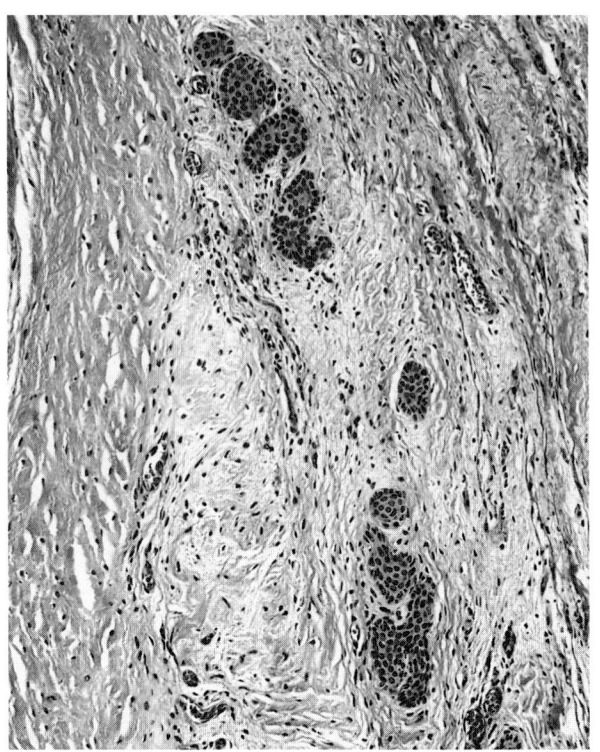

Figure 11-8
CYSTIC TUMOR OF THE
ATRIOVENTRICULAR NODE

Not all of the cell nests form cysts; in this example, they resemble transitional cells.

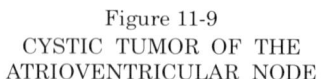

Figure 11-9
CYSTIC TUMOR OF THE
ATRIOVENTRICULAR NODE

Higher magnification of tumor shown in figure 11-5 demonstrating squamous differentiation and calcification of luminal debris.

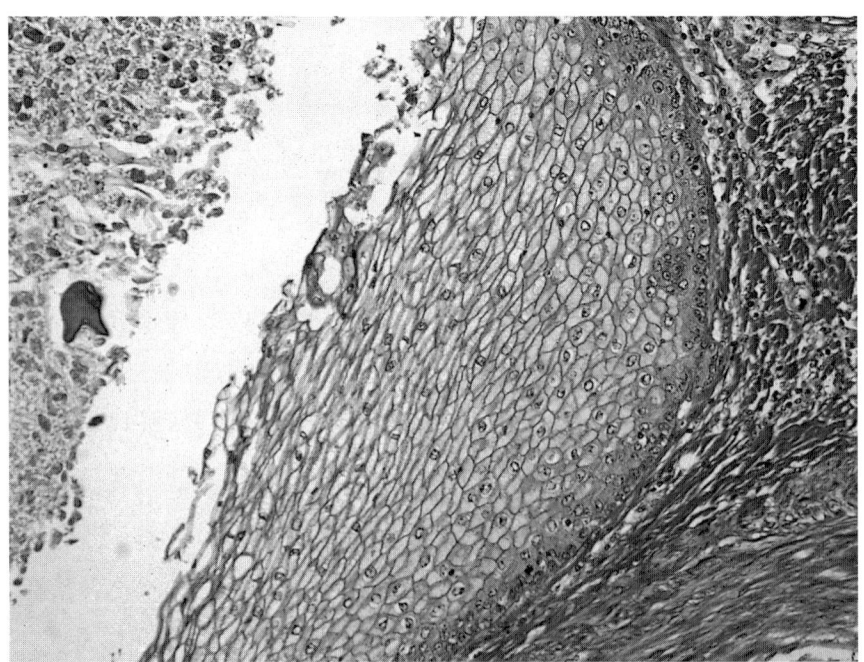

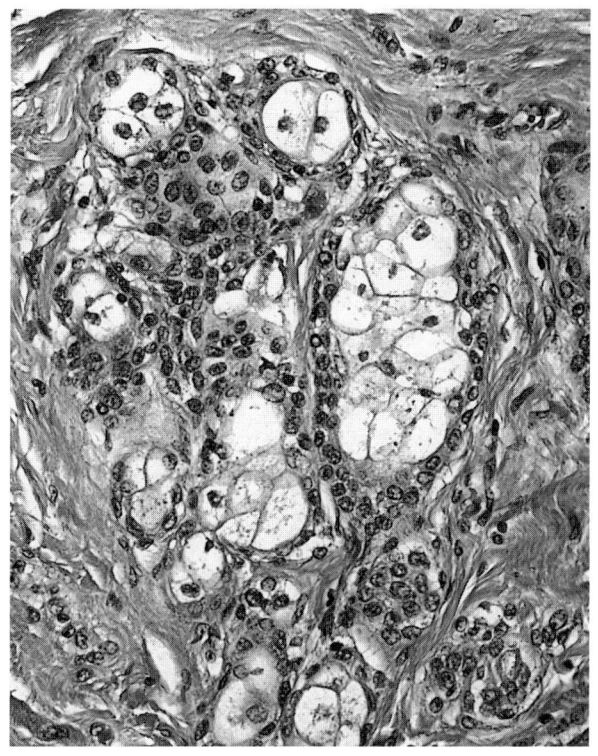

Figure 11-10
CYSTIC TUMOR OF THE
ATRIOVENTRICULAR NODE
Higher magnification of tumor shown in figure 11-5
demonstrates a two-cell population, composed of clear, seba-
ceous-appearing cells and cuboidal cells.

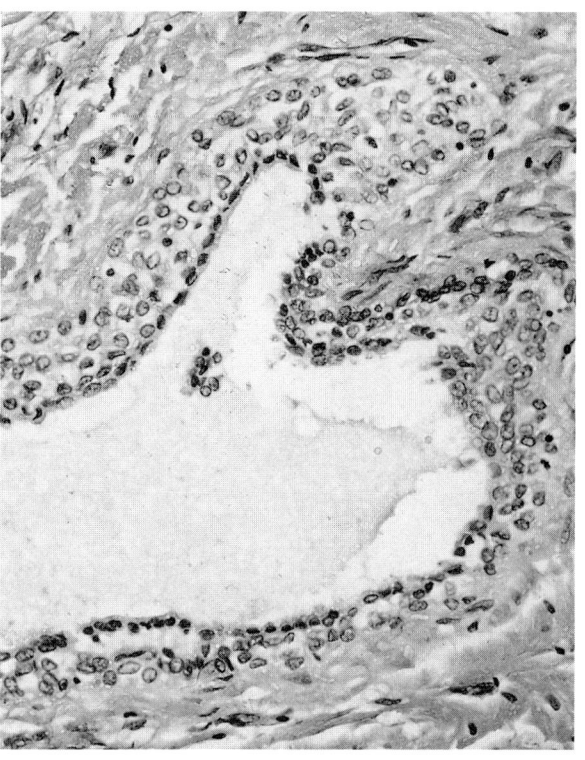

Figure 11-11
CYSTIC TUMOR OF THE
ATRIOVENTRICULAR NODE
The cyst lining can form a two-cell layer, the innermost lining
composed of a single layer of smaller cuboidal cells.

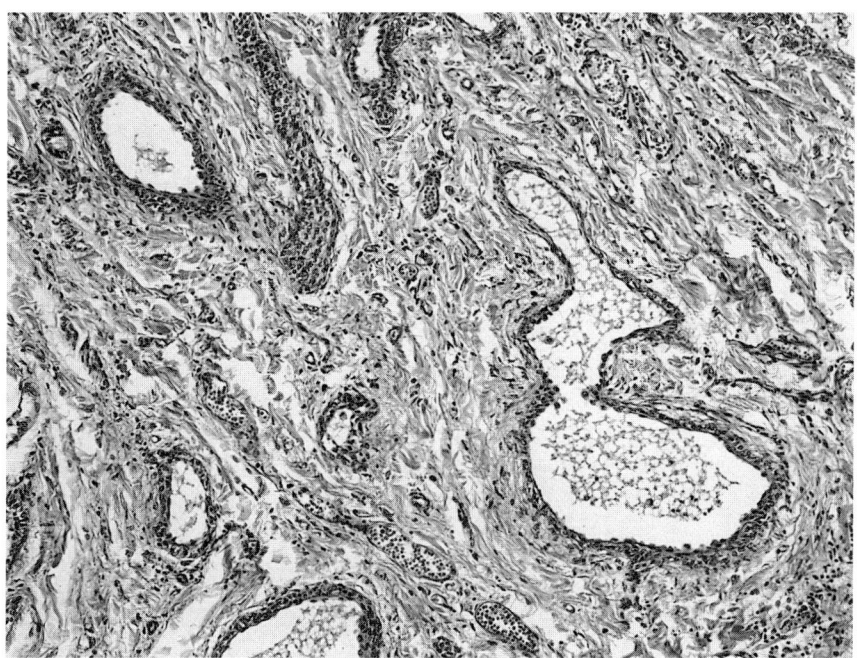

Figure 11-12
CYSTIC TUMOR OF THE
ATRIOVENTRICULAR NODE
The cysts can assume irregular
shapes and be surrounded by a fi-
brous reaction.

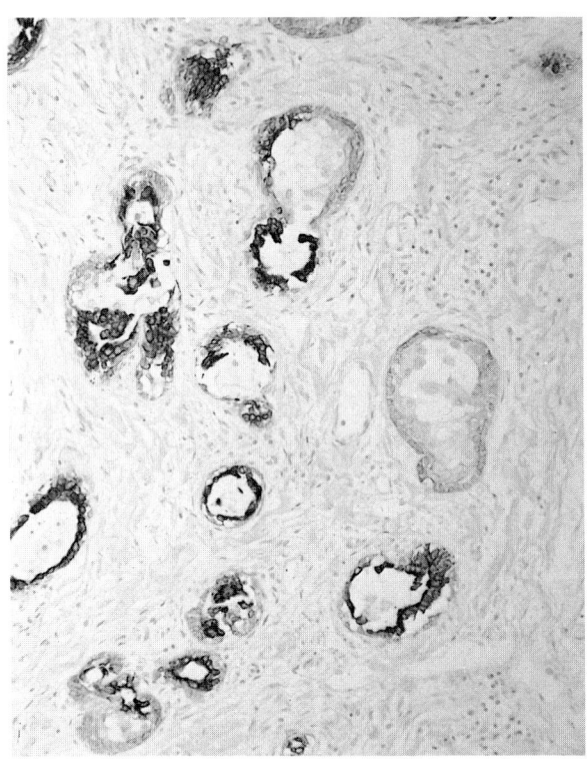

Figure 11-13
CYSTIC TUMOR OF THE ATRIOVENTRICULAR NODE
This tumor was positive for carcinoembryonic antigen. (Fig. 2 from Burke AP, Anderson PG, Virmani R, James TN, Herrera GA, Ceballos R. Tumors of the atrioventricular node. Arch Pathol Lab Med 1990;114:1057–62.)

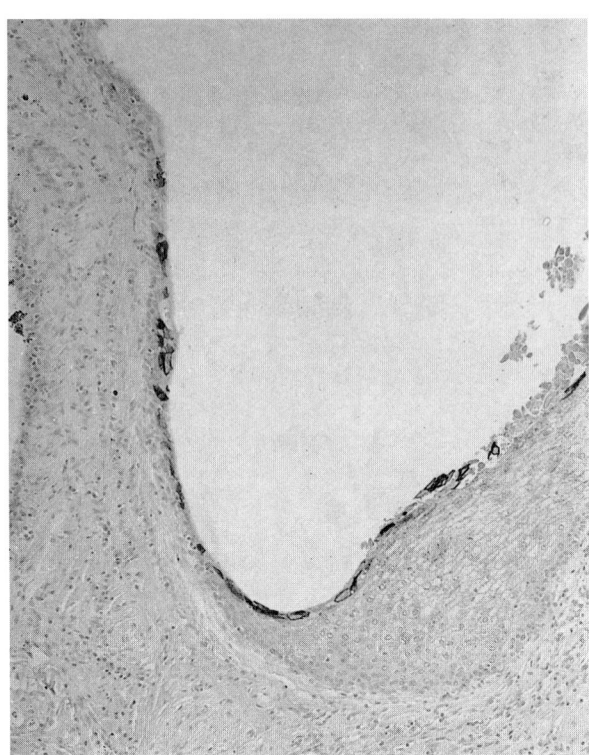

Figure 11-14
CYSTIC TUMOR OF THE ATRIOVENTRICULAR NODE
Immunohistochemical stain of tumor shown in figure 11-4 demonstrating positivity for B72.3 antigen. (Fig. 3 from Burke AP, Anderson PG, Virmani R, James TN, Herrera GA, Ceballos R. Tumors of the atrioventricular node. Arch Pathol Lab Med 1990;114:1057–62.)

The ultrastructural appearance of tumors of the AV node has been described as typical of mesothelioma (14). This conclusion has been based on limited material. In our experience, long microvilli characteristic of mesotheliomas are absent and the ultrastructural appearance is nonspecific and compatible with epithelial rests. Two cell types are identified: in one, the cells form solid nests, have a well-formed basement membrane, possess cytoplasmic tonofilaments, and are joined by desmosomes; in the other, the cells are also connected by desmosomes, and form glands. These often contain electron-dense material and have short microvilli (fig. 11-15), which have erroneously been described as indicative of mesothelial differentiation.

Differential Diagnosis. There are few entities in the pathologic differential diagnosis of cystic tumor of the AV node. Bronchogenic cysts are larger, usually single cysts, that tend to occur

on the epicardial surface, remote from the atrial septum. Teratomas may occur in a similar location, but are easily distinguished by the presence of neural and other ectodermal structures. Mesothelial cysts are generally larger and unilocular, and occur on the surface of the heart. An early example of an AV nodal tumor, originally misdiagnosed as metastatic clear cell carcinoma, was subsequently reported as a cystic tumor of the AV node (17). Unlike metastatic carcinoma, cystic tumors of the AV node lack mitotic figures and cellular pleomorphism. One AV nodal tumor reported as an "intracardiac endodermal heterotopia" appears to represent a myxoma with glandular structures (16). Although the cysts of AV nodal tumors may occasionally contain mucin, the myxoid background and extensive intracavitary growth characteristic of myxoma are absent. The tumors can be overlooked on gross

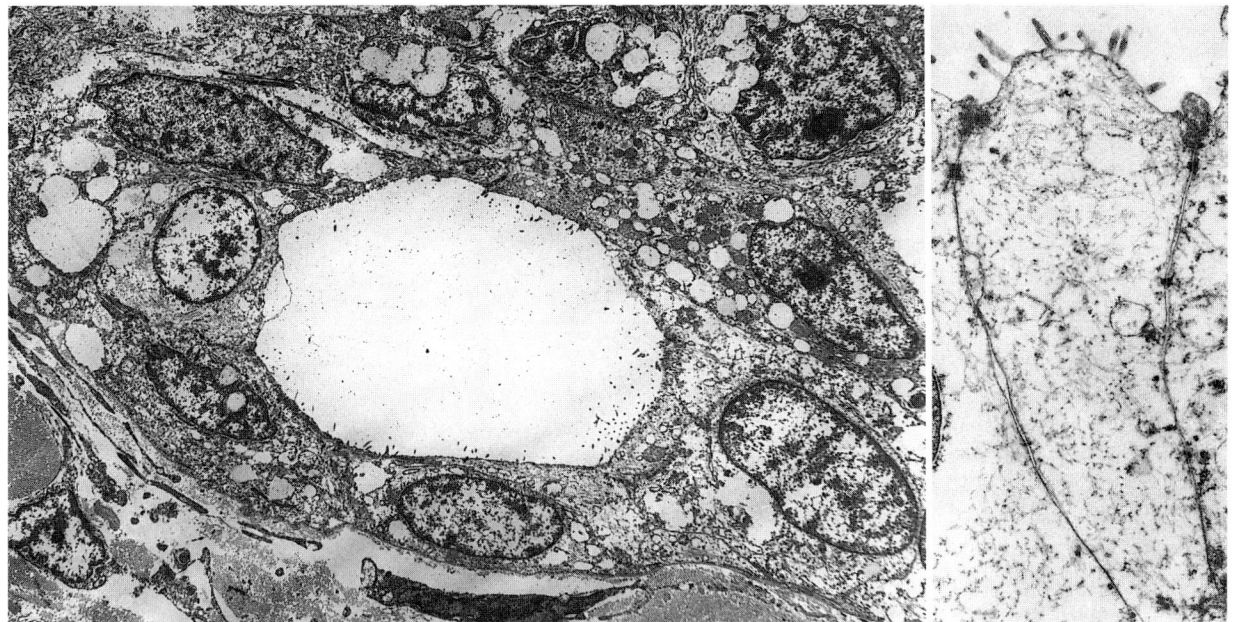

Figure 11-15
CYSTIC TUMOR OF THE ATRIOVENTRICULAR NODE
Electron micrograph demonstrates short microvilli. (X1000; insert X6000) (Fig. 4 from Burke AP, Anderson PG, Virmani R, James TN, Herrera GA, Ceballos R. Tumors of the atrioventricular node. Arch Pathol Lab Med 1990;114:1057–62.)

inspection, necessitating histologic examination of the conduction system in all cases of sudden death, especially for those with a history of arrhythmia or heart block.

Treatment. The treatment of congenital heart block consists of pacemaker implantation for treatment of Stokes-Adams attacks (25) and antiarrhythmic drugs to suppress ventricular tachycardias. Treatment with pacemakers does not always prevent terminal arrhythmias in patients with AV nodal tumors, however. It has even been suggested that electrical pacing can precipitate arrhythmias in these patients (17). As has been mentioned, there is a single report of successful surgical removal of one of these tumors (10). The degree of persistent damage to the conduction system related to surgical removal remains to be determined.

CARDIAC GERM CELL TUMORS (TERATOMAS)

Definition. A germ cell tumor is a neoplasm of germ cell origin that is classified by histologic type into seminoma (dysgerminoma), embryonal carcinoma, yolk sac tumor (endodermal sinus tumor), choriocarcinoma, and teratoma. The majority of cardiac germ cell tumors are teratomas, which contain endodermal, mesodermal, and ectodermal elements. Most reports of intrapericardial teratoma describe the presence of only one or two germ cell layers, and are therefore possibly bronchogenic cysts. Synonyms and related terms for teratoma include *intrapericardial teratoma, pericardial teratoma,* and *intrapericardial dermoid cyst.*

Histogenesis. According to the germ cell theory, the cell of origin of extragonadal teratoma, including cardiac teratoma, is the primordial germ cell. Although normal germ cells migrate from the yolk sac to the gonad, it is hypothesized that they may lodge, early in embryogenesis, in midline structures such as the mediastinum and central nervous system. These ectopic germ cells may give rise to germ cell tumors indistinguishable from those that occur in the testes and ovaries. For a further discussion of the histogenesis of these tumors, the reader is referred to a discussion of the subject by Gonzalez-Crussi (33).

Incidence. The first reported case of intrapericardial teratoma was in 1890 (30). In 1983, 57 cases were compiled in a review of the literature (30), 10 of which involved the myocardium. By 1993, at least 5 more cases had appeared in the literature (28–37).

Clinical Features. In McAllister and Fenoglio's series of 14 patients with intrapericardial teratoma, the patients' ages ranged from 1 day to 42 years (34). The majority of patients are infants (31); over 75 percent of cardiac teratomas occur in children under age 15. Two thirds of patients are female (31,34). Patients present with respiratory distress, pericardial tamponade, and cyanosis; cardiac murmurs are rarely heard. In adults, pericardial teratoma is usually discovered as an incidental radiographic finding, although chest pain and friction rubs from rapidly growing tumors or from hemorrhage within the tumor (32) have been reported. Pericardial effusion is usually present and is serous, yellow, and clear.

Only five entirely intramyocardial teratomas have been reported (36), and there is one recent case in the AFIP files; these have all occurred in newborns or during the first 6 years of life. Most patients are symptomatic and present with congestive heart failure; rarely, a patient is asymptomatic. Sudden death may be the first symptom, due to acute arrhythmia caused from the tumor's interventricular location (36).

With the advent of fetal echocardiography, an increasing number of cardiac tumors, including rhabdomyomas and teratomas, are being diagnosed in second and third trimester fetuses (29). To date, five cases of cardiac teratoma have been positively identified before birth (36). Of these, two patients died at birth from cardiac tamponade and cardiac compression (29). The three live-born infants underwent successful surgery in the neonatal period. Pericardial effusion is not uncommon in a fetus with intrapericardial teratoma, and cardiac tamponade is a common cause of fetal death; however, intrauterine pericardiocentesis has been successful in averting fetal death (29).

Pathologic Findings. Intrapericardial teratomas may be massive, measuring up to 15 cm, especially in adults (32). They have a smooth surface and are lobulated. On cut surface, the tumor is multicystic with intervening solid areas. The tumors usually displace the heart and rotate it along its longitudinal axis. Intrapericardial teratomas are usually located on the right side of the heart (fig. 11-16), displacing the organs to the left and posteriorly; those located on the left side produce the opposite effect. Teratomas are usually attached by a pedicle to one of the great vessels, with arterial supply directly from the aorta.

Intracardiac teratomas are almost always located in the interventricular septum and extend into the right ventricle; however, they occasionally bulge into the left ventricular cavity. Intracardiac teratomas are multicystic with interspersed solid areas. The size of these tumors ranges from 2 to 15 cm.

Grossly and microscopically, teratomas of the heart are similar to extrapericardial teratomas. In addition to squamous or mucous-lined cysts, there may be cartilage, calcified neuroglial tissue, smooth muscle, mucous glands, intestine, pancreas, respiratory mucosa, ependyma, and bone. A myxoid stroma is often present. The major entity in the differential diagnosis is bronchogenic cyst; the presence of elements of ectodermal origin, such as hair, teeth, or neurogenic elements, favor the diagnosis of teratoma (figs. 11-17, 11-18).

Pure cardiac teratomas are benign lesions. When other germ cell tumor elements are present, the tumor is malignant. McAllister and Fenoglio (34) reported four malignant pericardial germ cell tumors; the malignant foci were histologically composed of either embryonal carcinoma, squamous cell carcinoma arising in a teratoma, or choriocarcinoma. Three of these tumors metastasized to the lungs, and one was locally infiltrative. We recently saw a malignant germ cell tumor of the heart with large areas of yolk sac tumor (infantile embryonal carcinoma, endodermal sinus tumor) (figs. 11-19, 11-20).

Treatment. Surgical excision is the only effective treatment for cardiac teratoma. Since the blood supply is usually from the root of the ascending aorta, the surgeon must perform a careful dissection and ligation of these vessels to prevent massive hemorrhage. Intracardiac teratomas, because of their location in the interventricular septum, are more difficult to remove than pericardial teratomas. However, even incomplete excision has been shown to be beneficial (32).

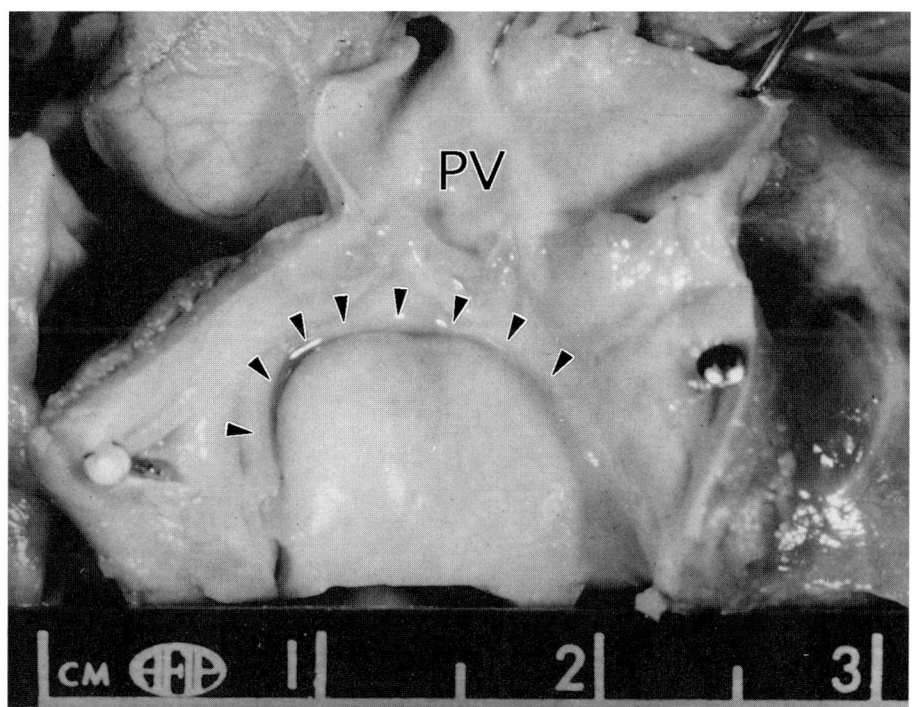

Figure 11-16
TERATOMA
Patient was a newborn child born at 37 weeks gestation who died minutes after birth. Note the bulging mass in the right ventricular outflow tract (arrowheads). PV = pulmonary valve.

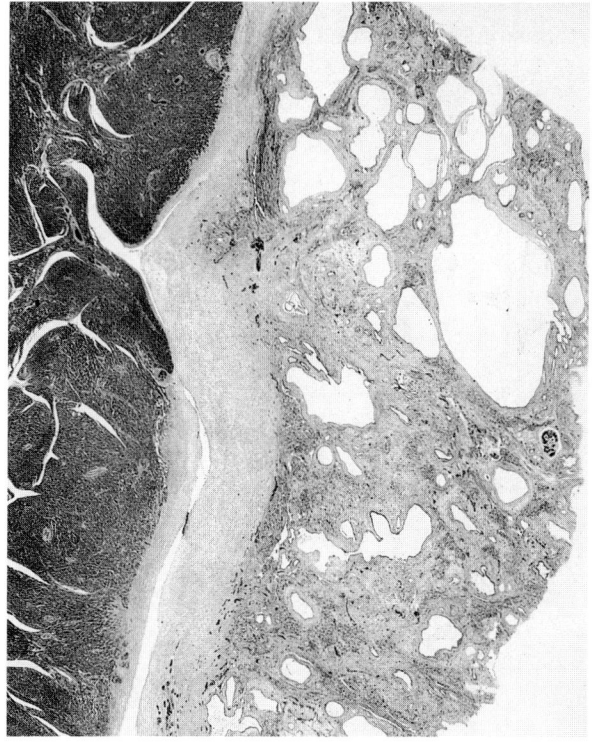

Figure 11-17
TERATOMA
A histologic section of the case shown in figure 11-16 shows cysts on the endocardial surface. (Masson trichrome stain)

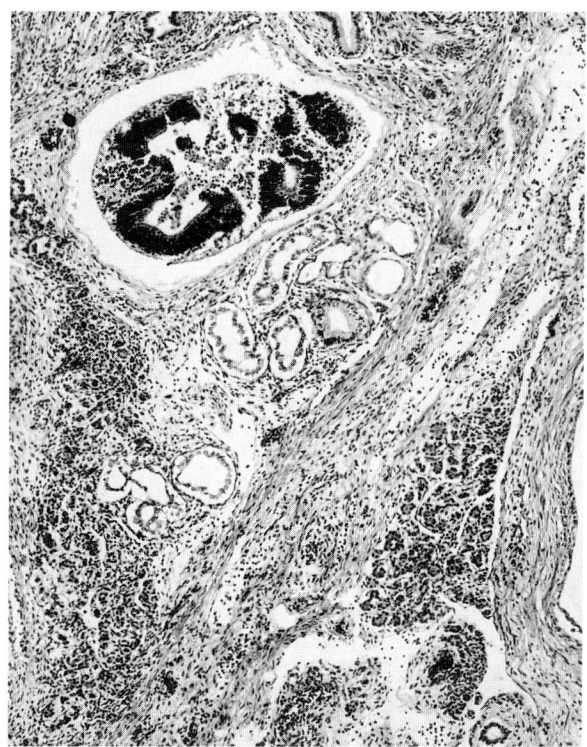

Figure 11-18
TERATOMA
A higher magnification of figure 11-17 demonstrates neural, glandular, and stromal structures.

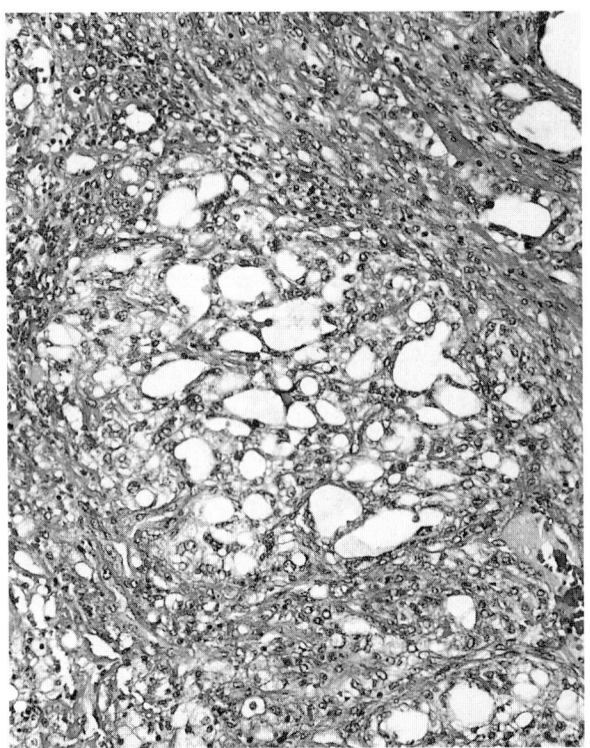

Figure 11-19
YOLK SAC (ENDODERMAL SINUS) TUMOR

The patient was a 14-month-old girl with a clinical diagnosis of atrial septal defect. Echocardiography demonstrated a pericardial mass attached to the ascending aorta. Histologically, there are irregular spaces of various sizes in the center of the tumor.

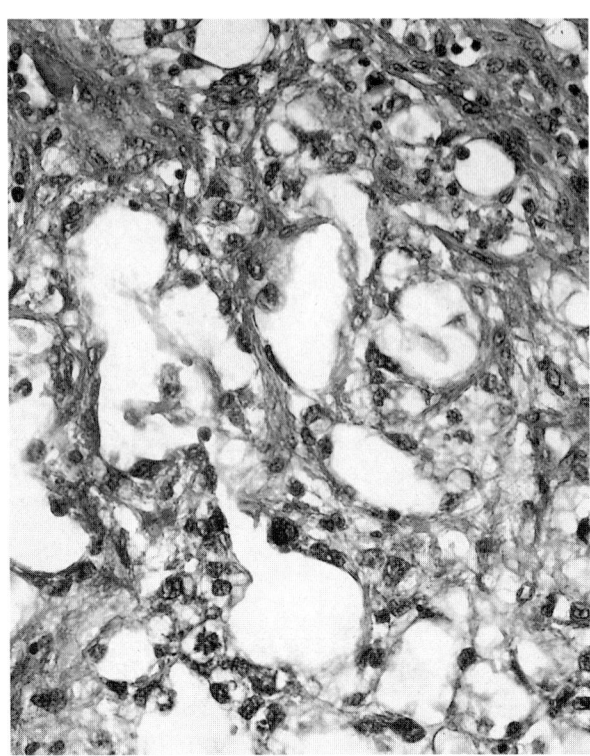

Figure 11-20
YOLK SAC TUMOR

Higher magnification of tumor in figure 11-19 demonstrates irregular spaces lined by flattened cells that were positive for alpha-fetoprotein by immunohistochemistry (not shown).

THYROID HETEROTOPIA

Heterotopic thyroid tissue may be incidentally discovered in the parietal pericardium (39). Ectopic thyroid tissue is usually found between the base of the tongue and the normal thyroid gland, and is a result of a migration failure along the pathway of the thyroglossal duct. The mechanism for thyroid tissue migration inferior to the thyroid gland is less clear, but may be a result of excessive migration in combination with traction of hyperplastic tissues (43). Ectopic thyroid tissue in the heart may be the consequence of the intimate relationship between the cephalic portion of the developing foregut, which contains the thyroid anlage in the foramen cecum of the tongue, and the cardiac primordia (see chapter 1).

Intracardiac thyroid is extremely rare, and is synonymously referred to as *struma cordis*. Approximately 12 cases of intracardiac ectopic thyroid, nearly all in the right ventricular outflow area, have been published in the English language literature (37,38,40–42).

Prior to the development of noninvasive technologies, cases of heterotopic cardiac thyroid tissue were discovered only at autopsy. Echocardiography has allowed antemortem diagnosis (38,41,42,44). In a middle-aged woman, a right ventricular mass, which may be obstructing the outflow tract causing a systolic murmur and right ventricular hypertrophy, should alert the clinician to the possibility of ectopic intracardiac thyroid tissue; a preoperative thyroid scan may be useful in such a patient. The clinical differential diagnosis includes metastatic disease since the right ventricular outflow tract may be a site of metastasis (see chapter 15), including metastasis from thyroid carcinoma.

Surgical removal is curative. Thyroid hormone replacement should be initiated prior to

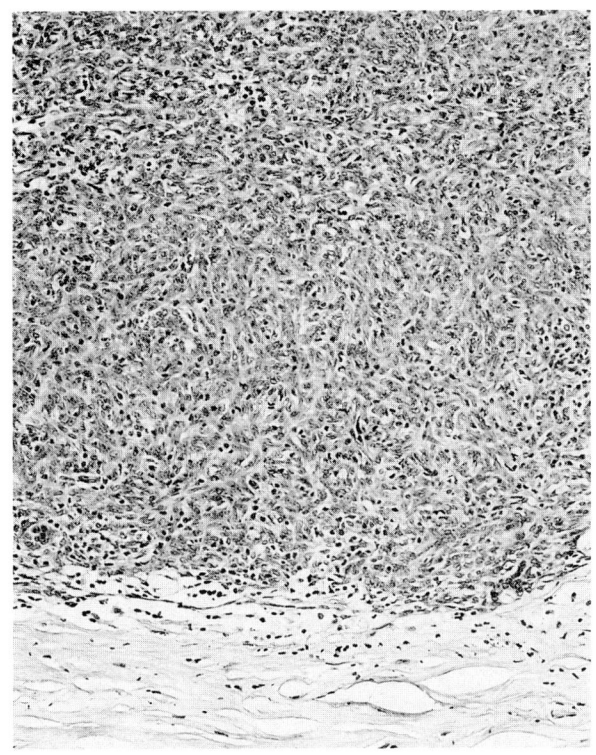

Figure 11-21
THYMOMA
The patient was a 40-year-old man with an incidental pericardial nodule found at autopsy. There is a proliferation of spindled cells with a sparse inflammatory background.

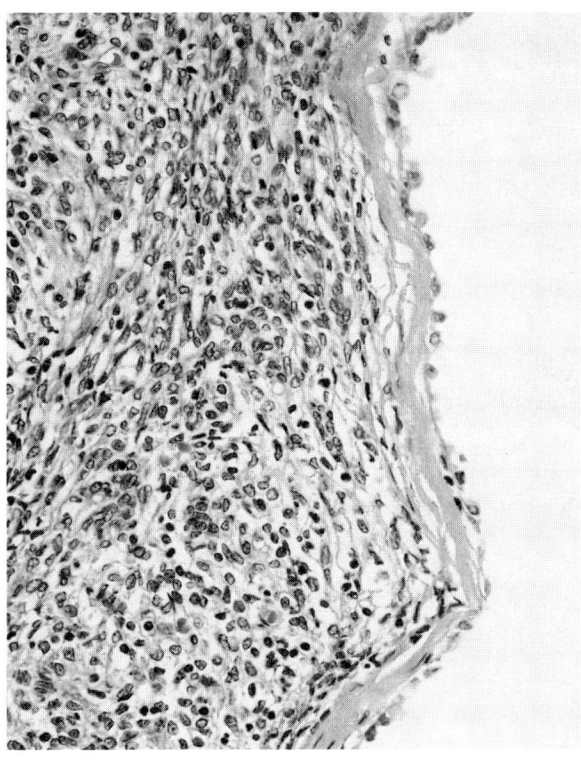

Figure 11-22
THYMOMA
A higher magnification of figure 11-21 shows tumor near the mesothelial layer. There was diffuse positivity for cytokeratin (not shown).

surgery, because the ectopic tissue may be the only functioning thyroid tissue (37).

PERICARDIAL THYMOMA

Thymomas involving the heart are usually extensions of primary mediastinal tumors. Approximately 20 percent of thymomas are locally infiltrative (50), and pericardial involvement represents a late stage of tumor spread (see chapter 15) (48). Compression of the pulmonary trunk may occur (49) in addition to pericardial infiltration. Occasionally, mediastinal thymomas present as pericardial effusions, and the diagnosis is made by examination of pericardial fluid or by pericardial biopsy (50).

Rarely, thymomas may be entirely intrapericardial; these tumors are believed to derive from pericardial thymic rests (figs. 11-21, 11-22) (47). Patients are often women (45–47). Pericardial effusions lead to symptoms of dyspnea or chest pain, and diagnosis is made by biopsy or fine-needle aspiration (45). The tumor may be an incidental autopsy finding (figs. 11-21, 11-22). Treatment is generally surgical, although chemotherapy may result in tumor regression in inoperable cases (46).

Histologically, intrapericardial thymomas have not been extensively described (45–47). They are generally epithelial, with a background of lymphoid cells.

REFERENCES

Bronchogenic Cyst

1. Deenadayalu RP, Tuuri D, Dewell RA, Johnson GF. Intrapericardial teratomas and bronchogenic cyst. Review of literature and report of successful surgery in infant with intrapericardial teratoma. J Thorac Cardiovasc Surg 1974;67:945–52.
2. DiLorenzo M, Collin PP, Vaillancourt R, Duranceau A. Bronchogenic cysts. J Pediatr Surg 1989; 24:988–91.
3. Hayashi AH, McLean DR, Peliowski A, Tierney AJ, Finer NN. A rare intrapericardial mass in a neonate. J Pediatr Surg 1992;27:1361–3.
4. Gould SE. Cysts of the myocardium and heart valves and diverticula. In: Gould SE, Thomas CC, eds. Pathology of the heart. Springfield, Illinois: Charles C. Thomas, 1960:883–6.
5. Machens G, Vahl CF, Hofmann R, Wolf D, Hagl S. Entodermal inclusion cyst of the tricuspid valve. Thorac Cardiovasc Surg 1991;39:296–8.
6. McAllister HA, Fenoglio JJ Jr. Tumors of the cardiovascular system. Atlas of Tumor Pathology, 2nd Series, Fascicle 15, Washington D.C.: Armed Forces Institute of Pathology, 1978:62–3.
7. Shimizu M, Takeda R, Mifune J, Tanaka T. Echocardiographic features of intrapericardial bronchogenic cyst. Cardiology 1990;77:322–6.
8. Thomas R, Van Wesep R. Intracardiac epithelial cyst in association with an atrioventricular canal defect. Am J Cardiovasc Pathol 1990;3:325–8.

AV Nodal Tumor

9. Armstrong H, Monckeberg JG. Herzblock bedingt durch primaren Herztumor, bei einem 5-jahrigen Kinde. Deutsch Arch Klin Med 1911;102:144–56.
10. Balasundaram S, Halees SA, Duran C. Mesothelioma of the atrioventricular node: first successful follow-up after excision. Eur Heart J 1992;13:718–9.
11. Burke AP, Anderson PG, Virmani R, James TN, Herrera GA, Ceballos R. Tumors of the atrioventricular nodal region. A clinical and immunohistochemical study. Arch Pathol Lab Med 1990;114:1057–62.
12. de Chatel A. Kongenitale epidermoid-cyste des Herzens. Frankfurt Z Ath 1933;44:426–34.
13. Duray PH, Mark EJ, Barwick KW, Madri JA, Strom RL. Congenital polycystic tumor of the atrioventricular node. Arch Pathol Lab Med 1985;109:30–4.
14. Fenoglio JJ Jr, Jacobs DW, McAllister HA Jr. Ultrastructure of the mesothelioma of the atrioventricular node. Cancer 1977;40:721–7.
15. Fine G, Raju U. Congenital polycystic tumor of the atrioventricular node (endodermal heterotopia, mesothelioma): a histogenetic appraisal with evidence for its endodermal origin. Human Pathol 1987;18:791–5.
16. Honey M, Axelrad MA. Intracardiac endodermal heterotopia. Brit Heart J 1962;24:667–70.
17. James TN, Galakhov I. De subitaneius mortibus. XXVI. Fatal electrical instability of the heart associated with benign congenital polycystic tumor of the atrioventricular node. Circulation 1977;56:667–78.
18. Leighton J, Hurst JW, Crawford JD. Squamous epithelial cysts in the heart of an infant, with coincident cystic changes in the ovaries and breasts. Arch Pathol 1950;50:632–43.
19. Lewman LV, Demany MA, Zimmerman HA. Congenital tumor of atrioventricular node with complete heart block and sudden death. Mesothelioma or lymphangio-endothelioma of atrioventricular node. Am J Cardiol 1972;29:554–7.
20. Linder J, Shelburne JD, Sorge JP, Whalen RE, Hackel DB. Congenital endodermal heterotopia of the atrioventricular node: evidence for the endodermal origin of so-called mesotheliomas of the atrioventricular node. Hum Pathol 1984;15:1093–7.
21. Monma N, Satodate R, Tashiro A, Segawa I. Origin of so-called mesothelioma of the atrioventricular node. An immunohistochemical study. Arch Pathol Lab Med 1991;115:1026–9.
22. Morris AW, Johnson IM. Epithelial inclusion cysts of the heart. Arch Pathol 1964;77:36–40.
23. Prichard RW. Tumors of the heart. Arch Pathol 1951;51:98–128.
24. Sachs LJ, Angrist A. Congenital cyst of the myocardium. Am J Pathol 1945;21:187–93.
25. Scully RE, Mark EJ, McNeely BU. Case records of the Massachusetts General Hospital (#1-1982). N Engl J Med 1982;306:32–9.
26. Subramanian R, Flygenring B. Mesothelioma of the atrioventricular node and congenital complete heart block. Clin Cardiol 1989;12:469–72.
27. Travers H. Congenital polycystic tumor of the atrioventricular node: possible familial occurrence and critical review of reported cases with special emphasis on histogenesis. Hum Pathol 1982;13:25–35.

Cardiac Teratoma

28. Arciniegas E, Hakimi M, Farooki ZQ, Green EW. Intrapericardial teratoma in infancy. J Thorac Cardiovasc Surg 1980;79:306–11.
29. Benatar A, Vaughan J, Nicolini U, Trotter S, Corrin B, Lincoln C. Prenatal pericardiocentesis: its role in the management of intrapericardial teratoma. Obst Gynecol 1992;79:856–9.
30. Cox JN, Friedli B, Mechmeche R, Ben Ismail M, Oberhaensli I, Faidutti B. Teratoma of the heart. A case report and review of the literature. Virchows Arch [A] 1983;402:163–74.
31. Deenadayalu RP, Tuuri D, Dewell RA, Johnson GF. Intrapericardial teratomas and bronchogenic cyst. Review of literature and report of successful surgery in infant with intrapericardial teratoma. J Thorac Cardiovasc Surg 1974;67:945–52.
32. Garcia Cors M, Mulet J, Caralps J, Oller G. Fast-growing pericardial mass as first manifestation of intrapericardial teratoma in a young man [Letter]. Am J Med 1990;89:818–20.

33. Gonzalez-Crussi F. Extragonadal teratomas. Atlas of Tumor Pathology. 2nd Series, Fascicle 18. Washington, D.C.: Armed Forces Institute of Pathology, 1982:9–12.

34. McAllister HA, Fenoglio JJ Jr. Tumors of the cardiovascular system. Atlas of Tumor Pathology, 2nd Series, Fascicle 15, Washington D.C.: Armed Forces Institute of Pathology, 1978:62–3.

35. Meissner A, Kirch W, Regensburger D, Mayer-Eichberger S, Ohnhaus EE. Intrapericardial teratoma in an adult. Am J Med 1988;84:1089–90.

36. Swalwell CI. Benign intracardiac teratoma. A case of sudden death. Arch Pathol Lab Med 1993;117:739–42.

Ectopic Thyroid

37. Ansani L, Percoco G, Zanardi F, Peranzoni P, Gamba G, Antonioli G. Intracardiac thyroid heterotopia. Am Heart J 1993;86:227–35.

38. Kon ND, Headley RN, Cordell AR. Successful operative management of struma cordis obstructing the left ventricular outflow tract. Ann Thorac Surg 1988;46:244–5.

39. McAllister HA, Fenoglio JJ Jr. Tumors of the cardiovascular system. Atlas of Tumor Pathology, 2nd Series, Fascicle 15, Washington D.C.: Armed Forces Institute of Pathology, 1978:62–3.

40. Pollice L, Caruso G. Struma cordis. Ectopic thyroid goiter in the right ventricle. Arch Pathol Lab Med 1986;110:452–3.

41. Polvani GL, Antona C, Porpueddu M, et al. Intracardiac ectopic thyroid: conservative surgical treatment. Ann Thorac Surg 1993;55:1249–51.

42. Richmond I, Whittaker JS, Deiraniya AK, Hassan R. Intracardiac ectopic thyroid: a case report and review of published cases. Thorax 1990;45:293–4.

43. Rosai J, Carcangiu ML, DeLellis RA. Tumors of the thyroid gland. Atlas of Tumor Pathology, 3rd Series, Fascicle 5. Washington, D.C.: Armed Forces Institute of Pathology, 1992:317–20.

44. Swalwell CI. Benign intracardiac teratoma. A case of sudden death. Arch Pathol Lab Med 1993;117:739–42.

Pericardial Thymoma

45. Eglen DE. Pericardial based thymoma: diagnosis by fine needle aspiration. Indiana Med 1986;79:526–8.

46. Iliceto S, Quagliara D, Calabrese P, Rizzon P. Visualization of pericardial thymoma and evaluation of chemotherapy by two-dimensional echocardiography. Am Heart J 1984;107:605–6.

47. McAllister HA, Fenoglio JJ Jr. Tumors of the cardiovascular system. Atlas of Tumor Pathology, 2nd Series, Fascicle 15, Washington D.C.: Armed Forces Institute of Pathology, 1978:62–3.

48. Masaoka A, Monden Y, Nakahara K, Tanioka T. Follow-up study of thymomas with special reference to their clinical stages. Cancer 1981;48:2485–92.

49. Nishimura T, Kondo M, Miyazaki S, Mochizuki T, Umadome H, Shimono Y. Two-dimensional echocardiographic findings of cardiovascular involvement by invasive thymoma. Chest 1982;81:752–4.

50. Venegas RJ, Sun NC. Cardiac tamponade as a presentation of malignant thymoma. Acta Cytol 1988;32:257–62.

12
PRIMARY CARDIAC SARCOMAS

OVERVIEW

Definition. Primary cardiac sarcomas are malignant neoplasms of mesenchymal cells. To be designated a primary tumor, the neoplasm must be confined to the heart or pericardium at the time of presentation, or the bulk of the tumor must be within the pericardial cavity.

The majority of sarcomas that are first detected in the heart are primary. Because there are rare exceptions (7), an occult primary, especially in the soft tissues, skeleton, and retroperitoneum, should always be ruled out radiologically or at autopsy before making the diagnosis of primary cardiac sarcoma. A tumor is likely a metastasis if it is in the right atrium and if the histologic type is not angiosarcoma. Angiosarcomas, unlike all other primary cardiac sarcomas, are typically found in the right atrium.

Histogenesis and Classification. The cell of origin of cardiac sarcomas is presumed to be an undifferentiated, pluripotential mesenchymal cell. The molecular basis for the wide range of differentiation of these tumors is unknown. Although there is no logical explanation for the intracardiac distribution of sarcomas by tissue type, several generalizations can be made. Cardiac tumors with fibrous, smooth muscle, and osteogenic differentiation are often intracavitary left atrial lesions that clinically mimic cardiac myxoma. Angiosarcomas, on the other hand, generally arise in the right atrium, often spread along epicardial surfaces, and metastasize to the lung early in the course of disease. Rhabdomyosarcomas are scattered throughout the heart without any apparent predilection for site. They and liposarcomas are not the most common cardiac tumors even though the bulk of the cardiac tissue is composed of modified striated muscle and fat.

Virtually all types of soft tissue sarcomas have been described in the heart, and the classification follows guidelines established for extracardiac sarcomas (11). However, it is impossible to classify up to 20 percent of cardiac sarcomas, for a variety of reasons. In earlier reports, and even today, immunohistochemical and ultrastructural studies were not done. In some cases, only portions of the tumor demonstrate areas of differentiation; if these areas are not sampled, a specific diagnosis cannot be rendered. There are some tumors that defy classification despite exhaustive immunohistochemical and ultrastructural analysis, because antigenic expression and ultrastructural findings are not always specific for a given sarcoma type. Finally, the diagnostic criteria for malignant fibrous histiocytoma (MFH) are not entirely uniform and reproducible because of the wide variety of morphologic patterns encountered.

There are, to our knowledge, no known cases of familial or environmentally induced cardiac sarcomas. The molecular basis for the histogenesis of these tumors is essentially unexplored, although chromosomal translocations typical of synovial sarcoma have been occasionally demonstrated (see below). A cardiac rhabdomyosarcoma in a patient with von Recklinghausen's disease has been reported (16), and we have encountered a cardiac MFH in a patient with Noonan's syndrome, but these may be chance occurrences.

Role of Immunohistochemistry in the Classification of Cardiac Sarcomas. Specialized techniques for classifying cardiac sarcomas are in a state of infancy compared to their use in soft tissue neoplasms. There are only a handful of reports on immunohistochemical findings in a series of cardiac sarcomas (7,32). For this reason, the role of immunohistochemistry in the diagnosis of cardiac sarcomas must be largely inferred from its role in extracardiac soft tissue tumors. Routine light microscopy forms the cornerstone for the classification of these lesions, and specialized techniques are helpful after a specific differential diagnosis has been formulated on the basis of gross and histologic features.

The immunohistochemical antibodies and antisera that are routinely employed in the differential diagnosis of sarcomas include endothelial markers, intermediate filaments, muscle antigens, and neural markers. For the diagnosis of vascular malignancies, specifically angiosarcoma, factor VIII–related antigen is relatively specific for endothelial differentiation, but lacks sensitivity. *Ulex europaeus,* a lectin that binds endothelial cells, is also relatively insensitive and not entirely specific for endothelial differentiation. Although anti-CD34 is more sensitive in the diagnosis of endothelial differentiation, its specificity has also been questioned. Recently, CD31 has been shown to be a more specific vascular tumor marker.

Several intermediate filaments have been used to classify soft tissue tumors. The cytokeratins are strongly expressed by mesothelial and epithelial malignancies, and only focally, if at all, by cardiac sarcomas. Vimentin is an ubiquitous intermediate filament that is of little use in the differential diagnosis of sarcomas, although strong coexpression of this filament and cytokeratin is suggestive of mesothelioma. Desmin, an intermediate filament found within skeletal and smooth muscle, is a relatively specific marker for myoid differentiation and is useful in two settings: the presence of cells that express desmin in a fascicular spindle cell tumor of the heart is quite suggestive of leiomyosarcoma and desmin positivity in an embryonal or small cell tumor is diagnostic of rhabdomyosarcoma. Unfortunately, the specificity of other myoid markers, such as muscle-specific actin (HHF35), smooth muscle actin, and myosin, is questionable; we detect staining for actin, irrespective of the tissue type, in a frequency that nearly equals that of vimentin staining.

The application of neural markers, especially S-100 protein, is occasionally helpful for differentiating fibrosarcoma and neurofibrosarcoma from malignant peripheral nerve sheath tumor. The histologic appearance of these lesions can be quite similar, and we have seen at least one case in which the diagnosis of cardiac neurofibrosarcoma was made on the basis of immunohistochemical stains. Occasionally, glial fibrillary acidic protein may be expressed in peripheral nerve sheath tumors, and neurofilament protein may be useful in the differential diagnosis of small cell malignancies. Theoretically, primitive neuroectodermal tumor, a small cell neoplasm that may histologically resemble Ewing's sarcoma and embryonal rhabdomyosarcoma, might occur in the heart; for this reason, application of this marker to small cell malignancies of the heart may be indicated.

There are several pitfalls in the interpretation of immunohistochemical stains of cardiac sarcomas. Entrapped myocytes may stain for a muscle-specific antigen and should not be mistaken for tumor cells. Similarly, mesothelial cells entrapped within a tumor near the epicardium express cytokeratin. Langerhans macrophages, found in a variety of soft tissue tumors, mark strongly for S-100 protein and are not indicative of neural differentiation.

A further discussion of immunohistochemical and ultrastructural findings, as pertaining to specific entities, is presented below.

Incidence. Primary cardiac sarcomas are the second most common primary cardiac tumor, after myxoma. However, they are quite rare: 112 cases were reported by 1951 (26), and less than 300 have been reported since then. In a French autopsy series, 12 cardiac sarcomas were identified in 7,200 autopsies, representing a 0.07 percent incidence, or a 0.16 percent incidence in autopsies performed on patients with malignant disease (9). This incidence rate, however, is much higher than that reported in the United States, which is generally less than 0.01 percent (see chapter 1). Approximately 10 percent of surgically resected cardiac tumors are primary sarcomas (see Table 1-2) (6,10,23,25,28,32).

Sarcomas metastatic to the heart are found in approximately 0.6 percent of autopsies performed on patients with malignancy (see chapter 15). This is about a 60-fold increase over primary sarcomas of the heart. In surgical series, primary sarcomas are more frequent than metastatic sarcomas, at a ratio of approximately 3 to 1 (23,25).

Clinical Features. The mean age of patients with cardiac sarcomas is approximately 41 years of age at presentation (7). There is no sex predilection (5,7,23,25). Sarcomas in children and infants are extremely rare, and are usually undifferentiated sarcomas, myxosarcomas, or rhabdomyosarcomas (2,7,12,19,21,22,25,27,32). There was a single rhabdomyosarcoma among 75 cardiac tumors in a large series of pediatric tumors (8).

The mean duration of symptoms before diagnosis is about 5 months (23). Because 50 percent of cardiac sarcomas are located in the left atrium, the most common presenting symptom is dyspnea secondary to venous obstruction or mitral stenosis (Table 12-1) (30). Other modes of presentation include pericardial tamponade

Table 12-1

PRIMARY CARDIAC SARCOMAS PRESENTING SIGNS AND SYMPTOMS IN 141 PATIENTS: AFIP EXPERIENCE

Dyspnea/shortness of breath	57
Chest pain	20
Cardiac tamponade	11
Palpitations	9
Syncope	7
Weight loss	6
Peripheral edema	5
Fever of unknown origin	5
Cerebrovascular accident	4
Hemoptysis	3
Peripheral emboli	3
Bronchopneumonia	3
Sudden death	2
Seizures	1
Incidental finding, autopsy	1
Incidental finding, surgery	1
Rib fracture (from metastasis)	1
Chest wall mass (metastasis)	1
Changing murmur	1

(23), embolic phenomena resulting in cerebrovascular accidents (5), chest pain (25), syncope, sudden death, fever of unknown origin, arrhythmias (25), and peripheral edema. Rare examples are incidental findings, either at autopsy or cardiac surgery for other reasons (7). Rarely, there is asymmetric septal hypertrophy (17) or metastatic deposits (pathologic fractures, skin masses) (15).

Radiologic Findings. The diagnosis of cardiac sarcoma is often first considered at two-dimensional echocardiography (30). With a technically adequate study, two-dimensional echocardiography will delineate a mass in at least 75 percent of patients; in the remaining cases large pericardial effusions may obscure the tumor echos. In most of these instances, computerized tomography (CT) and magnetic resonance imaging (MRI) will differentiate fluid from tumor. With diffuse pericardial tumors, which do not form a discrete mass, the tumor may be first diagnosed at surgery.

In atrial tumors, the clinical and radiologic distinction between cardiac myxoma and sarcoma can be difficult (3,29). Cardiac sarcomas are misdiagnosed as myxomas on the basis of two-dimensional echocardiography (7,23) or cardiac catheterization in up to one third of cases. Transesophageal echocardiography is especially useful in the delineation of atrial lesions (4). MRI and CT scan, in some instances, suggest the diagnosis of sarcoma over myxoma based on infiltration at the base of the tumor into myocardium. However, because occasional sarcomas are pedunculated, and many are myxoid with similar densities as myxomas, pathologic samplings may be needed to distinguish between benign and malignant cardiac tumor.

Occasionally, the MRI features of primary cardiac sarcomas suggest a specific diagnosis. For example, the signals of angiosarcoma are heterogeneous, probably related to thrombosis or hemorrhage; are found over the epicardium; and are somewhat different from the signals of cardiac MFH (18).

Gross Findings. Most cardiac sarcomas are bulky, infiltrating, nodular masses with irregular margins (figs. 12-1–12-4); occasionally, however, they are discrete masses that are pedunculated and mimic myxoma (fig. 12-5). Although typically firm and white, areas of hemorrhage or calcification can impart a variegated and gritty surface.

Tissue Sampling. Until recently, the diagnosis of cardiac sarcoma occurred either at autopsy, at surgical excision, or at open surgical biopsy. In most cases cardiac bypass is required for tumor excision. In some patients, pericardial or epicardial biopsy is performed without attempt at resection; many of these tumors are angiosarcomas, because of their propensity for pericardial infiltration.

Within the last 3 years there have been reports of cardiac malignancies biopsied with transvenous catheters (fig. 12-6) (13,14). Because the majority of cardiac sarcomas are left-sided, transarterial biopsy of the left ventricle may be necessary (14); this is technically more difficult than right ventricular endomyocardial biopsy. Classification of sarcomas is very difficult if there is limited tissue, and occasionally, even distinguishing benign and malignant soft tissue neoplasms is hard.

The diagnosis of a primary heart sarcoma may also be made on the basis of cytologic examination of fine needle aspirates (24).

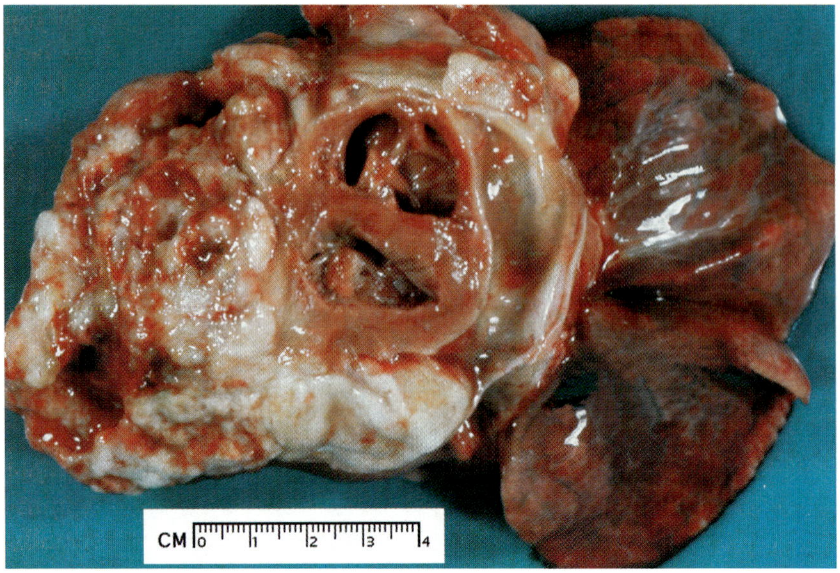

Figure 12-1
UNDIFFERENTIATED SARCOMA
This specimen is from the autopsy of a 1-year-old girl who died of congestive heart failure. Note the bulky tumor which histologically was undifferentiated (not shown).

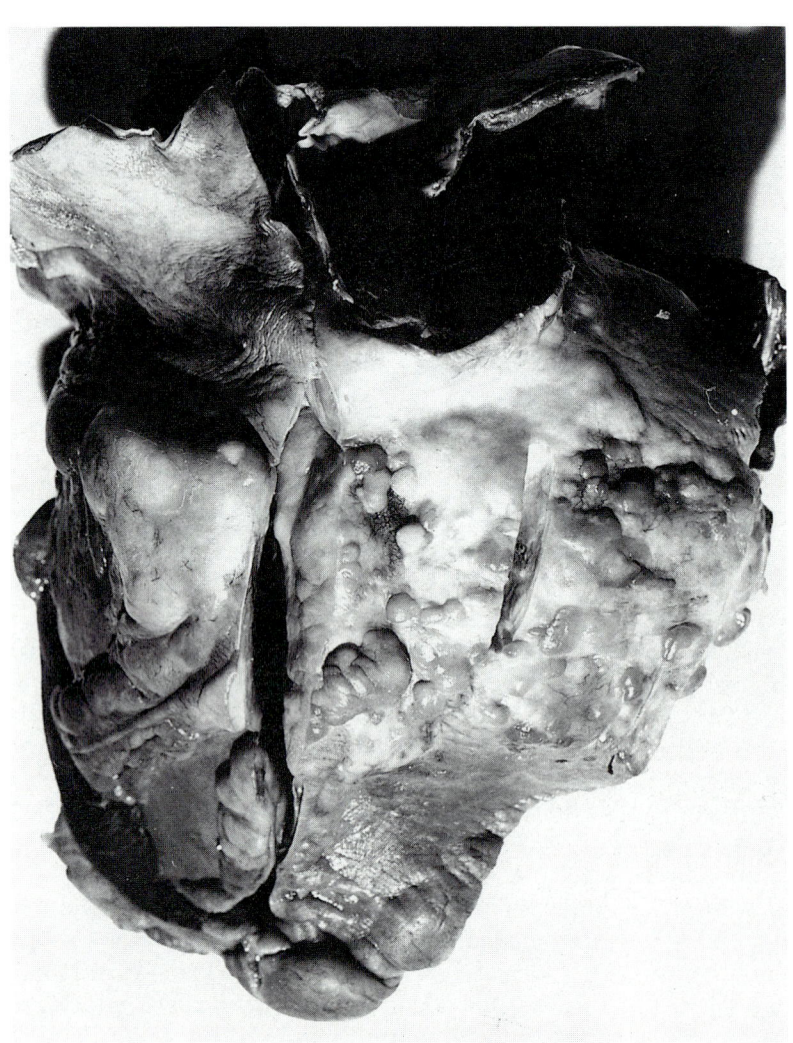

Figure 12-2
LIPOSARCOMA
Gross specimen demonstrates the posterior wall of the heart studded with multiple epicardial nodules over the right and left ventricles.

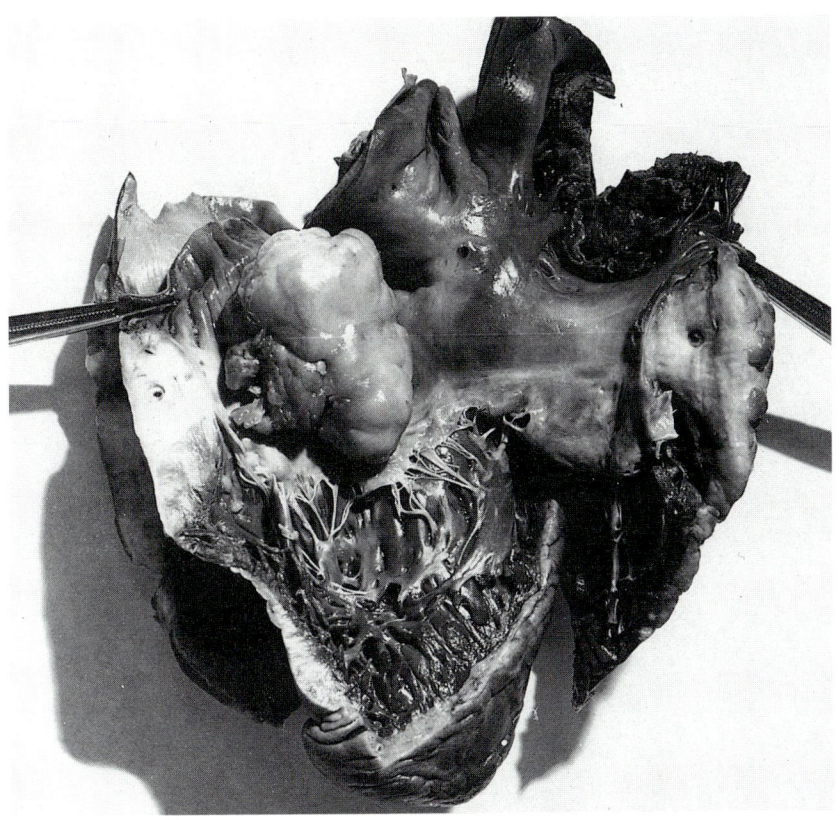

Figure 12-3
LIPOSARCOMA
The right side of the heart has been opened to demonstrate a large right atrial mass overlying the septal leaflet of the tricuspid valve. No metastases were demonstrated at autopsy.

Figure 12-4
UNDIFFERENTIATED SARCOMA
This left atrial tumor involved the mitral valve and filled the left atrial appendage (arrowheads).

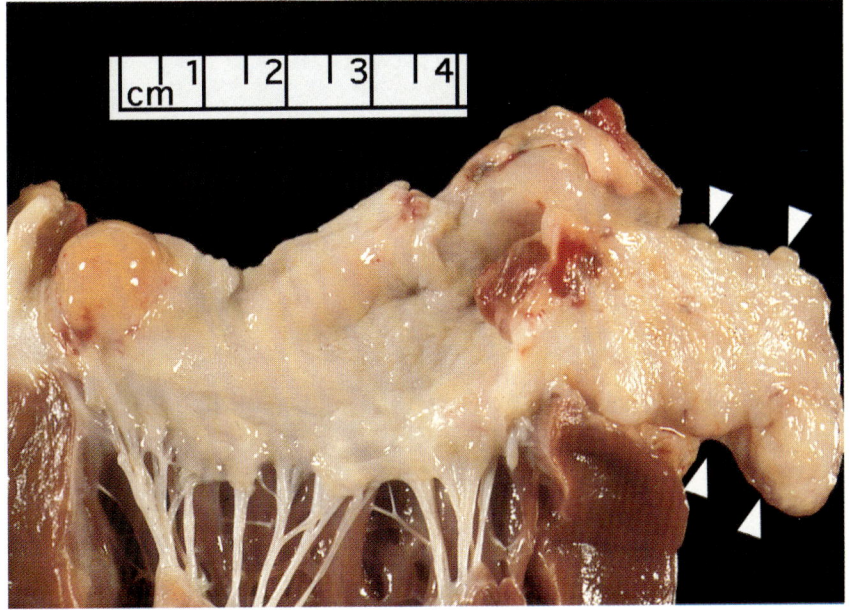

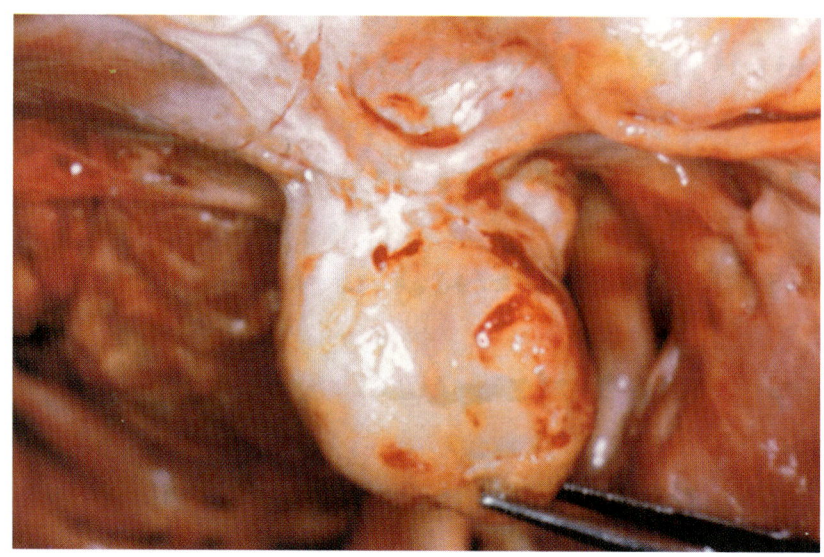

Figure 12-5
UNDIFFERENTIATED SARCOMA
This 70-year-old man presented with syncope and right ventricular outflow tract obstruction. Autopsy demonstrated a pedunculated mass attached to the infundibulum. Cardiac sarcoma may have a gross and radiologic appearance that mimics myxoma.

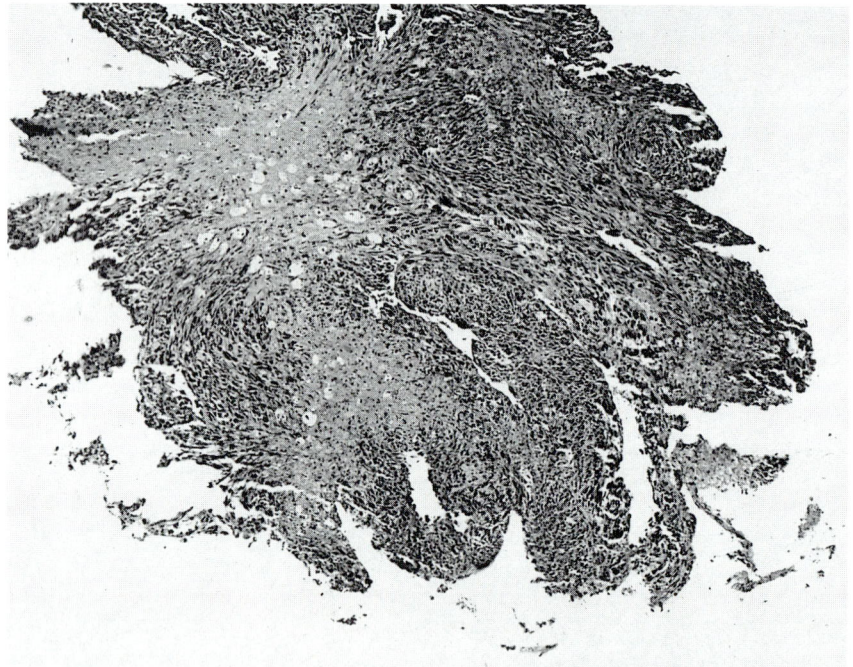

Figure 12-6
ANGIOSARCOMA
Endomyocardial biopsy of a right atrial mass in a 20-year-old woman with chest pain of pericardial origin.

Spread and Metastasis. Cardiac sarcomas are usually confined to the heart at the time of diagnosis. However, cardiac angiosarcomas often present with pulmonary metastases, possibly because of their right-sided location in most instances (see below). Occasionally, cardiac sarcomas have invaded lungs, diaphragm, and venae cavae at the time of diagnosis, making complete excision difficult. Of 115 primary cardiac sarcomas with clinical data in the Armed Forces Institute of Pathology (AFIP) files, 35 (30 percent) had documented metastatic disease at the time of diagnosis. Metastatic sites in these cases were lung (24 cases), vertebrae (6 cases), liver (5 cases), brain (3 cases), jejunum (2 cases), long bones (2 cases), spleen (2 cases), adrenal (1 case), and skull (1 case). In several cases, multiple metastatic sites were present, and in two instances, the metastatic deposits were responsible for the presenting symptoms.

Table 12-2

CLINICAL AND MORPHOLOGIC CHARACTERIZATION OF SURGICALLY RESECTED CARDIAC SARCOMAS: RESULTS OF SEVEN INSTITUTIONAL SERIES*

Histologic Type	Mean Age, Range (yrs)	Male: Female	LA**	RA	Other Sites	Survival Until Death, Mean (mos)	Survival Until Last Follow-up, Mean (mos)
Angiosarcoma (n=25)(37%)	45 (26-80)	13:12	10%	90%	0%	6.6 (n=17)	16 (n=1)
MFH (n=16) (24%)	44 (24-74)	8:8	86%	0	14%[†]	14.9 (n=11)	16 (n=2)
Leiomyosacoma (n=6)(9%)	37 (20-61)	4:2	80%	0	20%[‡]	6.8 (n=6)	0
Rhabdomyosarcoma (n=5)(7%)	30 (0-63)	3:2	50%	25%	25%	3 (n=2)	87[§] (n=2)
Unclassified (n=5)(7%)	16 (0-59)	2:3	67%	33%	0	4.5 (n=2)	21 (n=3)
Fibromyxosarcoma (n=4)(6%)	46 (46-56)	0:4	67%	0	33%	4.0 (n=4)	0
Myxosarcoma (n=3)(4%)	28 (28-28)	0:3	100%	0	0	8.6 (n=3)	0
Fibrosarcoma (n=2)(3%)	43 (26,60)	1:1	0	0	100%	9.5 (n=2)	0
Osteosarcoma (n=2)(3%)	25 (18,31)	1:1	100%	0	0	17 days (n=1)	24 (n=1)
Totals: (n=68)	44 (3 mos-80 yrs)	32:36	53%	35%	12%	8 mos (n=48)	35 mos (n=9)

*Data derived from the following references: 27 (21 tumors), 25 (13 tumors), 5 (8 tumors), 32 (7 tumors), 23 (7 tumors), 10 (7 tumors), and 28 (5 tumors). Data were not available for all cases.
**LA = left atrium, RA = right atrium, MFH = malignant fibrous histiocytoma.
[†]Two tumors in the right ventricle.
[‡]Left ventricular tumor.
[§]One patient alive 10 years at last follow-up.

Histologic Grading. Although there are no specific guidelines for the grading of cardiac sarcomas, the presence of necrosis and numerous mitotic figures indicates decreased survival (fig. 12-7). Because small biopsies are often all that is obtained, and grading schemes have not been adapted to specific histologic types of cardiac sarcoma, the amount of prognostic information available from a biopsy specimen is limited. In general, if tumor necrosis or numerous mitotic figures are present, then the tumor is high grade (7): necrosis must be present in groups of cells with an inflammatory infiltrate or there must be 5 mitotic figures per X400 field, with a mean of 10 fields in the most mitotically active area. Because cardiac sarcomas are rare, more precise measures of grading, such as Ki-67 antigen expression or DNA ploidy, have

not been used. However, it is likely that these techniques are as valid for cardiac sarcomas as they are for extracardiac sarcomas.

Treatment and Survival. Complete excision is possible in less than half of patients (5,23,25), and reconstruction of cardiac chambers with synthetic patches is often required (23, 25). Mitral valve replacement or coronary artery bypass grafting may also be necessary (5,28). Most patients die of their disease within 2 years (23,25); a mean survival is 7 months to 2 years (Tables 12-2, 12-3) (6,10,25). Although resection of cardiac sarcomas is rarely curative, short-term palliation is possible. Features that are associated with increased survival include left-sided tumors, a mitotic rate of less than 10 mitoses per high-powered field, and the absence

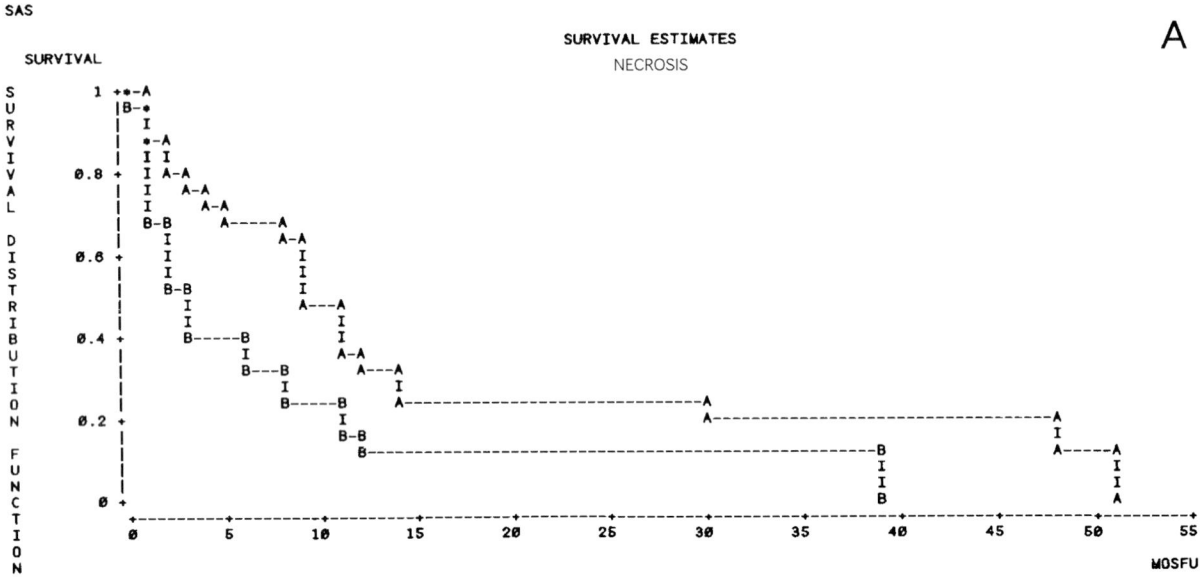

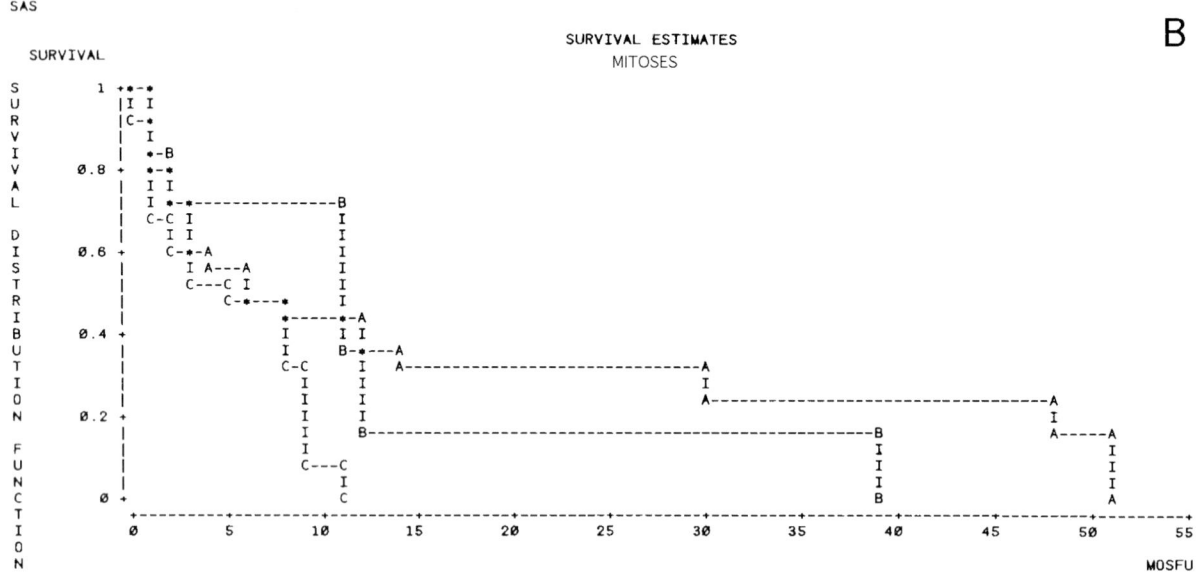

Figure 12-7
SURVIVAL: CARDIAC SARCOMA

A: Survival curves compare tumors with necrosis (A) and tumors without necrosis (B).

B: A comparison of tumors with <5 mitotic figures per 490 µm-diameter field (A), tumors with 5 to 10 mitotic figures per 490 µm-diameter field (B), and tumors with 10 mitotic figures per 490 µm-diameter field (C).

C: Comparison of left sided tumors (L), right sided tumors (R), and tumors involving both atria or ventricles (O).

D: Comparison of tumors apparently localized to the heart (A) and those with metastasis at the time of presentation (B). Note adverse affect on survival by mitotic rate, presence of necrosis, right sided tumors, and tumors with metastases. MOSFU= months of follow-up. (Figure 6 from Burke AP, Cowan D, Virmani R. Cardiac sarcomas. Cancer 1992;69:387–95.)

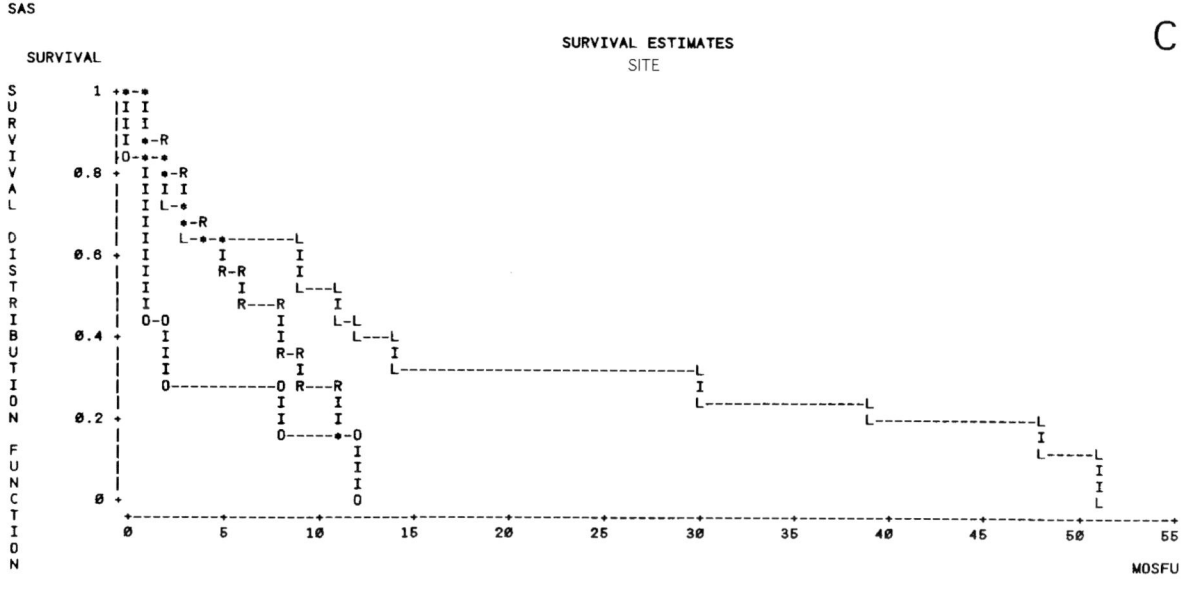

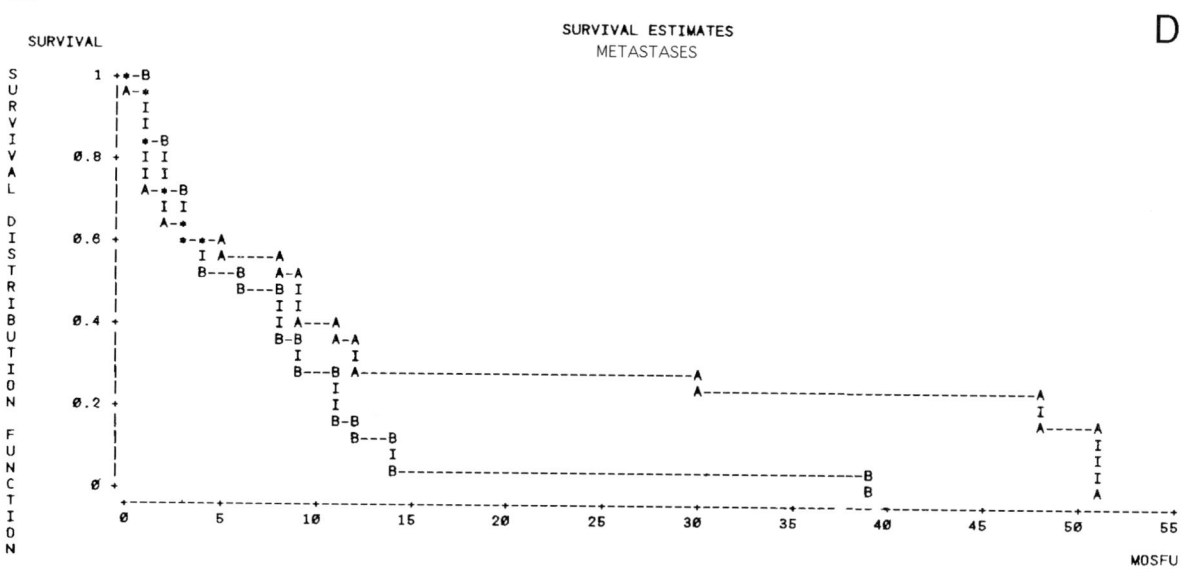

Figure 12-7 (continued)
SURVIVAL: CARDIAC SARCOMA

of necrosis (fig. 12-7) (7). The histologic type does not seem to affect the outcome. One report suggests that angiosarcomas may have a relatively good prognosis (6); this is not supported by other series (5,7,23,25,28). Some recent studies suggest that some patients with cardiac rhabdomyosarcoma may have a good short-term prognosis, although most patients die soon after diagnosis (16). Even with sarcomas of low mitotic rate that lack necrosis, the long-term outlook is poor and few patients survive 5 years (7).

Both chemotherapy and radiation therapy have been used in conjunction with surgery for the treatment of cardiac sarcoma (5,7,10,23,25). Prolongation of life has not been clearly demonstrated, however. Recommendations for chemotherapy

Table 12-3

CLINICAL AND MORPHOLOGIC CHARACTERIZATION OF SARCOMAS OF THE HEART AND PERICARDIUM: AFIP EXPERIENCE

Histologic Type	Mean Age, Range (yrs)	Male: Female	LA*	RA	Ventricals, Diffuse	Peri-card-ium	Survival Until Death Mean (mos)	Survival Until Last Follow-up, Mean (mos)
Angiosarcoma (n=37)(26%)	42 (15-70)	29:8	5%	68%	16%	11%	3 (n=19)	22 (n=2)
Unclassified (n=35)(24%)	45 (1-88)	19:16	49%	13%	32%	6%	3 (n=14)	12 (n=2)
MFH (n=16)(11%)	43 (12-86)	5:11	81%	13%	6%	0	5 (n=9)	8 (n=2)
Osteosarcoma (n=13)(9%)	35 (16-67)	6:7	100%**	0	0	0	6 (n=11)	8 (n=2)
Leiomyosarcoma (n=12)(8%)	30 (1-58)	5:7	76%	16%	8%	0	9 (n=3)	0
Fibrosarcoma (n=9)(6%)	44 (2-68)	4:5	45%	0	33%	22%[†]	5 (n=3)	5 (n=1)
Myxosarcoma (n=8)(6%)	42 (2-66)	3:5	76%	12%	12%	0	50 (n=1)	6 (n=3)
Rhabdomyosarcoma (n=6)(4%)	14 (0-24)	2:4	33%	17%	50%	0	4 (n=3)	0
Synovial sarcoma (n=5)(3%)	39 (30-48)	4:1	40%	0	40%	20%	56 (n=2)	8 (n=1)
Liposarcoma (n=2)(1%)	67 (64,70)	1:1	0	100%	0	0	9 (n=2)	no data
MPNST (n=2)(1%)	52 (48,55)	2:0	0	0	50%	50%	no data	no data
Totals (n=145)	41 (0-88)	80:65	46%	26%	21%	7%	6.6 (n=67)	10 (n=13)

*Abbreviations: LA = left atrium; RA = right atrium; MFH = malignant fibrous histiocytoma; MPNST = malignant peripheral nerve sheath tumor (malignant schwannoma).
**One tumor arose on the anterior leaflet of the mitral valve.
[†]Alternately classified as malignant fibrous tumor of pericardium (see text).

and radiation therapy essentially follow those for extracardiac sarcomas (20), with certain exceptions for cardiotoxic drugs. In rare instances, patients without distant metastases are treated with heart or heart-lung transplantation because of the dismal prognosis with conventional treatment (1,31).

ANGIOSARCOMA

Definition. Angiosarcoma is a malignant tumor demonstrating endothelial differentiation, which is characterized by vascular channels lined by atypical endothelial cells or cellular vacuoles containing red blood cells. Synonyms include *hemangiosarcoma, hemangioendothelioma, malignant hemangioendothelioma, angioendothelial sarcoma, hemangioendotheliosarcoma,* and *malignant hemangioma.* Currently, the term hemangioendothelioma is reserved for distinctive tumors of low-grade malignancy (see chapter 7).

Incidence. Angiosarcoma is the most common type of cardiac sarcoma in surgical series: a review of seven reports showed a 37 percent incidence (Table 12-2). Glancy et al. (36) reviewed 41 cases in 1968, and 46 additional cases were compiled by Janigan et al. in 1986 (38). Since that time, at least 50 cases have been reported (34,37,39-41). In 1992, 161 cardiac angiosarcomas were reviewed from the literature (37).

Clinical Features. Janigan et al. (38) reported a mean age of 40 years among 87 patients with cardiac angiosarcoma. The age range at the time of presentation is 9 to 80 years (37). Unlike other cardiac sarcomas, there is a male predominance of approximately 2.5 to 1 (38), and a marked predominance in the right atrium of 60 percent (38). In a recent surgical series of six cases, all were in the right atrium (37). Presenting clinical symptoms are most often related to obstruction of right ventricular blood flow, hemopericardium, or pericardial constriction (42,45). Because of the propensity for pericardial involvement, cardiac tamponade occurs more frequently than with other types of cardiac sarcomas. In AFIP data accumulated since the writing of the second series Fascicle, tamponade occurred in 4 patients (12 percent) (Table 12-3). Metastases occur in 66 to 89 percent of patients, most often to the lungs; other sites include bone, liver, adrenal gland, and spleen (37,38).

Gross Findings. Angiosarcoma is typically a large, multilobular mass replacing the right atrial wall and either protruding into, or filling, the chamber. The mass or masses are typically dark brown or black, resembling melanoma. Invasion of the venae cavae and tricuspid valve is common, but the atrial septum and pulmonary artery are usually spared. The pericardium is frequently involved and is sometimes diffusely infiltrated. Rarely, it is the only site of tumor without myocardial infiltration (see chapter 14) (38,43).

Histologic Findings. Two thirds of cardiac angiosarcomas are composed of malignant endothelial cells that form papillary structures or vascular channels (fig. 12-8). The diagnosis of such tumors, some of which have been misdiagnosed as atypical cavernous hemangiomas in the past, is relatively straightforward. Unlike hemangiomas, the lining cells are atypical and form irregular anastomosing sinusoidal structures (38). Cells of angiosarcoma may form compressed capillary channels without recognizable lumina; unlike capillary hemangioma, mitoses and atypia are present (figs. 12-9, 12-10).

The remaining one third of cardiac angiosarcomas are focally or largely composed of anaplas-

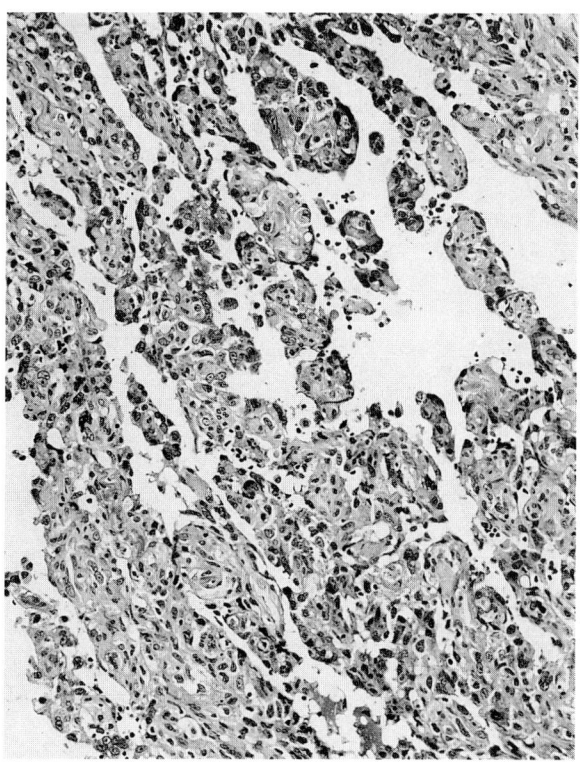

Figure 12-8
ANGIOSARCOMA
Note the atypical papillary fronds lined by hyperchromatic endothelial cells. The tumor was removed from the base of the right ventricle of a 70-year-old man with recurrent hemopericardium.

tic or spindle cells with poorly formed vascular channels and large numbers of extravascular erythrocytes (figs. 12-11, 12-12). In these cases, the identification of vacuoles with red blood cells may help in diagnosis, and extensive sampling of the tumor usually reveals diagnostic areas. Metastatic deposits are often more vasoformative than the primary lesions (fig. 12-13) (38), and occasionally, the histologic appearance of the metastasis is more diagnostic than the primary tumor.

Immunohistochemical studies indicate that factor VIII–related antigen, although a specific marker, is not particularly sensitive. Herrmann et al. (37) found that this antigen stained only one of six cases, and one of two cases for Tazelaar et al. (46). Of the angiosarcomas in the AFIP files, 5 of 10 tumors with adequate material for immunohistochemical studies contained cells that expressed this antigen and staining was often focal (figs. 12-10, 12-12). *Ulex europaeus* and CD34 are

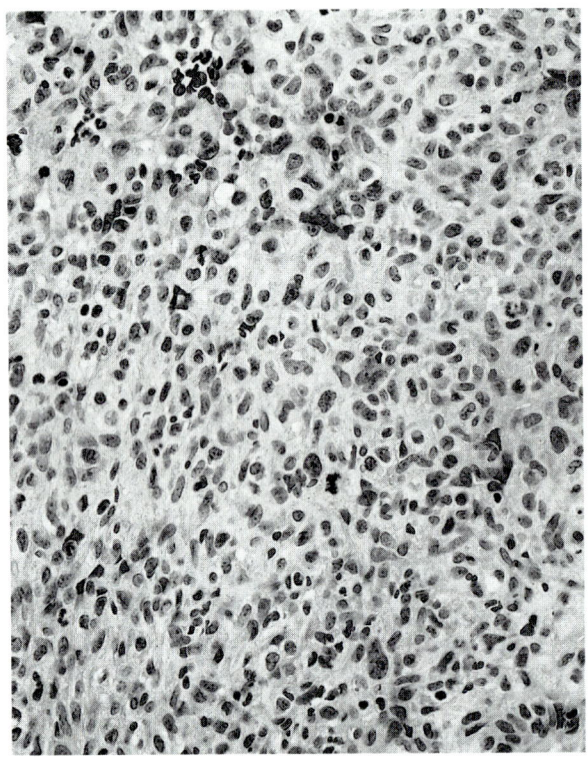

Figure 12-9
ANGIOSARCOMA
Cellular area without obvious vascular channels. There are plump, atypical endothelial cells with occasional mitotic figures.

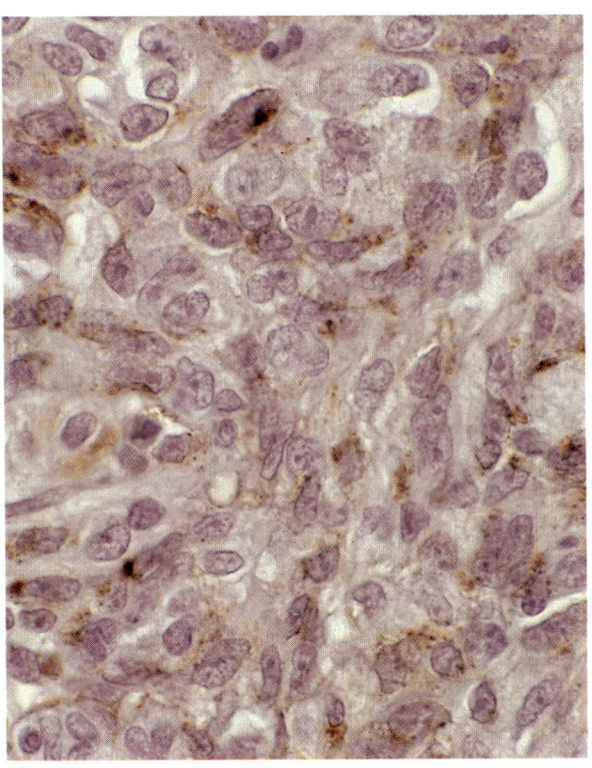

Figure 12-10
ANGIOSARCOMA
Immunohistochemical stain for factor VIII–related antigen demonstrates fine punctate positivity within the cytoplasm. (Same tumor as shown in figure 12-9.)

Figure 12-11
ANGIOSARCOMA
This is a spindle cell tumor with extravasated erythrocytes and poorly formed vascular structures. Extravasated red blood cells are not specific but should prompt a search for diagnostic areas of angiosarcoma.

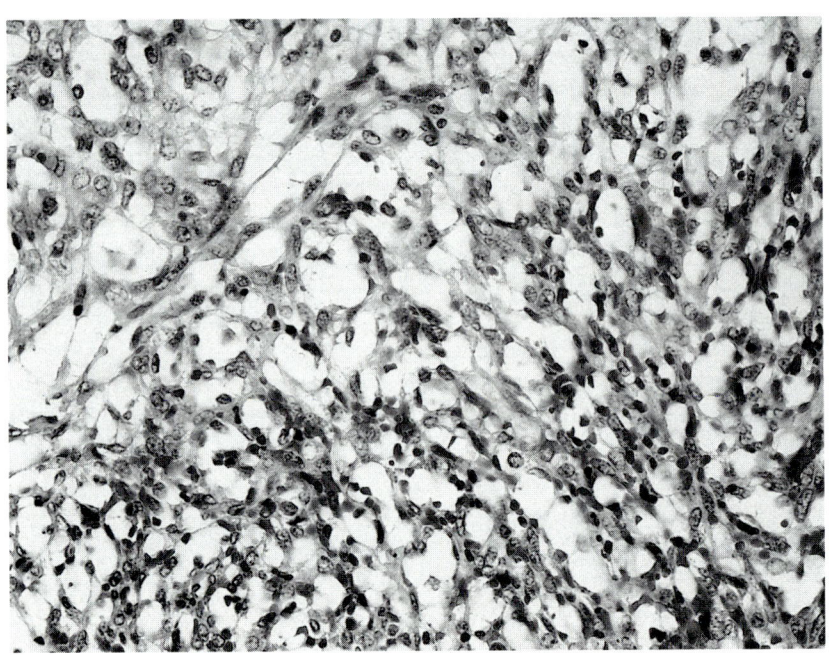

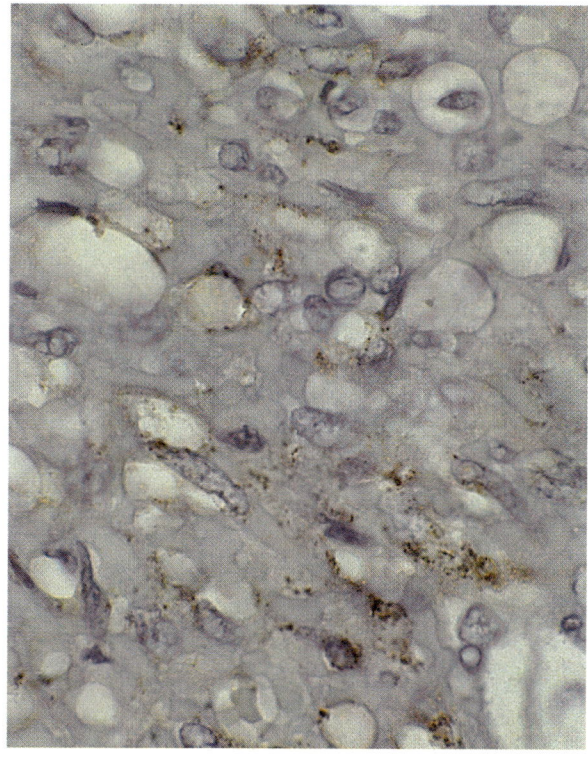

Figure 12-12
ANGIOSARCOMA
Immunohistochemical stain for factor VIII–related antigen demonstrates positive cells in the same tumor as shown in figure 12-11.

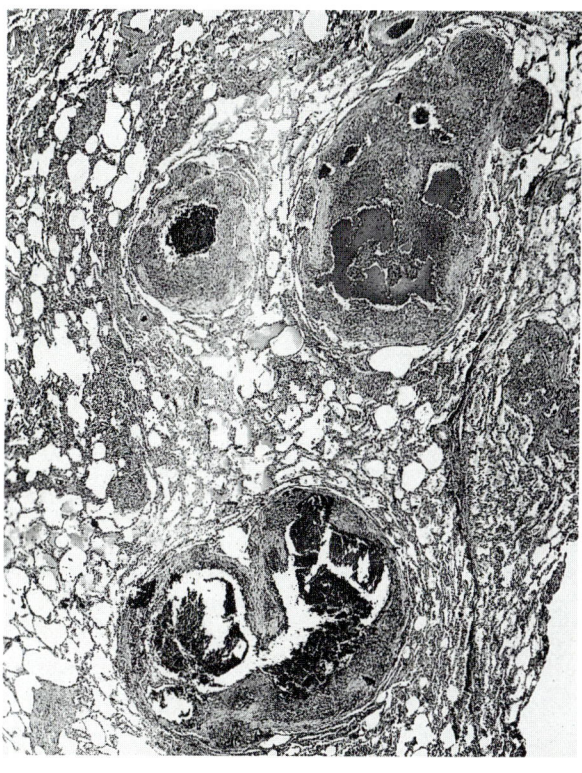

Figure 12-13
ANGIOSARCOMA: METASTATIC TO LUNG
The sections were taken at an autopsy of a 30-year-old man who presented with syncope and pericardial effusion.

not entirely specific markers for endothelial cells and may be detected in cardiac angiosarcoma (46). Weibel-Palade bodies, which are specific for endothelial differentiation, are unfortunately rarely present.

Differential Diagnosis. The spindle cell areas of angiosarcoma may be difficult, if not impossible, to distinguish from unclassifiable spindle cell sarcomas, fibrosarcomas, or MFH. In such tumors, extensive sampling is important to detect endothelial vacuoles or diagnostic papillary structures. Reticulin stains highlight vascular lumina (35,44).

Kaposi's sarcoma may also be difficult to distinguish from spindle cell areas of angiosarcoma. However, angiosarcoma differs clinically and pathologically from Kaposi's sarcoma (see section on Kaposi's sarcoma). Kaposi's sarcoma forms small nodules that coat the pericardial surface infiltrates only minimally within the myocardium, and is virtually always a form of multi-

systemic disease, including multiple skin lesions in immunocompromised patients.

Angiosarcomas of the pericardium can be quite difficult to diagnose in pericardial biopsies (43), and may be mistaken for mesothelioma. Nests of reactive mesothelial cells may become incorporated into the sarcoma and be mistaken for malignant cells. Immunohistochemical stains for cytokeratin and factor VIII–related antigen help delineate the two populations of cells.

Papillary endothelial hyperplasia may be present in cardiac hemangiomas (see chapter 7), and superficially resembles the papillary growths of angiosarcoma. However, marked cellular atypia and mitoses are absent, and the unequivocally benign structures of hemangioma are present elsewhere within the tumor.

Prognosis. The prognosis of patients with angiosarcoma of the heart is poor. In our series, follow-up data on 12 patients showed a mean survival of only 3 months. Herrmann et al. (37) found a similar life expectancy of 4 months in six patients. Combined data from seven institutional series show a mean survival in 17 patients of 6.6 months, and only one patient alive at 16 months (Table 12-2). Blondeau et al. (33) reported a mean survival of 2.14 years in 11 French patients; the reason for this disparity in survival is unclear.

UNCLASSIFIABLE AND UNDIFFERENTIATED SARCOMAS

Definition. Sarcomas without specific histologic patterns, ultrastructural features, or immunohistochemical findings are considered undifferentiated or unclassifiable. Occasionally, nonspecific terms such as *spindle cell sarcoma* (53,54), *round cell sarcoma*, or *pleomorphic sarcoma* are used as descriptive terms, especially in the older literature (61).

Incidence. The incidence of unclassifiable cardiac sarcomas was as high as 50 percent before a classification scheme for soft tissue sarcomas was developed (61). In recent series of primary cardiac tumors, the proportion that was unclassifiable was 0 (49,57), 12 percent (52,60), 16 percent (58), and 24 percent (50). In the recent AFIP files, 24 percent of primary cardiac sarcomas were unclassifiable (Table 12-3). This high incidence may reflect a bias towards difficult and unclassifiable cases referred to the AFIP, inadequate sampling, and a lack of adequate material for complete immunohistochemical and ultrastructural analysis.

Clinical Features. In the 35 unclassifiable tumors in the AFIP files, the mean age at presentation was 45 years, with a range of 1 to 88 years. The presenting symptom was usually related to congestive heart failure; other symptoms were a result of cardiac tamponade (1 patient), coronary insufficiency (1 patient), bronchopneumonia (1 patient), superior vena cava obstruction (2 patients), sudden death (1 patient), and syncope (2 patients). The majority of tumors were left-sided (Table 12-3). Twenty-six tumors were diagnosed premortem: at total resection in 15 cases, at partial resection in 7 cases, at open biopsy in 3 cases, and at endomyocardial biopsy in 1 case. All 12 patients with follow-up information died; mean survival was 3 months. Sites of metastatic spread for undifferentiated cardiac sarcomas were, in order of decreasing frequency, lung, lymph node, central nervous system, bone, liver, and adrenal gland.

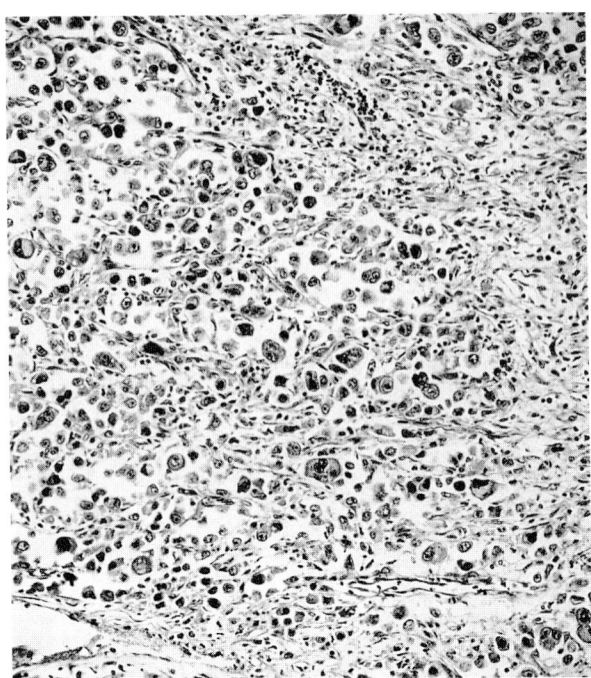

Figure 12-14
UNDIFFERENTIATED SARCOMA
There are undifferentiated pleomorphic and giant cells. The tumor was resected from the left ventricle of a 52-year-old man. Immunohistochemical studies (not shown) did not support a specific diagnosis.

Histologic Findings. Histologically, there are pleomorphic (fig. 12-14), epithelioid (fig. 12-15), and small cell types of undifferentiated and unclassifiable tumors (figs. 12-16, 12-17). Immunohistochemical stains for epithelial, neural, and endothelial markers are generally negative: reported cases of unclassifiable cardiac sarcomas have demonstrated a lack of expression of factor VIII–related antigen, muscle-specific actin, S-100 protein, HAM-56, desmin, and cytokeratin (56,60); other studies have demonstrated expression of multiple antigens (54). Vimentin filaments are typically present (56,60). In the AFIP cases focal smooth muscle actin or muscle-specific actin was detected in most. Because actin filaments may be produced by a wide variety of mesenchymal neoplasms (59), these markers are not considered specific for leiomyosarcoma. Ultrastructurally, differentiation along a specific cell line, eg., desmosomes, well-developed basal lamina, abundant pinocytotic vesicles, and

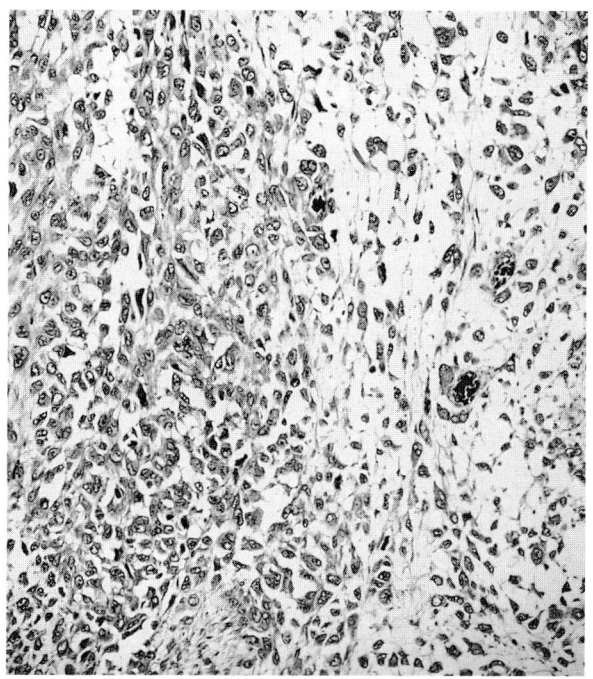

Figure 12-15
UNDIFFERENTIATED SARCOMA
This figure illustrates a left atrial sarcoma in a 24-year-old man who died 2 months postoperatively despite chemotherapy and radiation therapy. The tumor has an epithelioid appearance, and metastatic carcinoma must be considered in the differential diagnosis.

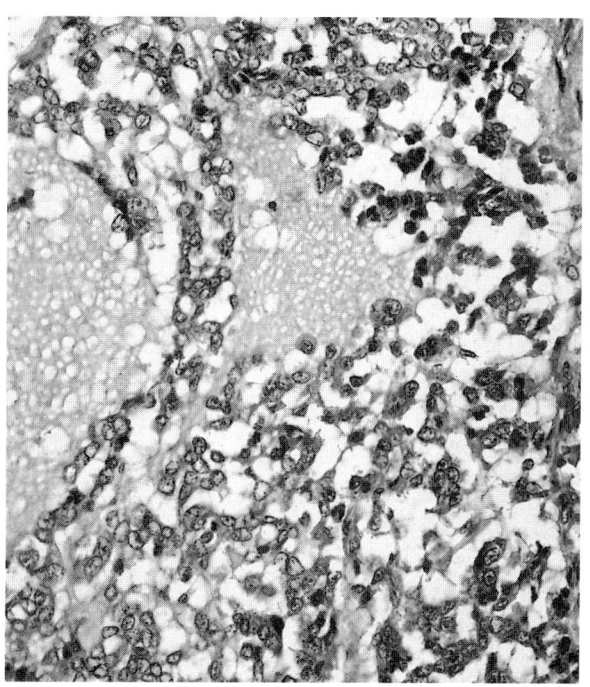

Figure 12-16
UNDIFFERENTIATED SARCOMA
A higher magnification of the tumor in figure 12-15 demonstrates small round cells in a focally myxoid background. Histologic and immunohistochemical features of embryonal rhabdomyosarcoma or round cell liposarcoma were absent.

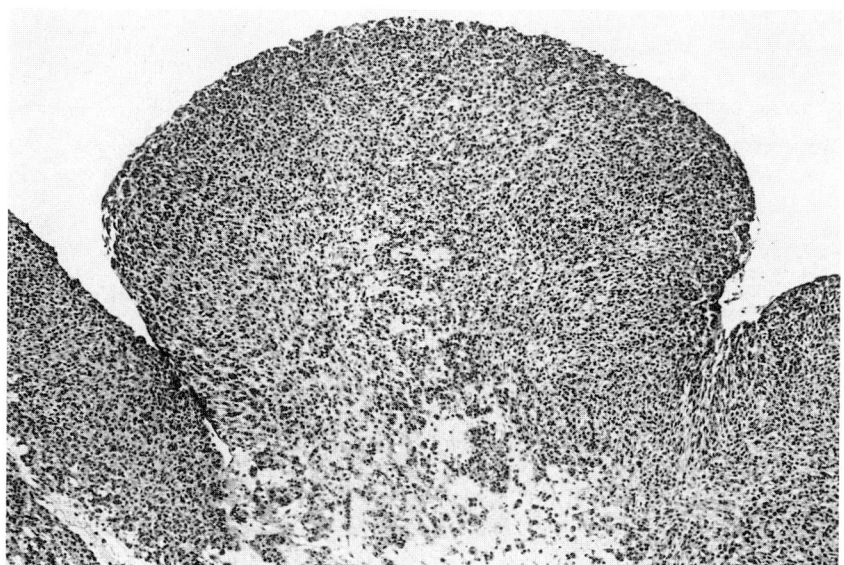

Figure 12-17
UNDIFFERENTIATED SARCOMA
This figures illustrates a small round cell neoplasm removed from the right atrium of a 71-year-old woman with right heart failure and a clinical diagnosis of atrial myxoma.

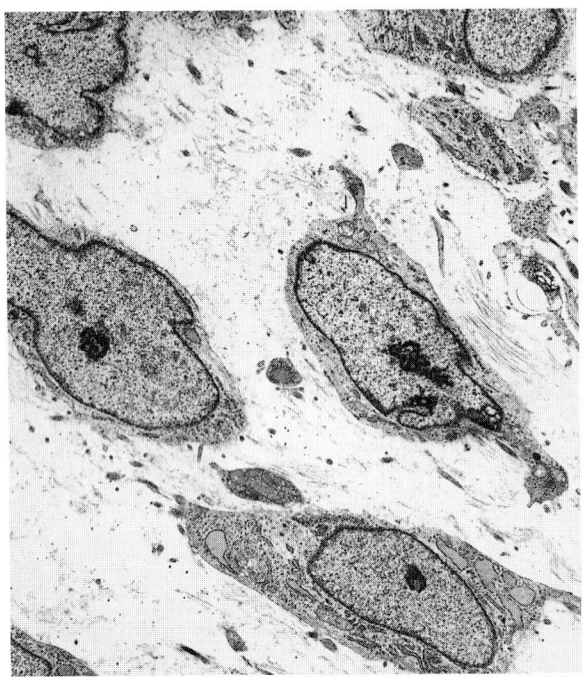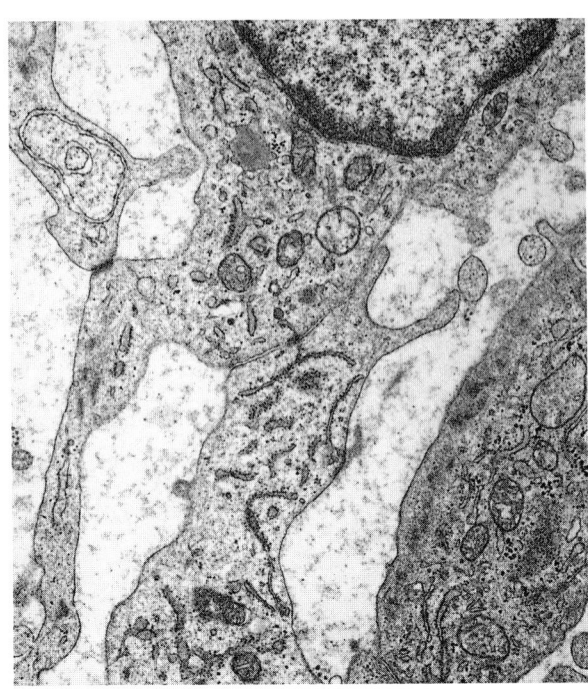

Figure 12-18
UNDIFFERENTIATED SARCOMA

This tumor was removed from the left atrium of a 28-year-old man. The light microscopic features (not shown) of an undifferentiated tumor favor sarcoma. Ultrastructural features were not helpful in further diagnosis and include bipolar cells with tapering cell processes (left). There are abundant rough endoplasmic reticuli and well-formed intercellular junctions (right).

tonofilaments, is generally not seen in undifferentiated sarcoma (fig. 12-18) (54).

In the differential diagnosis of pleomorphic undifferentiated cardiac sarcomas are metastatic carcinoma, metastatic melanoma, and mesothelioma. Immunohistochemical studies and a thorough clinical or autopsy search for primary tumors are important for differentiation. Cytokeratin is generally, but not always (51,55), absent in sarcomas and diffusely positive in carcinomas and mesotheliomas; melanoma-specific markers help diagnose metastatic melanoma. We have seen rare examples of spindle cell carcinoma that present as metastatic cardiac masses simulating primary sarcoma.

Undifferentiated sarcomas with a small cell or embryonal pattern may be confused with hematologic malignancies, embryonal rhabdomyosarcoma, primitive neuroectodermal tumor, extraosseous Ewing's sarcoma, and metastatic small cell carcinoma. Embryonal rhabdomyosarcoma often expresses desmin or myoglobin (see section on rhabdomyosarcoma), and hematologic

markers are usually present in lymphomas and leukemias. The other lesions rarely, if ever, occur initially in the heart.

MALIGNANT FIBROUS HISTIOCYTOMA

Definition. Malignant fibrous histiocytoma (MFH) is a malignant tumor of fibroblasts and pleomorphic histiocytoid cells that assume a characteristic storiform growth pattern in areas of the tumor.

Histogenesis. The histogenesis of the histiocytoid cells in MFH has been debated. Lysosomal enzymes (acid phosphatase, nonspecific esterase) and oxidative enzymes (succinic dehydrogenase) have been demonstrated in cells resembling histiocytes within the tumor, similar to normal histiocytes. The presence of alpha-1-antitrypsin and alpha-1-antichymotrypsin, as demonstrated by immunohistochemistry (75), was interpreted as evidence for histiocytic differentiation of these cells, as was the presence of complement and immunoglobulin receptors in pleomorphic cells (75). However, lysosomal enzymes and membrane receptors for complement and immunoglobulin are not specific for histiocytic tumors (63). More specific antibodies for monocyte-derived macrophages (histiocytes) such as Leu-M1 (CD-15) and Leu-M3 (CD-14) have not been demonstrated in MFH (65). Cultured cells grown from human MFH demonstrate functional markers of histiocytes, such as lysosomal enzymes, immunoglobulin receptors, and immunophagocytosis (65); however, they lack monocyte markers and express a mesenchymal antigen (FU3). These results indicate that the histiocyte-like MFH cell belongs to the mesenchymal cell-fibroblastic lineage and is not a true monocyte-macrophage.

Although radiation is considered a possible etiologic factor in some cases of soft tissue MFH (63), we are unaware of such an association in cardiac MFH.

Incidence. MFH is the second most common cardiac sarcoma in most series (Table 12-2) and the third most common in the AFIP files (Table 12-3), accounting for 11 to 24 percent of cardiac sarcomas. By 1987, seven cases were reported (69); by 1992, however, 27 cases were tabulated by Korbmacher et al. (67).

Clinical Features. The mean age at presentation is approximately 44 years, and there is no sex predilection. Cardiac MFH rarely occurs in children, and we are not aware of any occurrence in an infant. Over 90 percent arise in the left atrium, most commonly on the posterior wall. Because of this location, the symptoms are related to pulmonary congestion due to pulmonary vein obstruction, mitral stenosis, mitral regurgitation, and right ventricular failure (64,66). The tumor often adheres to the posterior leaflet of the mitral valve or mitral valve annulus, but is rarely located on the mitral valve. The initial symptoms may also be secondary to peripheral arterial insufficiency secondary to tumor emboli (67). Tumor masses are invariably noted on two-dimensional echocardiography (69,71,72), but are often misdiagnosed as cardiac myxoma (64,71). Metastatic sites in AFIP cases include lung, skeleton, lymph node, serosal surfaces, kidney, thyroid, and skin. Cerebral aneurysms may result from intracranial hematogenous metastases (70).

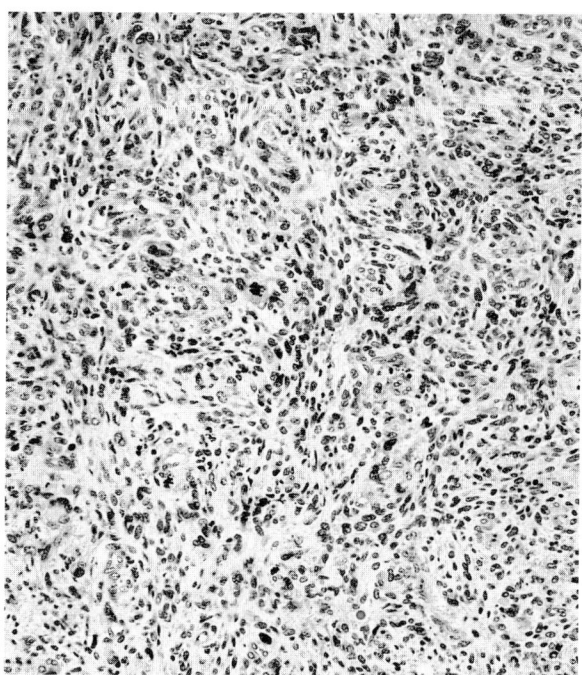

Figure 12-19
MALIGNANT FIBROUS HISTIOCYTOMA
Note the "storiform" appearance as well as fibrohistiocytic cells. The tumor was removed from the left atrium of a 31-year-old woman.

Pathologic Findings. Grossly, cardiac MFHs are lobulated, polypoid masses that are often multiple: up to 10 tumors have been identified in a single case (64). Like cardiac myxoma, they may be sessile (67) or pedunculated (64); one tumor we have seen had a narrow pedicle 4 cm in length. In most reports, they are described as soft or even creamy in texture (64). The tumors are large, often filling and distending the atrium and measuring up to 10 cm in diameter.

Histologically, cardiac MFH is similar to histiocytoma of extracardiac soft tissue (63). Of the five histologic subtypes of MFH (storiform-pleomorphic, myxoid, giant cell, inflammatory, and angiomatoid types) (63), the storiform-pleomorphic and myxoid forms have been reported in the heart. Giant cell MFH is probably synonymous with "osteoclastoma" of the heart (see Osteosarcoma). Typically, there is a cellular proliferation of spindled and pleomorphic cells, often with a storiform pattern (fig. 12-19). Collagen fibers are usually sparse, but may be prominent. Pleomorphic cells are frequently present, and may

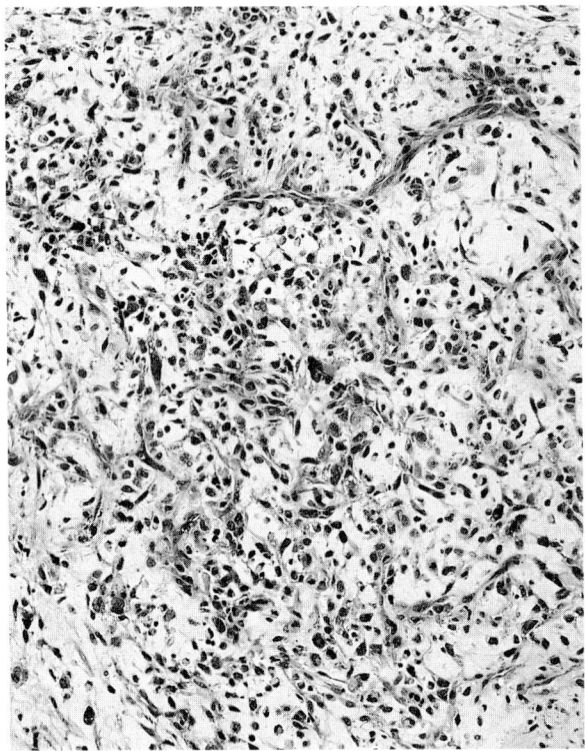

Figure 12-20
MALIGNANT FIBROUS HISTIOCYTOMA
There is prominent vascularity and myxoid changes in the stroma.

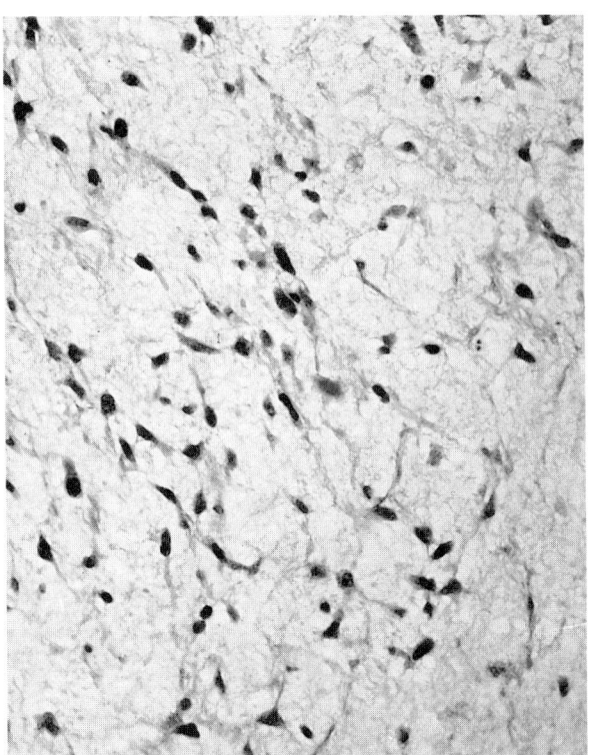

Figure 12-21
MYXOID MALIGNANT FIBROUS HISTIOCYTOMA
This area is nondiagnostic and shows a myxoid background with interspersed hyperchromatic spindled cells. In contrast to myxoma, there are no cords or ring structures. (Figures 12-21–12-23 are from the same tumor.)

represent foamy xanthoma or histiocytoid cells, or pleomorphic giant cells. Histiocytoid cells are oil red O positive (69,71). There may be multinucleated giant cells and a sparse background of inflammatory mononuclear cells, and scanty reticulum fibers may surround tumor cells (71). A myxoid background is common (66,76), and is typically accompanied by a prominent vascular network (fig. 12-20). Paucicellular and fibrotic areas of tumor appear deceptively benign; the presence of muscular infiltration and extensive sampling for diagnostic areas facilitate diagnosis (figs. 12-21–12-25).

Ultrastructurally, MFH is characterized by two tumor cell types (69,71): histiocytoid and fibroblastic cells. The histiocytoid cells demonstrate scattered lysosomes, lipid inclusions, cytoplasmic membranes with blunt pseudopodia, and no junctional structures. In contrast, fibroblastic cells have dilated endoplasmic reticulum, intracytoplasmic filaments, and poorly formed dense bodies with peripheral attachment plaques (75). Glycogen is generally absent in MFH.

Immunohistochemically, MFH is generally negative for cytokeratin, myoglobin, desmin, and S-100 protein (67,71,74), and positive for vimentin (67). Of five cases stained immunohistochemically at the AFIP, all were positive for vimentin and negative for desmin, factor VIII–related antigen, S-100 protein, and cytokeratin. Rarely, the latter antigen is expressed in extracardiac MFH (63). Three of these five tumors showed partial staining with antiactin antibodies.

Differential Diagnosis. The most common misdiagnosis of left atrial MFH, both clinically and pathologically, is myxoma. The difficulty distinguishing these two lesions occurs when there is a prominent myxoid background in MFH. The characteristics that distinguish myxoma from myxoid MFH are similar to those that distinguish myxoma from myxosarcoma (see section on myxosarcoma). Unlike the cells in MFH, myxoma cells are ovoid or polygonal, and form characteristic cords and

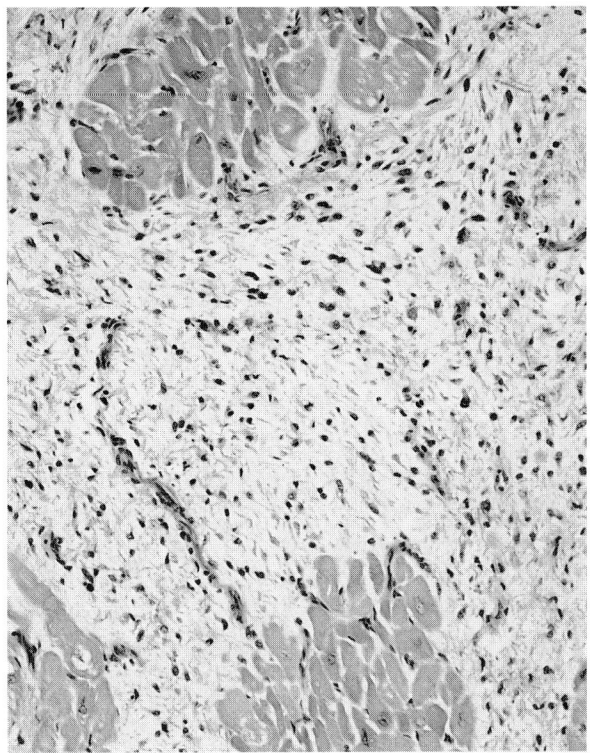

Figure 12-22
MYXOID MALIGNANT FIBROUS HISTIOCYTOMA
There is focal infiltration of atrial muscle.

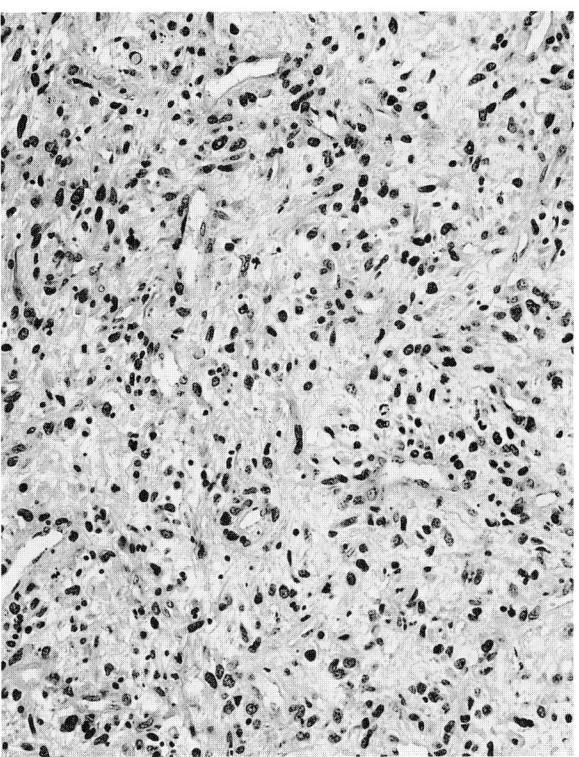

Figure 12-23
MYXOID MALIGNANT FIBROUS HISTIOCYTOMA
This field demonstrates an area of tumor that is relatively cellular, compared to those shown in the previous two figures.

ring structures that are often infiltrated by mononuclear inflammatory cells. In general, myxomas lack the degree of cellularity and pleomorphism that characterizes MFH. However, there is great overlap in this feature, as areas of myxoid MFH may be quite acellular. The vascular pattern of the tumor helps classify it: myxoid MFH typically has an orderly and extensive background of branching, relatively thick-walled vessels; in contrast, the vessels in myxoma are delicate capillaries that merge imperceptibly with myxoma cells.

A less clinically relevant distinction is that between MFH and leiomyosarcoma. The bundles or fascicles of leiomyosarcoma cells are more compact than those of MFH, and are often oriented at right angles to one another. In addition, intracellular glycogen is usually present, as well as longitudinal fuchsinophilic fibers seen with trichrome stain. Perinuclear vacuoles are rarely present in cardiac leiomyosarcoma, but, when present, are quite suggestive of the diagnosis. Although desmin has been

reported in MFH (73,68), we believe that this marker is fairly specific for muscle differentiation and consider desmin positivity as strong evidence for myoid differentiation.

Treatment. Surgical excision is the mainstay of treatment for cardiac MFH. Some patients are given radiation therapy and chemotherapy after surgery (69). Chemotherapy regimens are similar to those used for extracardiac soft tissue tumors, and often include cyclophosphamide, doxorubicin, dacarbazine, and vincristine (69). The mean postoperative survival period is 15 months for patients from several series (Table 12-2), 18 months in a review by Laya et al. (69), 18 months in a report by Korbmacher et al. (67), and only 5 months in our experience at the AFIP (Table 3). The cause of death may be related to metastatic disease (62), bulky intracardiac recurrences (64,71), or general debilitation. There may be up to five local recurrences before evidence of extracardiac disease is discovered (67), supporting the role of surgical treatment for cardiac MFH.

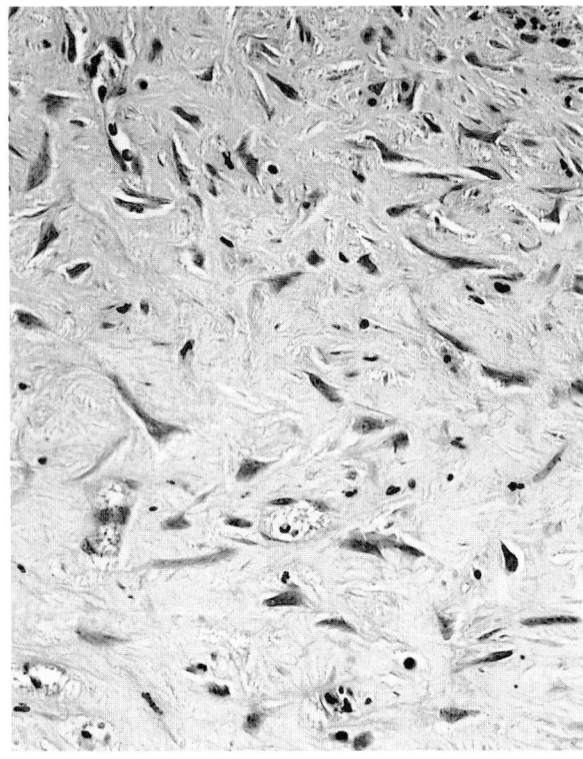

Figure 12-24
MYXOID MALIGNANT FIBROUS HISTIOCYTOMA
There are atypical spindled cells in a hyalinized background. Such areas may appear deceptively bland, but other foci of this tumor were more cellular and pleomorphic.

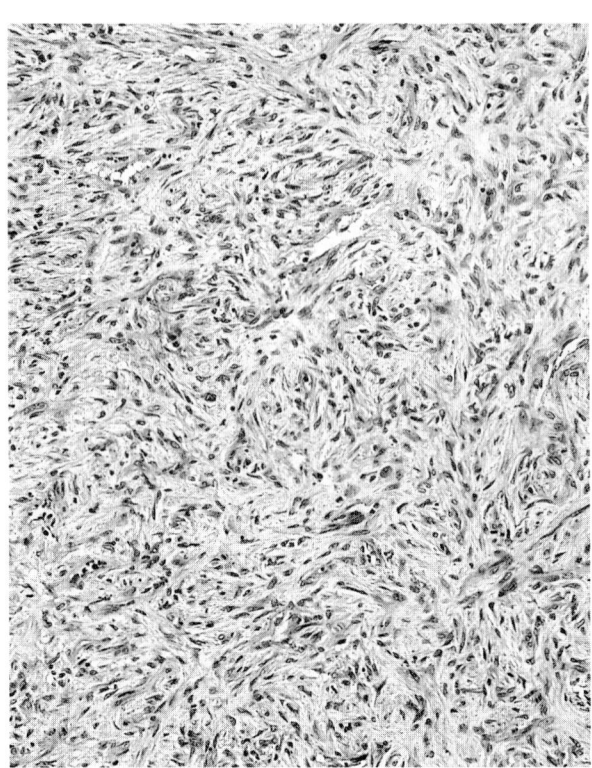

Figure 12-25
MALIGNANT FIBROUS HISTIOCYTOMA
Cellular area from tumor shown in figure 12-24.

OSTEOSARCOMA

Definition. Osteosarcoma is comprised of malignant bone-forming cells within a spindle cell or pleomorphic cardiac sarcoma. If chondroid areas are present in the absence of osteoid, a separate classification of *chondrosarcoma* has been used (79); *osteoclastoma* has been used for cardiac sarcomas with numerous osteoclast-like giant cells (78). Extraosseous osteoclastoma is essentially synonymous with giant cell type of MFH. Because of the great clinical and histologic overlap between cardiac osteosarcoma, chondrosarcoma, and osteoclastic giant cell tumor, and for simplicity, we group these tumors together under the term "osteosarcoma."

Incidence. From 3 to 9 percent of primary cardiac sarcomas have areas indistinguishable from osteosarcoma or chondrosarcoma of bone (Tables 12-2, 12-3). In a review of surgically resected atrial tumors, only 1 of 21 lesions was an osteosarcoma (80).

Clinical Features. Because cardiac osteosarcomas are invariably present within the left atrium, dyspnea is the most common symptom (83–85). Complications of cardiac osteosarcoma include recurrent pneumonitis, congestive heart failure, mitral stenosis (82,87), pulmonary hypertension, and syncope. In most cases, the echocardiographic diagnosis is atrial myxoma. Because the site of attachment is usually remote from the fossa ovalis, the diagnosis is usually atypical myxoma. Treatment is surgical excision, and cardiac reconstruction may be necessary (87). The little follow-up data that is available suggests a poor prognosis (Tables 12-2, 12-3). Sites of metastatic spread include lymph nodes, thoracotomy incision, lung, thyroid, and skin.

Pathologic Findings. Osteosarcomas of the heart are bulky masses measuring 4 to 10 cm in diameter. They are generally attached to the wall of the left atrium as a sessile mass. Approximately 20 percent invade the atrial wall or

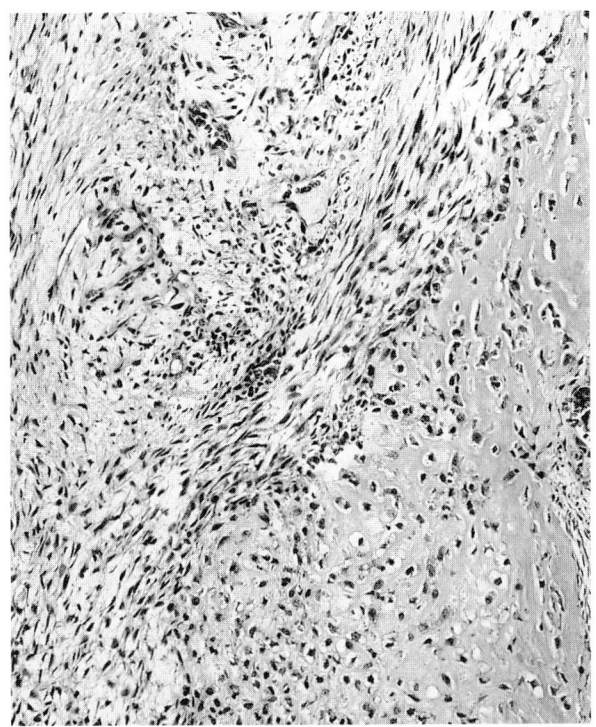

Figure 12-26
OSTEOSARCOMA
Most cardiac osteosarcomas have spindled areas in addition to differentiated osteosarcoma (note osteoid, lower portion of field). The patient was a 16-year-old boy with a left atrial mass; the tumor recurred in 13 months at the site of the chest wall incision.

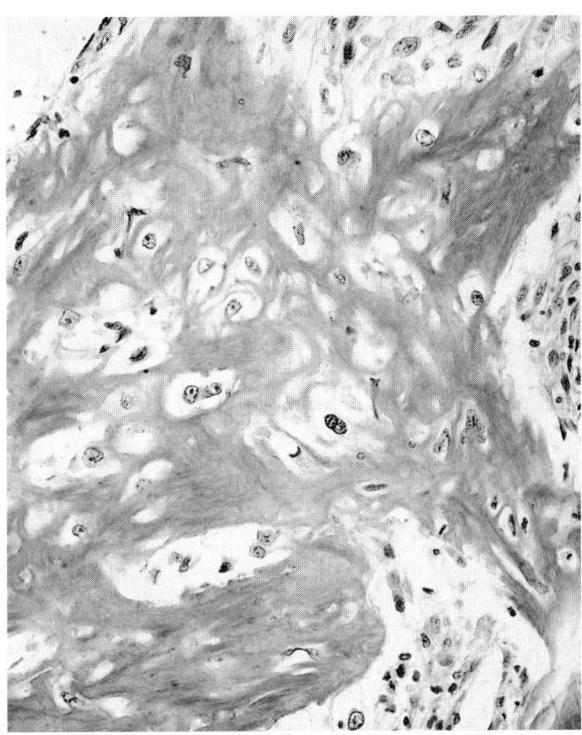

Figure 12-27
OSTEOSARCOMA
There are atypical cells within an osteoid matrix.

mitral valve. The surface may be mucoid or gelatinous, but sectioning reveals gritty and calcified areas, often with a variegated appearance.

Cardiac osteosarcomas are histologically heterogeneous (77). Most are composed of fibrosarcoma or MFH, with microscopic areas of osteosarcoma (figs. 12-26, 12-27) and chondrosarcoma (fig. 12-28) (79,86) among the spindle cell areas. Only four tumors in the AFIP files had large areas of mature bone formation; in three cases, portions of the tumor resembled giant cell tumor of bone, a feature that may be prominent (78). Cardiac sarcomas with prominent osteoclast-like giant cells may alternatively be classified as osteoclastoma or giant cell MFH. The metastatic deposits of cardiac osteosarcoma may histologically resemble any component of the primary tumor, such as the fibrosarcoma (fig. 12-29), osteosarcoma, or chondrosarcoma. Angiosarcoma, leiomyosarcoma, or rhabdomyosarcoma in tumors with osteosarcoma are diagnos-

tic of malignant mesenchymoma (see Malignant Mesenchymoma).

Immunohistochemically, the spindled areas of cardiac osteosarcoma are focally actin positive and diffusely vimentin positive. S-100 protein is expressed only by the chondrosarcomatous components of the tumor, if present.

Differential Diagnosis. The diagnosis of osteosarcoma depends on the recognition of osteoid and chondroid areas on routinely stained sections. Cardiac myxoma may also demonstrate calcified or ossified areas (see chapter 3). Unlike osteosarcoma, however, myxoma virtually never shows chondroid differentiation and possesses typical myxoma cells forming cords and rings. Two reported cases of cardiac chondrosarcoma containing myxoid areas were originally misdiagnosed as cardiac myxoma, based on the presence of a myxoid background (79,81). These cases underscore the fact that chondroid areas in a heart tumor should alert the pathologist to the strong likelihood of malignancy.

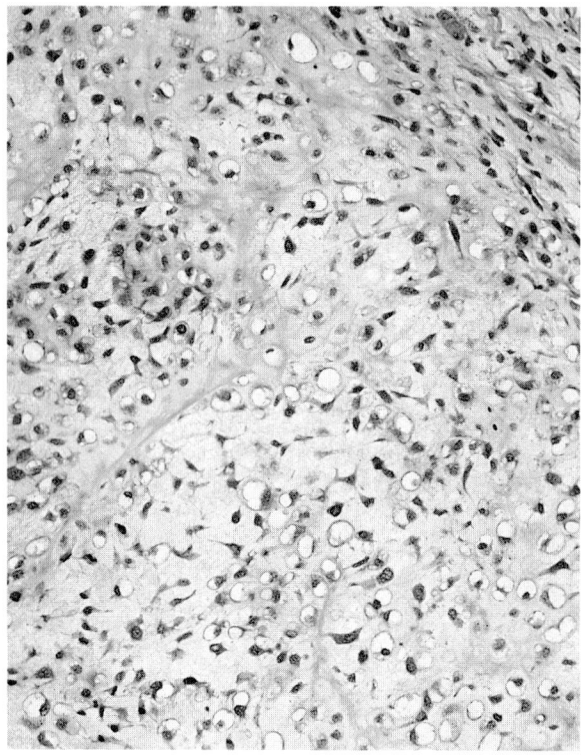

Figure 12-28
CHONDROSARCOMA
This is a cellular tumor composed of atypical cells within a chondroid matrix. Chondroid areas in a tumor of the heart are virtually diagnostic of malignancy.

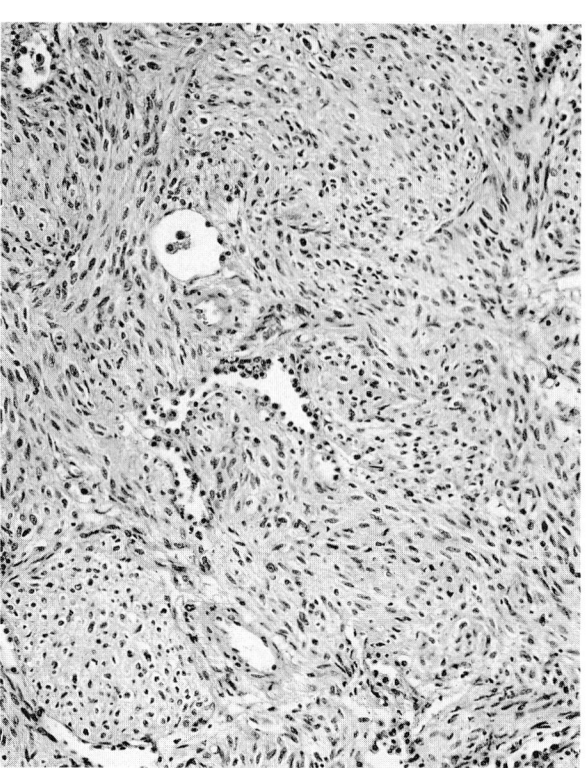

Figure 12-29
CARDIAC OSTEOSARCOMA:
METASTATIC TO LUNG
This spindle cell tumor resembles fibrosarcoma. Osteosarcoma and chondrosarcoma were present in the cardiac primary (not shown).

LEIOMYOSARCOMA

Definition and Histogenesis. Leiomyosarcoma is a malignant mesenchymal neoplasm composed of cells with structural or antigenic evidence of smooth muscle differentiation. The majority of cardiac leiomyosarcomas arise in the left atrium; at surgery, some appear to arise from a pulmonary vein. For these reasons, the cell of origin of cardiac leiomyosarcoma may reside in the smooth muscle media of pulmonary veins (90). However, it is likely that some leiomyosarcomas originate within the left atrium itself, because the left atrium is a preferred site of origin for most cardiac sarcomas, and because the subendocardial lining of the atrium normally contains bundles of smooth muscle cells. Their large size at the time of diagnosis makes assessment of precise site of origin impossible in most cases.

Incidence. Leiomyosarcoma is an uncommon cardiac tumor, representing 8 to 9 percent of cardiac sarcomas (Tables 12-2, 12-3).

Clinical Features. The mean age at presentation is within the fourth decade, 5 to 10 years younger than the mean age of patients with other cardiac sarcomas (90). There is no apparent sex predilection. Seventy-five to 80 percent of cardiac leiomyosarcomas occur in the left atrium and result in dyspnea; other signs and symptoms include pericardial effusions, chest pain, atrial arrhythmias, and congestive heart failure (87a,89). Budd-Chiari syndrome may occur in patients with right atrial leiomyosarcoma (92), and left ventricular outflow tract obstruction has been reported in a leiomyosarcoma of the ventricle (89).

Pathologic Findings. Grossly, leiomyosarcomas are typically sessile atrial lesions that may be grossly myxoid or mucoid. Unlike myxomas, the location is typically the posterior atrial wall, and tumors are multiple in 30 percent of cases. The pulmonary veins or mitral valve were infiltrated in 3 of 11 cases at the AFIP.

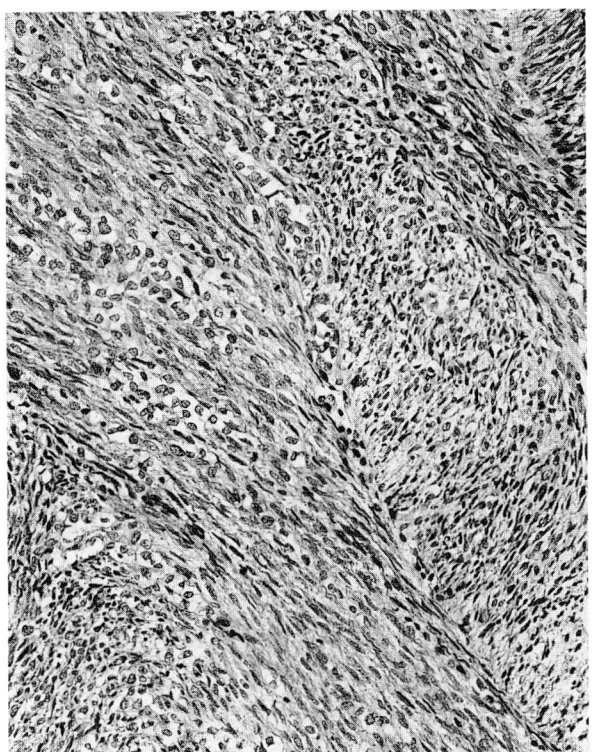

Figure 12-30
LEIOMYOSARCOMA
The cellular characteristics include blunt-ended nuclei and fascicles that course at sharp angles onto each other. The tumor was a left atrial mass (clinically diagnosed as myxoma) in a 35-year-old woman.

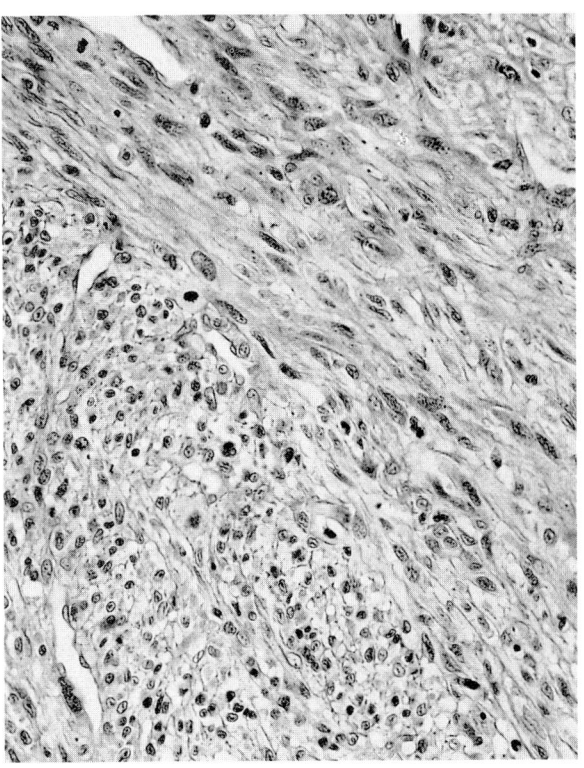

Figure 12-31
LEIOMYOSARCOMA
A higher magnification of the tumor shown in figure 12-30 shows characteristic fascicles and a slightly vacuolar appearance most prominent in cells cut in cross section. Well-formed perinuclear vacuoles are rarely present in cardiac leiomyosarcoma.

Histologically, leiomyosarcoma is composed of compact bundles of spindled cells that possess blunt-ended nuclei and are often oriented at sharp angles to one another (figs. 12-30, 12-31). Characteristic features include the presence of cytoplasmic glycogen (fig. 12-32), perinuclear vacuoles, and intracytoplasmic desmin; unfortunately, these features are not consistently demonstrated. Myxoid areas usually represent less than 25 percent of the tumor. In contrast to fibrosarcomas, pleomorphic and giant cells may be present. Zones of necrosis and mitotic figures are generally plentiful, and epithelioid areas may be identified (fig. 12-33) (91).

Immunohistochemically, 5 of 7 leiomyosarcomas at the AFIP showed focal positivity for desmin (fig. 12-34), actin was present in every case, and epithelial and neural markers were negative. A case report described strong staining for cytokeratin and desmin in an epithelioid leiomyosarcoma of the left atrium (89).

Ultrastructurally, features of leiomyosarcoma include an infolded or notched nucleus, thin actin filaments with focal densities, sparse mitochondria and endoplasmic reticulum, micropinocytotic vesicles, and a thin but distinct external lamina. Poorly differentiated tumors may lack these features, and myofilaments with dense bodies have been described in a variety of tumors (88).

Differential Diagnosis. Fibrosarcoma, in contrast to leiomyosarcoma, lacks intracytoplasmic glycogen, cellular pleomorphism, and intracytoplasmic desmin. The nuclei of leiomyosarcoma are described as blunt-ended and symmetric, unlike the tapered nuclei of fibrosarcoma and the asymmetric nuclei of neurofibrosarcoma. Differentiating between pleomorphic leiomyosarcoma and MFH may be more difficult, because some cardiac leiomyosarcomas have areas indistinguishable from MFH. We recommend

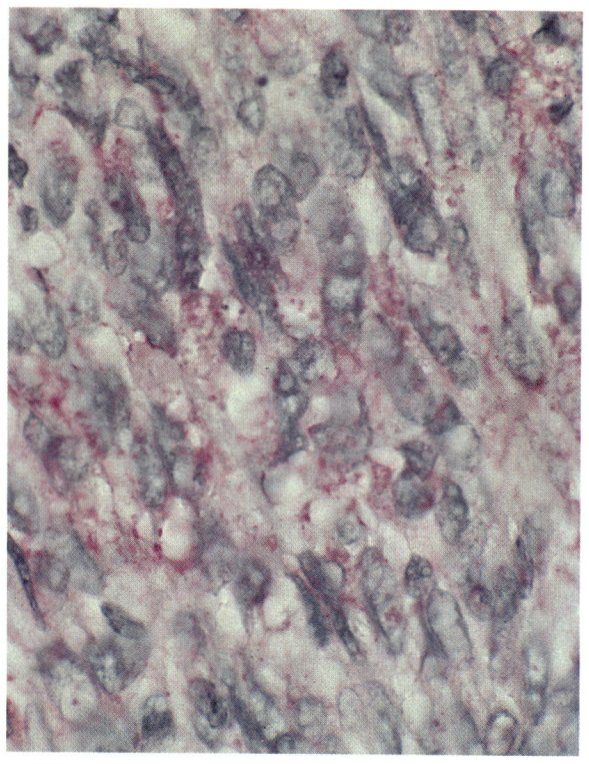

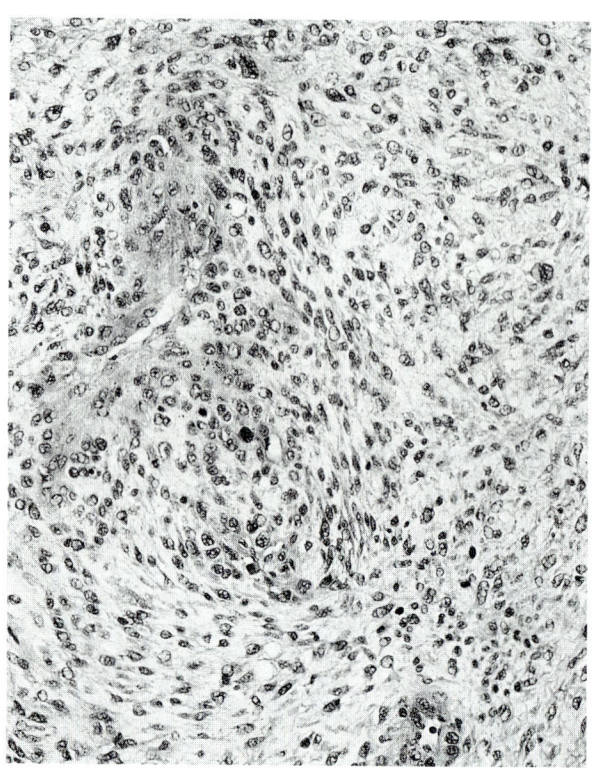

Figure 12-32
LEIOMYOSARCOMA
There is generally abundant glycogen in some areas of leiomyosarcoma, illustrated by diffuse punctate droplets stained with PAS.

Figure 12-33
LEIOMYOSARCOMA
This tumor has a somewhat epithelioid appearance, with rounded to ovoid nuclei.

Figure 12-34
LEIOMYOSARCOMA:
DESMIN POSITIVITY
This photomicrograph shows the tumor illustrated in figure 12-33. This degree of positivity is unusual in leiomyosarcoma.

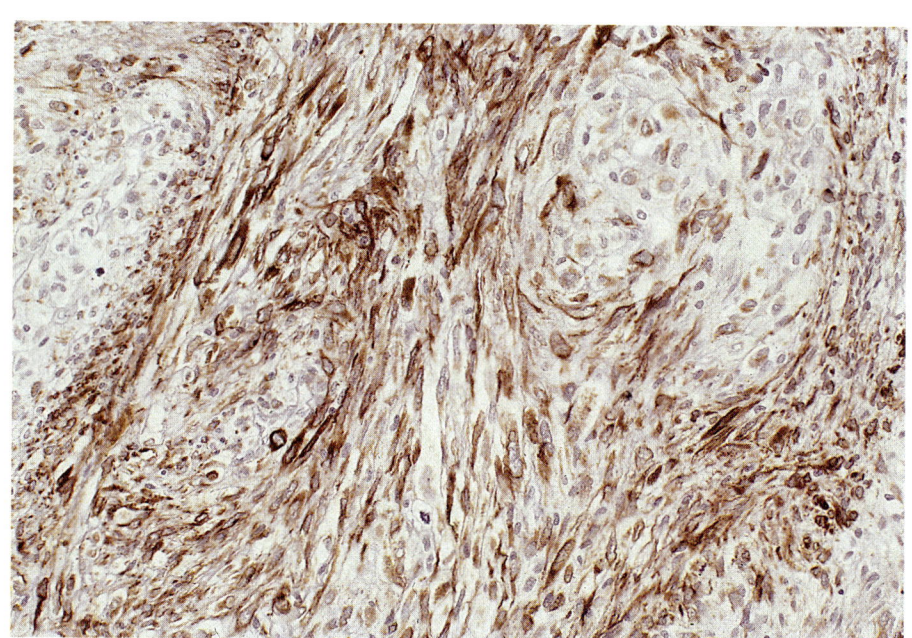

thorough sampling of undifferentiated or MFH-like cardiac sarcomas to identify areas of tumor that histologically and histochemically resemble leiomyosarcoma.

Treatment. Treatment consists of surgical excision; postoperative survival is measured in months (Tables 12-2, 12-3).

FIBROSARCOMA

Definition. Fibrosarcoma is a malignant tumor of mesenchymal cells with morphologic features of fibroblasts. In contrast to MFH, histiocytoid cells are absent and there is little cellular pleomorphism.

Solitary fibrous tumor of the serosal surface is believed to derive from subserosal mesenchymal cells that structurally resemble fibroblasts (96). Rare malignant fibrous tumors of the pericardium (94) and mediastinum near the pericardium (96) have been reported. Although these tumors clinically resemble mesotheliomas (see chapter 14), they are tumors of fibroblastic differentiation and therefore best considered sarcomas, not mesotheliomas.

Incidence. Fibrosarcoma is a rare cardiac tumor (93,95), representing about 5 percent of AFIP cases and recent series of cardiac sarcomas resected at surgery (Tables 12-2, 12-3).

Clinical Features. Because of their rarity, generalizations about cardiac fibrosarcomas are difficult to make. They are frequently located in the left atrium and result in symptoms of pulmonary congestion or mitral stenosis. They may be amenable to complete surgical excision (93). Like other cardiac sarcomas, however, the long-term prognosis is poor (Tables 12-2, 12-3).

Pathologic Findings. Fibrosarcomas are soft, polypoid tumors that may fill the atrium (93) or infiltrate the ventricles. Fibrosarcomas of the pericardium (malignant solitary fibrous tumor of the pericardium) diffusely infiltrate the pericardial space, grossly mimicking mesothelioma. Histologically, fibrosarcoma is composed of compact, spindled cells with little pleomorphism in a collagenized or myxoid matrix (figs. 12-35–12-37). Intracytoplasmic glycogen and perinuclear vacuoles are absent. Immunohistochemically, the tumors stain for vimentin, and variably for actin, but are negative for neural markers, desmin, and cytokeratin. Ultra-

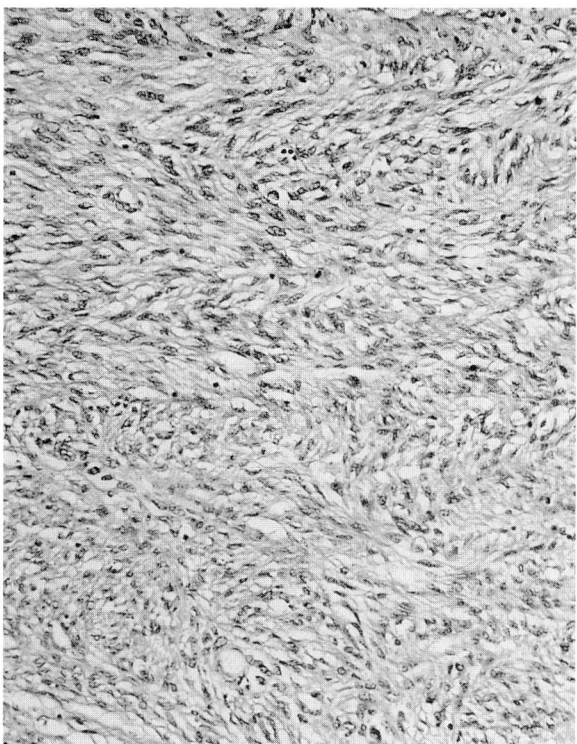

Figure 12-35
FIBROSARCOMA
This tumor, removed from a 60-year-old man with right ventricular outflow obstruction, shows a "herringbone" pattern characteristic of fibrosarcoma.

structurally, the tumor cells resemble fibroblasts. They are elongated with infrequent nucleoli; prominent, dilated rough endoplasmic reticulum; and granular or amorphous cytoplasmic material. Cytoplasmic organelles are sparse, and intracellular microfilaments and basal lamina may be identified. Extracellularly, mature and immature collagen may be present.

The histologic appearance of malignant solitary fibrous tumor of the pericardium is similar to fibrosarcoma. The distinction between these two lesions is made on the basis of gross appearance: the former infiltrates the pericardial space with little myocardial invasion (fig. 12-38). Fibrosarcomas are generally bland undifferentiated lesions of spindle cells (fig. 12-39), although pleomorphic areas may occur.

Differential Diagnosis. Areas indistinguishable from fibrosarcoma may occur in a variety of cardiac tumors. On the basis of routine

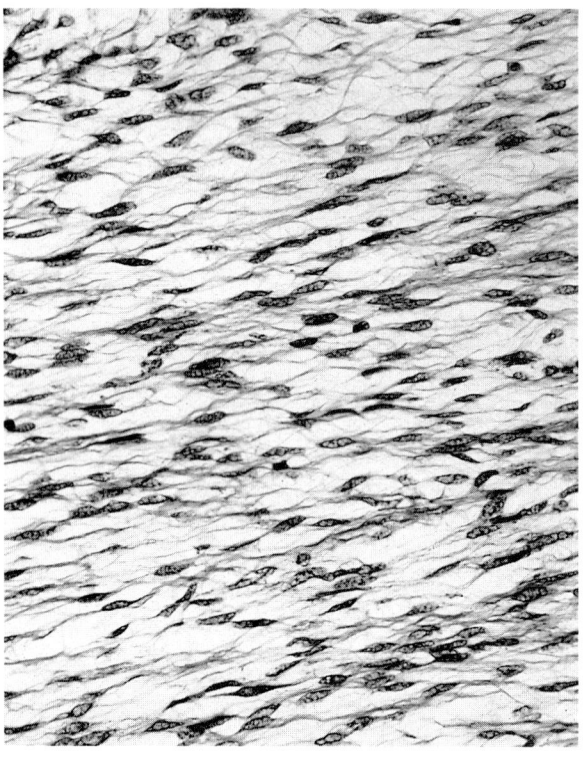

Figure 12-36
FIBROSARCOMA
The cells are spindled, with tapered nuclei and a fine collagenized background.

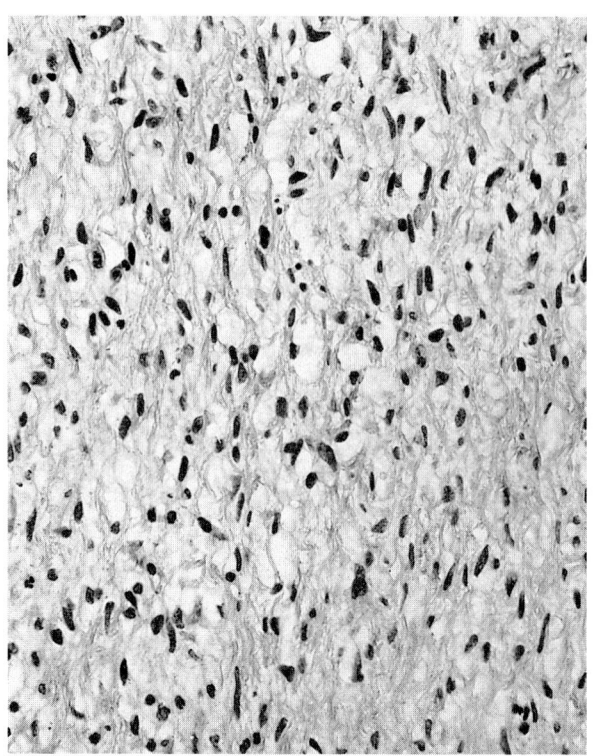

Figure 12-37
FIBROSARCOMA
There is a relatively monomorphous cell population in a collagenized background. The tumor was removed from the left atrium of a 60-year-old woman with recurrent "myxoma."

Figure 12-38
MALIGNANT FIBROUS TUMOR:
PERICARDIUM
Note the fleshy mass with small cysts along the epicardial surface.

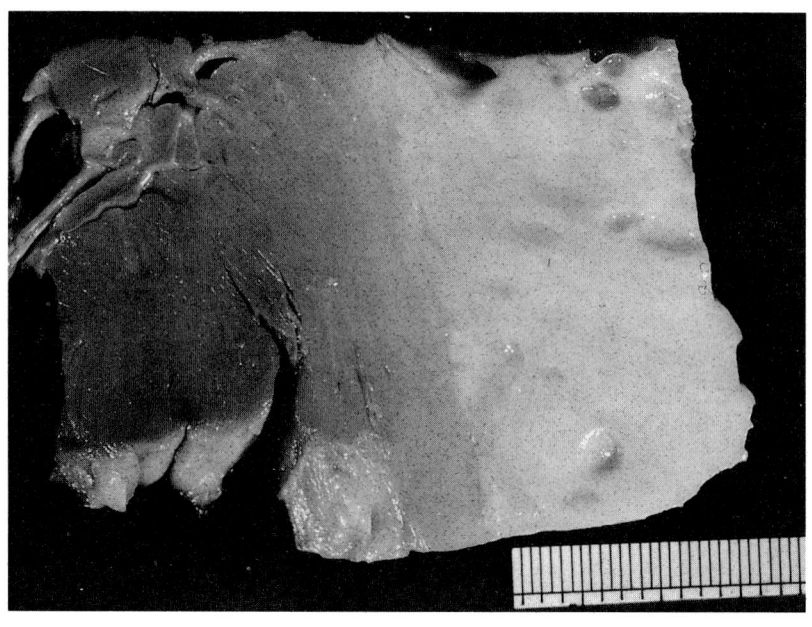

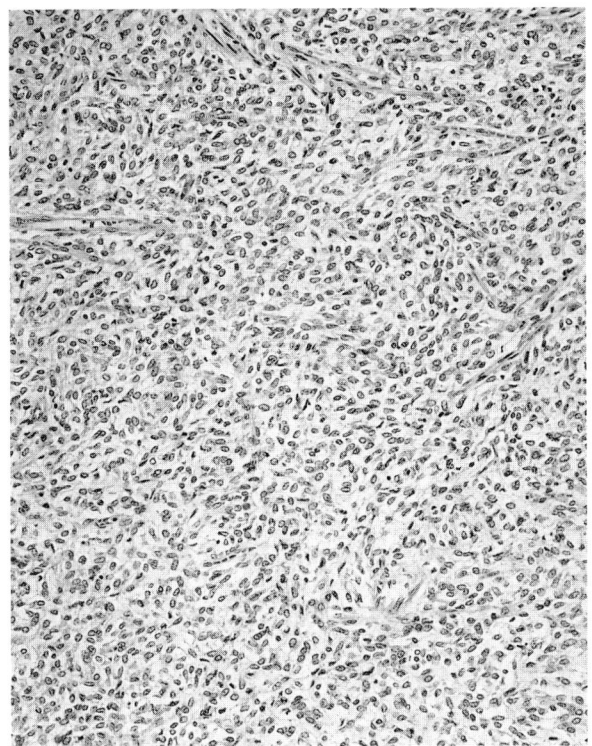

Figure 12-39
MALIGNANT FIBROUS TUMOR: PERICARDIUM
There is a cellular proliferation of bland, fibroblastic cells with rare mitotic figures (not shown). Microscopic illustration of tumor shown grossly in figure 12-38.

stains, neurofibrosarcoma is difficult to differentiate from fibrosarcoma; immunohistochemical stains for S-100 protein are helpful in this regard. The spindled areas of synovial sarcoma, which in our experience is more common in the heart than neurofibrosarcoma, are identical to fibrosarcoma; however, the tumor is usually biphasic and there are clumps or nests of cytokeratin-positive epithelioid cells. Osteosarcomas of the heart generally contain large areas of fibrosarcoma; if osteoid or chondrosarcoma is present, the tumor is classified by these features. Mesotheliomas may likewise mimic fibrosarcoma, but the spindle cells are generally cytokeratin positive and, like synovial sarcoma, they are generally biphasic tumors.

Leiomyosarcoma and fibrosarcoma may be similar histologically. Features favoring leiomyosarcoma are the presence of intracytoplasmic glycogen, perinuclear vacuoles, fascicles running at sharp angles to one another, and

multinucleated or giant cells. Intracytoplasmic desmin, when present, is diagnostic of leiomyosarcoma in a monomorphic spindle cell tumor. Ultrastructurally, leiomyosarcoma cells contain prominent myofilaments and basal lamina, unlike fibrosarcoma.

The distinction between fibrosarcoma and fibroma may be difficult in newborns and infants (see chapter 6). Fibromas in older children and adults, on the other hand, contain abundant collagen, are paucicellular, and are rarely confused with fibrosarcoma.

MYXOSARCOMA

Definition. The term "myxosarcoma" is currently not used in standard classifications for soft tissue tumors (98). Myxosarcoma, and a synonymous term "fibromyxosarcoma," have persisted in the cardiology and thoracic surgery literature because of the concept that benign cardiac myxomas undergo malignant "transformation" to myxosarcoma (101,103). The term myxosarcoma is useful only because it emphasizes that not all myxoid tumors of the atrium are benign myxomas. We restrict the use of the term myxosarcoma to cardiac tumors that are myxoid in all areas sampled, without cellular or vascular patterns diagnostic of MFH, fibrosarcoma, leiomyosarcoma, rhabdomyosarcoma, neurofibrosarcoma, or liposarcoma.

Histogenesis. Myxosarcoma and cardiac myxoma are sometimes considered to represent opposite ends of a biologic spectrum, because both are characterized by accumulations of extracellular proteoglycans and both are typically located in the left atrium. However, there are several reasons to doubt this relationship: there is no good evidence of a sequential transformation of cardiac myxoma to myxosarcoma (see chapter 3); composite tumors consisting of sarcoma and myxoma probably do not exist, and the propensity toward recurrence in cardiac myxoma is not a function of histologic appearance or atypia but depends on hereditary factors (see chapter 3); with the exception of angiosarcomas, most cardiac sarcomas, not only myxosarcomas, arise in the left atrium; and a myxoid background may occur in all types of cardiac sarcomas, and may be a consequence of intracavitary location rather than a reflection of histogenesis.

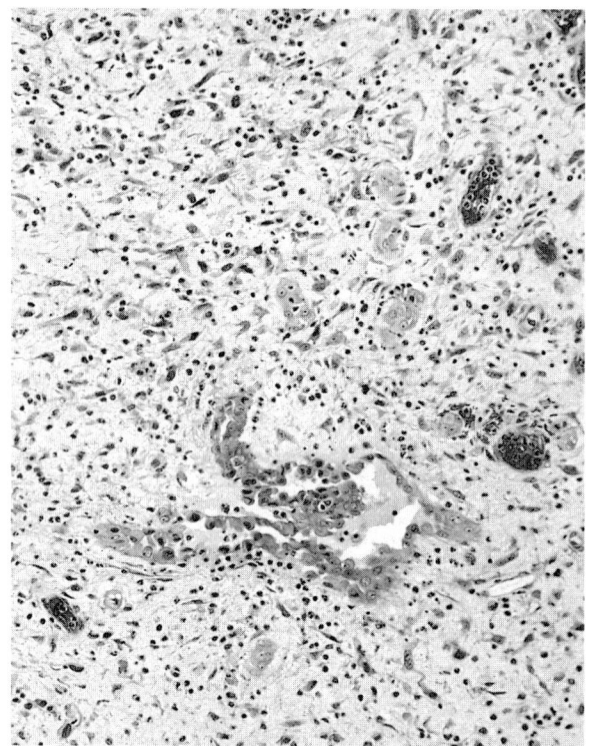

Figure 12-40
MYXOSARCOMA
This tumor was excised from a 27-year-old woman with a left atrial mass clinically diagnosed as myxoma. She died of widespread metastases 48 months postoperatively.

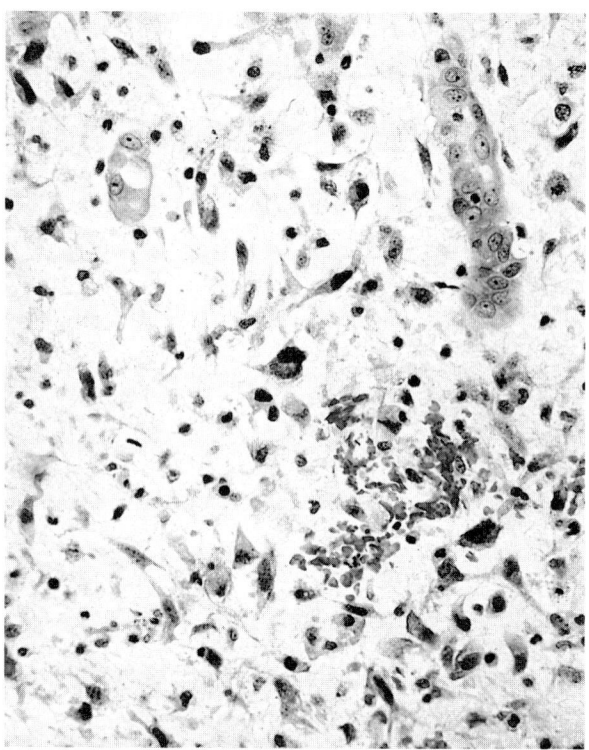

Figure 12-41
MYXOSARCOMA
A higher magnification of the tumor shown in figure 12-40 demonstrates atypical spindled cells with irregular, hyperchromatic nuclei. The atypia and hyperchromasia are not features of myxoma, and characteristic ring- and cord-like structures are absent.

Most cardiac myxosarcomas are indistinguishable from myxoid MFH as described in the soft tissue literature (106), and are probably descendants of the same precursor cell as cardiac MFH.

Clinical Features. Because of different terms and definitions used, it is difficult to interpret descriptions of cardiac myxosarcoma. Myxosarcoma or myxofibrosarcoma has been used to describe seven tumors in a recent series of surgical resections (Table 12-2). All of these patients were women, aged 28 to 56 years at the time of presentation; at the AFIP, a slight female preponderance is also evident (Table 12-3). Most myxosarcomas arise in the left atrium, but right ventricular tumors have also been described. Clinically, they are initially diagnosed as cardiac myxomas, and cause clinical signs and symptoms of mitral stenosis. Survival is generally poor (97,102, 104,105), although one patient in the AFIP files survived 50 months after several local recurrences.

Pathologic Findings. Myxosarcomas are gelatinous, multilobated tumors that are usually sessile endocardial growths. Although they may be grossly indistinguishable from myxoma, they are more likely to be multiple or infiltrate the myocardium. The largest myxosarcoma in the AFIP files measured 5.5 cm at the time of excision and reportedly filled and distended the left atrium.

By definition, myxosarcomas have a diffuse intracellular background of proteoglycans that are amphophilic when stained with hematoxylin and eosin. The cellular component is often quite bland, and is composed of single cells or cells in aggregates that may superficially resemble myxoma cells (figs. 12-40–12-42). More often, sarcoma cells are configured in a loose storiform pattern, with prominent arborizing vessels, and are indistinguishable from myxoid MFH (106). The degree of cellularity varies, but there are invariably foci with atypical hyperchromatic cells. Mitotic figures are

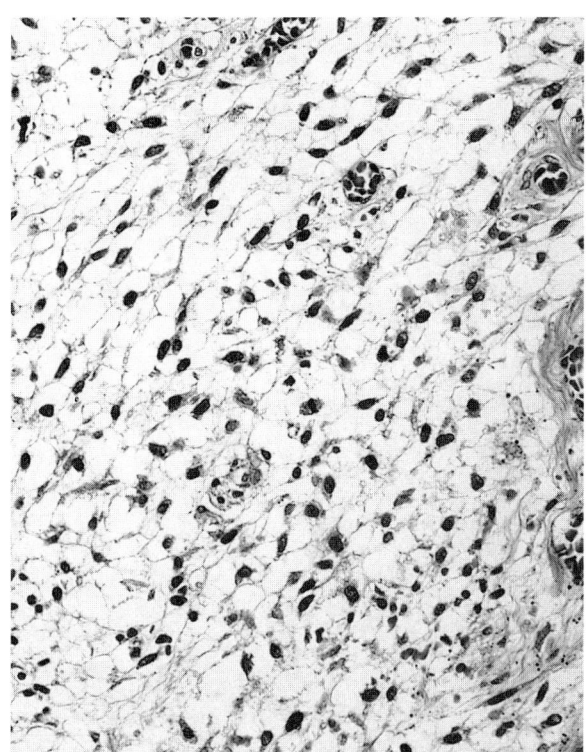

Figure 12-42
MYXOSARCOMA
This tumor consists of a monotonous proliferation of spindled cells in a myxoid matrix; no areas suggestive of MFH were present in several tumor sections. The patient was a 74-year-old woman with a mass obstructing the right ventricular outflow tract and infiltrating the pulmonary valve.

present, especially in atypical areas, and are not confined to the surface of the tumor.

Differential Diagnosis. Because of the gross and histologic similarities, myxosarcoma may be misdiagnosed as myxoma until the tumor recurs, often larger and more atypical than the initial lesion (99,100). The most important histologic criterion in identifying myxosarcoma is the absence of the typical cords, rings, and capillary structures formed by myxoma cells (see chapter 3). In those cases resembling myxoid MFH, arborizing vascular structures not found in myxoma identify the tumor as a sarcoma. Chondroid differentiation is extremely rare in myxoma and should immediately suggest myxoid sarcoma (99,100). Thorough sampling is more important than any special stain. If a myxoid tumor of the heart is not entirely typical of myxoma, the entire specimen should be sectioned to identify infiltration of myocardium or cellular areas diagnostic of a particular histologic type of sarcoma, such as a nonmyxoid type of MFH, osteosarcoma, synovial sarcoma, leiomyosarcoma, or rhabdomyosarcoma.

RHABDOMYOSARCOMA

Definition. Rhabdomyosarcoma is a malignant mesenchymal neoplasm with morphologic or antigenic features of striated muscle.

Incidence. Cardiac rhabdomyosarcoma is a rare neoplasm: in 1988, 77 cases were reviewed from the international literature (110). In current series, rhabdomyosarcoma constitutes 4 to 7 percent of cardiac sarcomas (Tables 12-2, 12-3). Whorton (119) compiled 100 cardiac sarcomas reported before 1948, 9 of which were rhabdomyosarcomas; of 35 sarcomas reported from 1948 to 1960, 8 (24 percent) were rhabdomyosarcomas, the most commonly occurring type of cardiac sarcoma in this time period (117). McAllister and Fenoglio (111) classified 20 percent of cardiac sarcomas in the AFIP files before 1976 as rhabdomyosarcomas. In contrast, no cardiac rhabdomyosarcomas were reported in the Mayo clinic series (118), which is the only series of cardiac sarcomas reported with detailed histologic data.

The reason for the apparent recent decrease in the incidence of cardiac rhabdomyosarcoma relative to other types of sarcoma is unknown. We suspect that in the past many sarcomas were diagnosed as rhabdomyosarcoma without strict documentation of muscle differentiation.

Histogenesis. Unlike cardiac sarcomas with fibrous or smooth muscle differentiation, cardiac rhabdomyosarcoma does not show a predilection for the left atrium. In infantile cases, 35 percent occur in the atrial or ventricular septum; it has been hypothesized that rhabdomyosarcomas in infants arise from congenital rests (110). Validation or further explanation of this theory is lacking, however, and it does not account for the origin of the remaining cases.

Clinical Features. Cardiac rhabdomyosarcoma is slightly more common in males than females, at a ratio of 1.4 to 1 (110). This male predominance is heightened in children: of 17 pediatric cases of cardiac rhabdomyosarcoma, 12 occurred in boys (110). Although it has been stated that no case of rhabdomyosarcoma has been reported in a female infant (110), the AFIP files have one case of a girl who died after 4 hours of life. The mean age at presentation in the second to third decade is earlier than that of other cardiac sarcomas.

Cardiac rhabdomyosarcoma may occur throughout the myocardium (108,112–114,116); either atrium or ventricle may be the primary site. Those in the left atrium may present as a "classic" atrial myxoma clinically and radiologically, and pulmonary symptoms and peripheral edema may occur. Other presenting symptoms include palpitations and symptoms related to pericardial effusion, congestive heart failure, and cerebral embolism (107). Preoperative assessment is facilitated by transesophageal echocardiography (107). Sites of metastatic spread are, in order of descending frequency: lung, regional lymph nodes, central nervous system, gastrointestinal tract, kidney, adrenal gland, thyroid, ovary, bone, and pancreas (110).

Pathologic Findings. Cardiac rhabdomyosarcomas are bulky, invasive tumors that can exceed 10 cm in greatest diameter. Like virtually any cardiac sarcoma, they may be grossly mucoid or gelatinous, similar to cardiac myxoma. However, they are more likely than myxoma to infiltrate the mitral valve and atrial wall.

Histologically, extracardiac rhabdomyosarcomas are divided into embryonal and adult forms. The former are small cell neoplasms with relatively easily identifiable rhabdomyoblasts, and occur primarily in infants, children, and young adults; the latter are more pleomorphic, and quite rare in the heart. Alveolar rhabdomyosarcoma has a characteristic collagenous stroma and a paucity of rhabdomyoblasts. Although relatively common in the soft tissues, it has been described in the heart generally as a metastatic lesion (115). Grape-like structures with a so-called cambium layer characteristic of sarcoma botryoides, another form of embryonal rhabdomyosarcoma, have been also described in cardiac embryonal rhabdomyosarcomas (109).

Embryonal rhabdomyosarcoma may be well differentiated with numerous tadpole-shaped rhabdomyoblasts (figs. 12-43, 12-44). By contrast, round cell tumors (fig. 12-45) have very few rhabdomyoblasts, which are only identified after extensive search. These rhabdomyoblasts contain abundant glycogen and are highlighted by

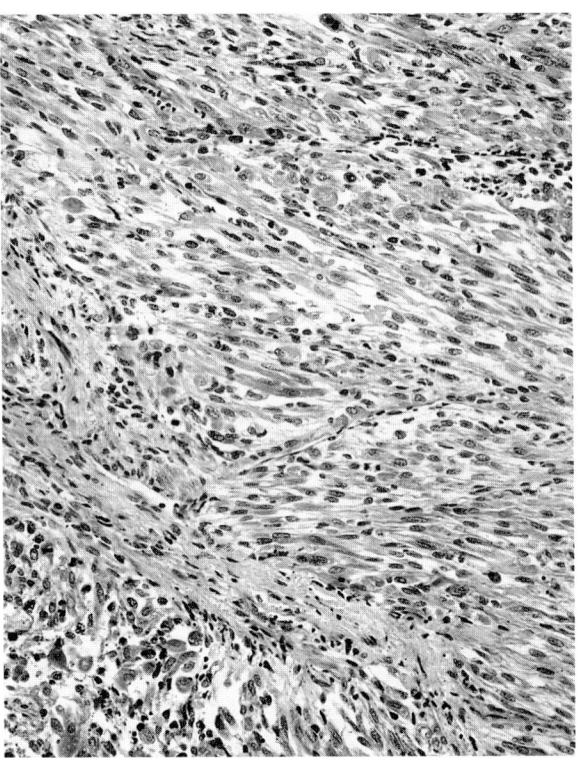

Figure 12-43
RHABDOMYOSARCOMA
Note the spindle cell tumor with abundant cytoplasm. This 24-year-old man had a clinical diagnosis of left atrial myxoma. At surgery, an infiltrative left atrial mass was removed.

periodic acid–Schiff (PAS) stain (figs. 12-46, 12-47). Although the identification of cross striations may be facilitated by histochemical stains (phosphotungstic acid hematoxylin, Masson's trichrome, for example), these stains have been superseded by immunohistochemical techniques. Staining with antibodies against desmin greatly facilitates the diagnosis (fig. 12-48). Myoglobin is also useful in documenting muscular differentiation, but the sensitivity of this antibody is inferior to that of desmin, unless microwave techniques are employed.

Cardiac rhabdomyosarcoma has been reportedly diagnosed by fine needle aspiration (114) and by the identification of cross striations or intracytoplasmic desmin or myoglobin on cytologic smears. Ultrastructurally, the diagnostic features are thick and thin filaments reminiscent of normal striated muscle. Internal A and I banding may or may not be present, but Z-bands are frequently well formed (fig. 12-49). Plentiful

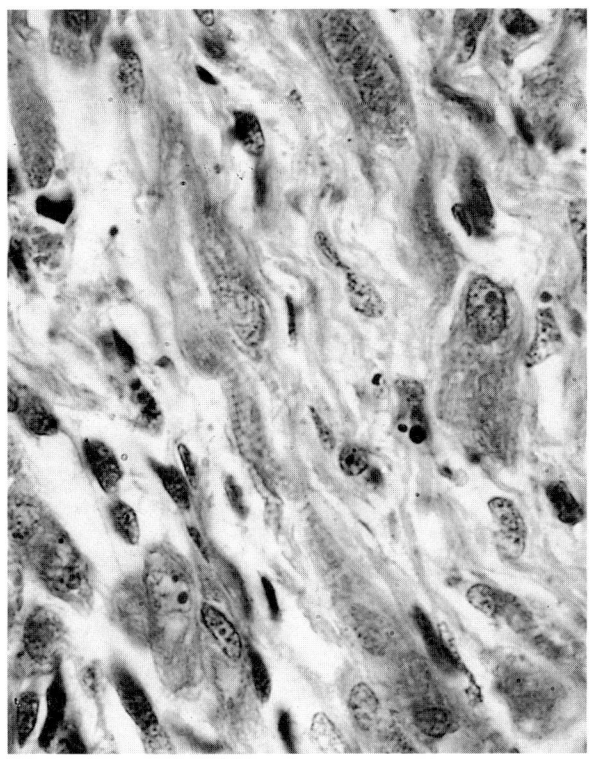

Figure 12-44
RHABDOMYOSARCOMA
Oil immersion photomicrography of the tumor seen in figure 12-43 demonstrates cross striations in some tumor cells.

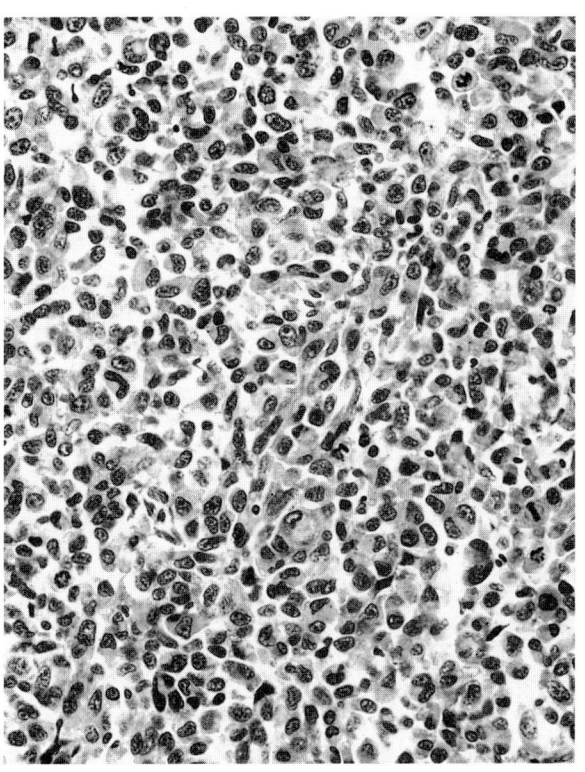

Figure 12-45
RHABDOMYOSARCOMA
This tumor, removed from a 1-year-old child, studded the epicardial surfaces and infiltrated both atria. Rhabdomyoblasts were scarce (not identified in this section).

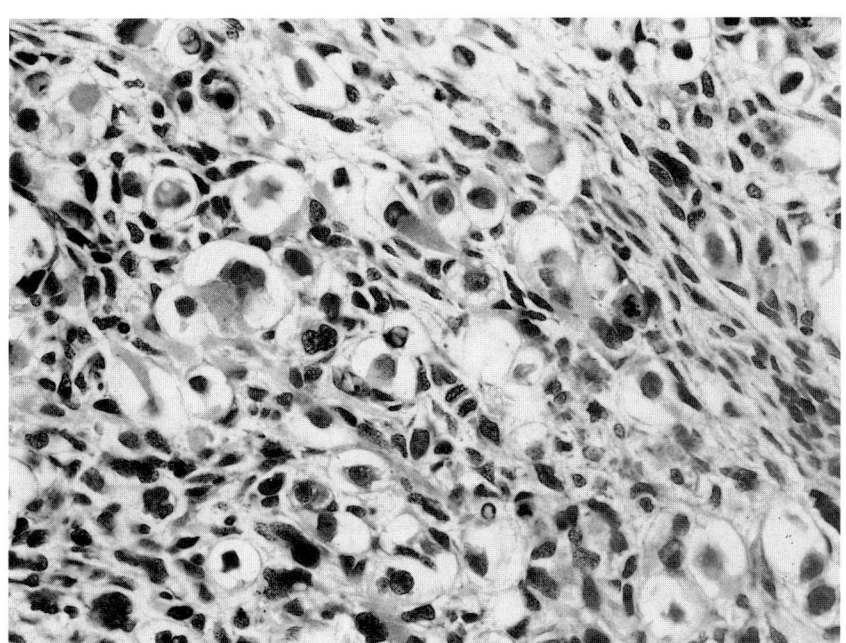

Figure 12-46
RHABDOMYOSARCOMA
Rhabdomyoblasts are identified as scattered cells with abundant cytoplasm within an otherwise undifferentiated embryonal sarcoma.

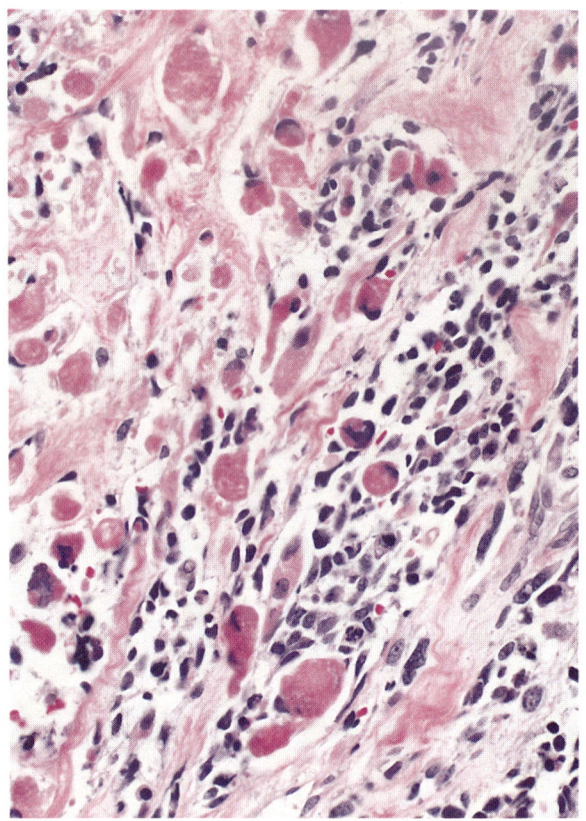

Figure 12-47
RHABDOMYOSARCOMA
In this field, rhabdomyoblasts with abundant eosino-philic cytoplasm are unusually numerous. This tumor was resected from the right atrium and superior vena cava of a young woman with superior vena cava syndrome.

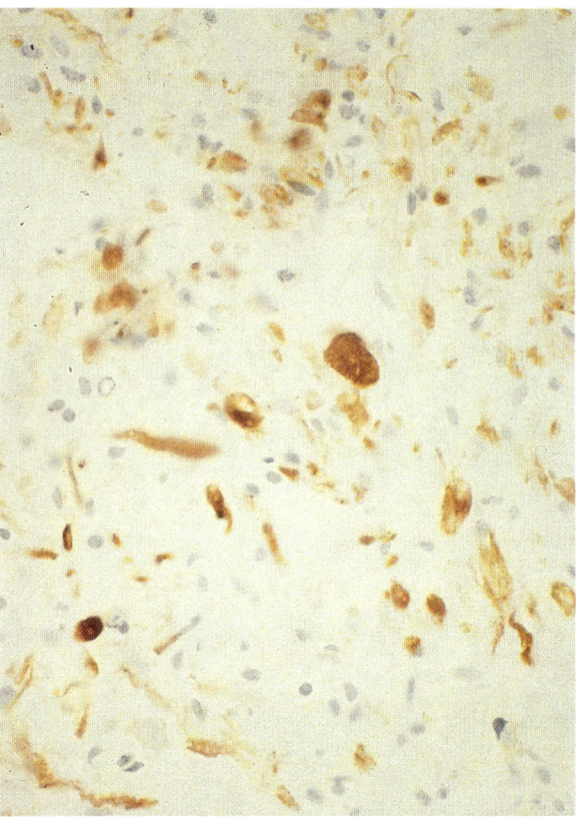

Figure 12-48
RHABDOMYOSARCOMA:
IMMUNOHISTOCHEMICAL STAIN FOR DESMIN
This photomicrograph demonstrates expression of desmin in the tumor cells illustrated in figure 12-47.

glycogen granules and abundant mitochondria are also present. Tumor nuclei are lobulated, containing variable amounts of condensed chromatin. Occasionally, several grids must be examined before rhabdomyoblasts are identified.

Differential Diagnosis. Rhabdomyosarcoma may be confused with undifferentiated sarcomas, especially the small cell type. Immunohistochemical detection of desmin identifies the rhabdomyoblasts, which are the key to the diagnosis. Leiomyosarcomas may also express desmin, but lack myoglobin and differ ultrastructurally from rhabdomyosarcoma (see section on leiomyosarcoma). Their morphologic appearance is usually quite different than rhabdomyosarcoma: they are composed of relatively well-differentiated, elongated spindled cells, with finely dispersed glycogen, rather than the clumped glycogen present in rhabdomyoblasts.

Treatment and Prognosis. Similar to surgical treatment for other cardiac tumors, atrial reconstruction with synthetic grafts may be necessary for complete tumor excision. Although there is little follow-up data in patients with cardiac rhabdomyosarcoma, there is a suggestion that prognosis is better than for other histologic types (Table 12-2). Combination chemotherapy, such as cytoxan, vincristine, and actinomycin D, may be given postoperatively.

SYNOVIAL SARCOMA

Definition. Synovial sarcoma is a biphasic tumor composed of spindled and epithelioid areas, and characterized by an X;18 chromosomal translocation. Although most are located near joint spaces, several synovial sarcomas in locations remote from synovial-lined spaces, including the

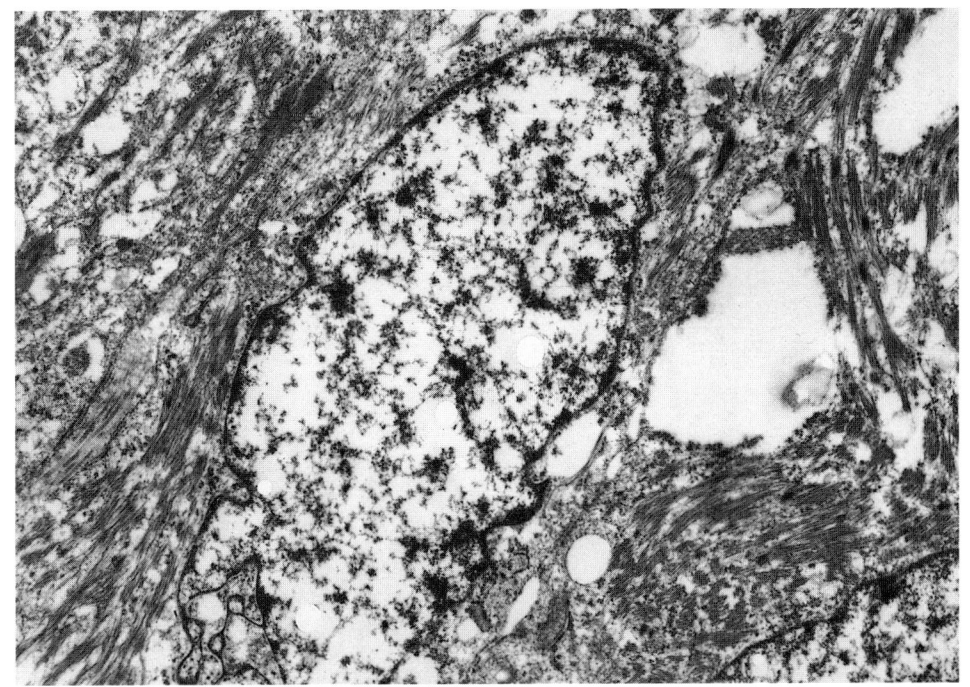

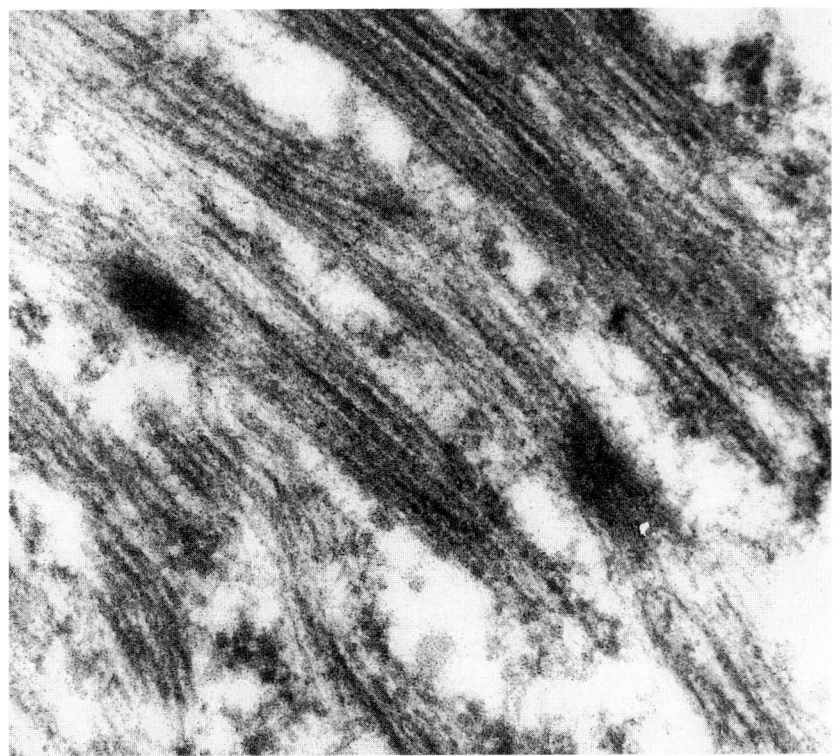

Figure 12-49
RHABDOMYOSARCOMA

Top: A 12-year-old boy had a right atrial mass. Routine histologic examination demonstrated an undifferentiated sarcoma that expressed myoglobin (not shown); electron microscopy demonstrated Z-bands indicative of myofibrils within tumor cells.
Bottom: A higher magnification demonstrates Z-bands.

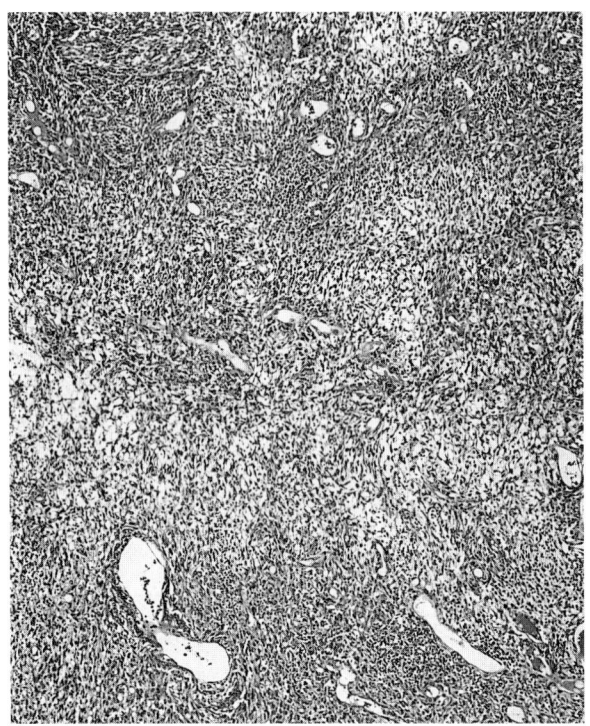

Figure 12-50
SYNOVIAL SARCOMA
This is a spindle cell tumor with cellular and hypocellular areas. This 48-year-old man had recurrent pericardial effusions. A circumscribed pericardial mass was removed; no other primary was found at autopsy 2 years later.

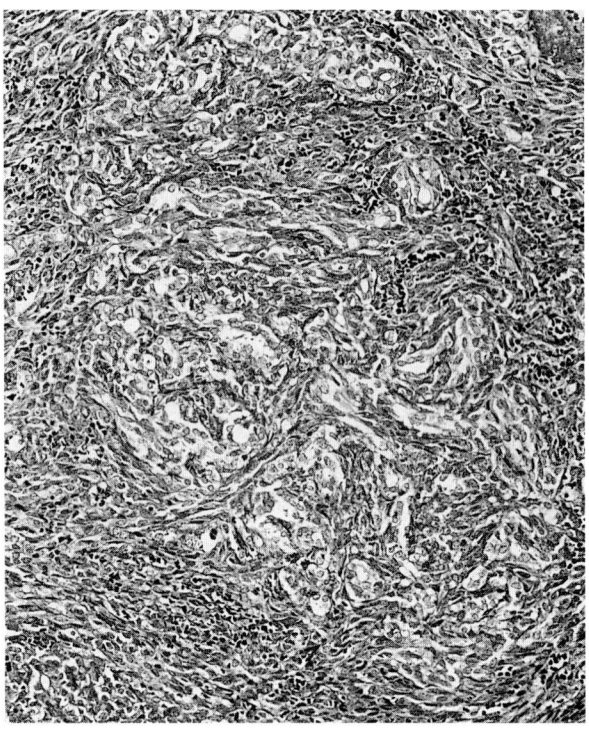

Figure 12-51
SYNOVIAL SARCOMA
This is a higher magnification of figure 12-50 demonstrating nests of epithelioid cells.

mediastinum, have been reported (123). The cell of origin is unknown.

Incidence. The existence of cardiac synovial sarcoma has only recently been recognized; there are but a handful of reported cases (120–122).

Clinical Features. Synovial sarcomas of the heart affect young and middle-aged adults of both sexes. Cardiac sites include the pericardium, right ventricle, right atrium, and left atrium (120–122); in the few cases reported, no particular cardiac site predominates.

Pathologic Findings. Synovial sarcomas are bulky tumors that infiltrate the myocardium and pericardial surfaces. Histologically, there is a biphasic pattern in synovial sarcomas reported in the heart. The spindle component is indistinguishable from fibrosarcoma, and alternating cellular and edematous areas are typical (fig. 12-50). The spindle cells are small, compact, and often infiltrated by sparse mononuclear lymphoid cells. The epithelioid cells form clusters

and nests (fig. 12-51), and occasionally larger branching structures. Histochemically, PAS-positive diastase-resistant mucin may be present within the epithelial areas. Immunohistochemically, cytokeratin is strongly expressed in the epithelial cells in a diffuse distribution (fig. 12-52); staining of the spindle cells with this antibody is weaker and more focal (123).

Differential Diagnosis. Differentiating between synovial sarcoma and mesothelioma of the heart is problematic. The characteristic X;18 translocation, presumptive evidence of synovial sarcoma, has been demonstrated in cardiac synovial sarcoma (121). Tumor cell cultures are rarely obtained for cytogenetic studies, however. In our experience in limited cases, mesothelioma diffusely infiltrates the pericardial space with little infiltration of myocardium whereas synovial sarcoma is a relatively circumscribed, solitary lesion which may or may not involve the pericardium. Staining for cytokeratin may reveal sharper demarcations between epithelioid and spindled areas in synovial sarcoma than in mesothelioma.

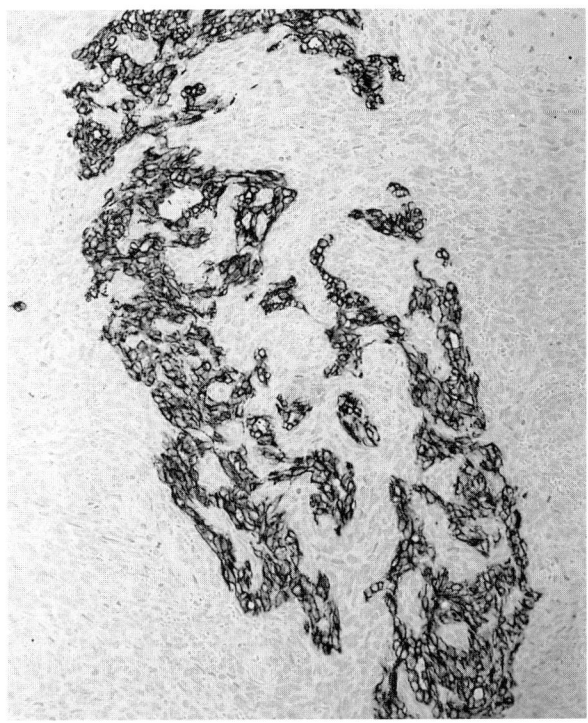

Figure 12-52
SYNOVIAL SARCOMA
Immunohistochemical preparation using antibodies to cytokeratin demonstrate positivity in epithelioid cells and a lack of positivity in surrounding spindle cells.

Finally, the spindled cells in most mesotheliomas are larger and more pleomorphic than those of synovial sarcoma. We agree with Witkin et al. (123) that synovial sarcomas near mesothelial-lined cavities are impossible to diagnose with certainty, but that the diagnosis is favored for a solitary mass with a histologic pattern identical to synovial sarcoma.

LIPOSARCOMA

Definition. Liposarcoma is a malignant mesenchymal neoplasm that contains lipoblasts.

Incidence. Liposarcomas of the heart are very rare and are not represented in most surgical series of cardiac tumors (Table 12-2). Approximately 12 cases have been reported (130).

Clinical Features. Cardiac liposarcoma is a tumor of adults: the mean age at presentation is approximately 53 years. There is no apparent sex predilection (130). Most cases are in the right or left atrium (124,125,127–129), although tumors of the mitral valve, right ventricle, and

pericardium have been described (124,130). The most common presenting symptoms are those related to congestive heart failure and atrial arrhythmias. Like virtually all types of cardiac sarcoma, cardiac liposarcoma can mimic myxoma clinically (129). Metastatic sites include liver, skeleton, lung, and central nervous system. The mean survival of reported cases is 8.3 months, with a range of 2 to 24 months.

Pathologic Findings. Grossly, cardiac liposarcomas are bulky tumors (see fig. 12-2) that often fill the atrium, may contain cysts, and are soft and bosselated. Tumors as large as 10 cm have been reported (128). Multiple tumor implants may be present on the surface of the great vessels, and extensive pericardial growth may result in cardiac tamponade (124).

Histologically, liposarcomas of the heart are similar to those of extracardiac soft tissue. Pleomorphic tumors contain cellular areas resembling MFH or fibrosarcoma and the lipoblasts have multiple vacuoles indenting the cell nuclei (figs. 12-53, 12-54). Approximately 50 percent of cardiac liposarcomas have been reported as myxoid liposarcoma: these tumors have a characteristic prominent plexiform maze of thin-walled capillaries. Lipoblasts of myxoid liposarcoma are signet ring cells; the single large fat vacuoles indent the nucleus, which forms a crescent (figs. 12-55, 12-56). In some cases, lipoblasts are scarce; in these cases, however, there is an easily recognized vascular pattern (126). In those tumors with a poorly developed capillary network, lipoblasts are plentiful (fig. 12-55). Several cardiac liposarcomas have areas of both myxoid and pleomorphic types, and the pleomorphism may increase in recurrent tumors (129).

Ultrastructurally, numerous nonmembrane-bound lipid droplets of variable size fill the cytoplasm and are associated with a large number of mitochondria (125). The nucleus is large, indented, and located at the cell periphery. Immunohistochemically, the lipoblasts may express S-100 protein.

Differential Diagnosis. Lipomatous hypertrophy of the interatrial septum may result in a large mass that, at surgery, suggests a liposarcoma. Histologically, however, the diagnosis is straightforward. In lipomatous hypertrophy, there are finely vacuolated cells resembling brown fat, and an absence of lipoblasts or a

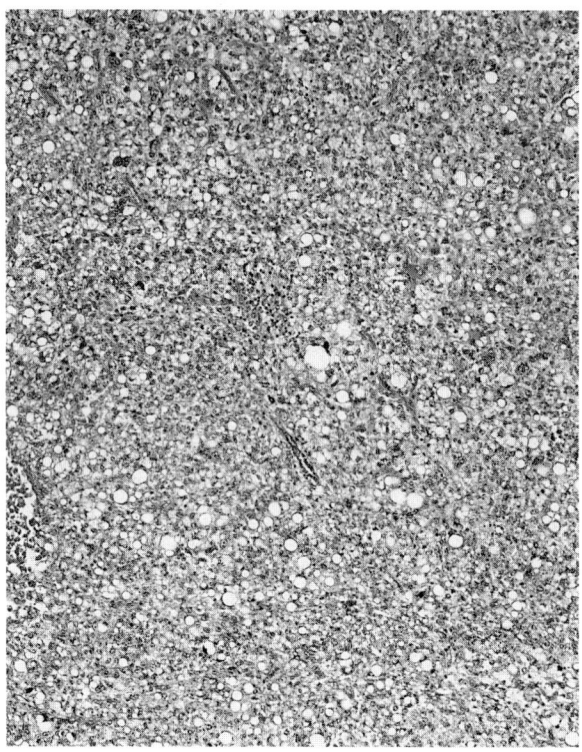

Figure 12-53
LIPOSARCOMA
A 64-year-old man with back pain had surgical excision of a right atrial mass. There was a pleomorphic sarcoma with vacuolated cells. The patient died with bony metastases.

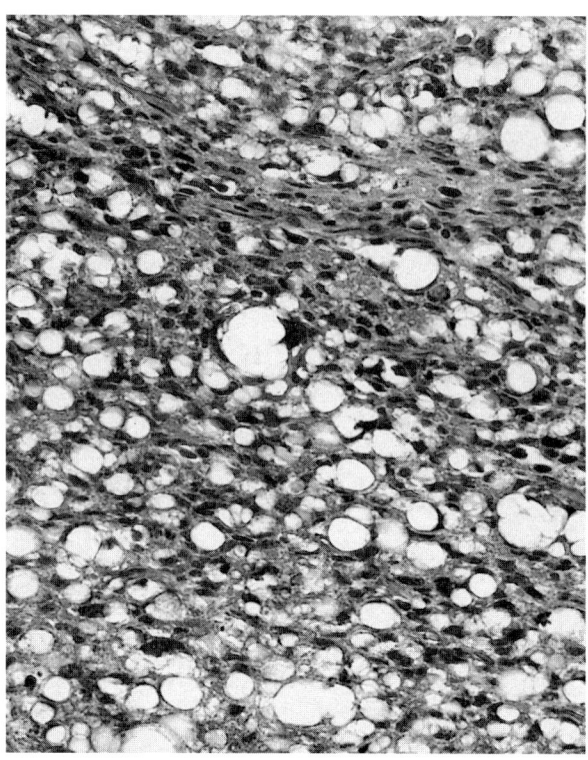

Figure 12-54
LIPOSARCOMA
A higher magnification of the tumor illustrated in figure 12-53 demonstrates large cytoplasmic vacuoles indenting the nuclear outline.

Figure 12-55
LIPOSARCOMA
There are numerous lipoblasts with vacuolated cytoplasm. This tumor was removed from the right atrium of a 70-year-old woman with congestive heart failure and pericardial effusion.

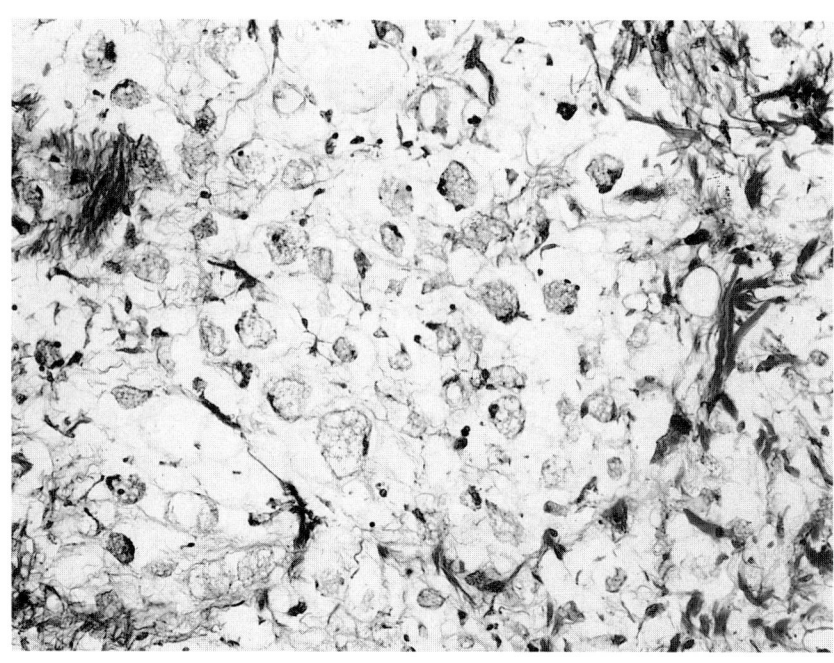

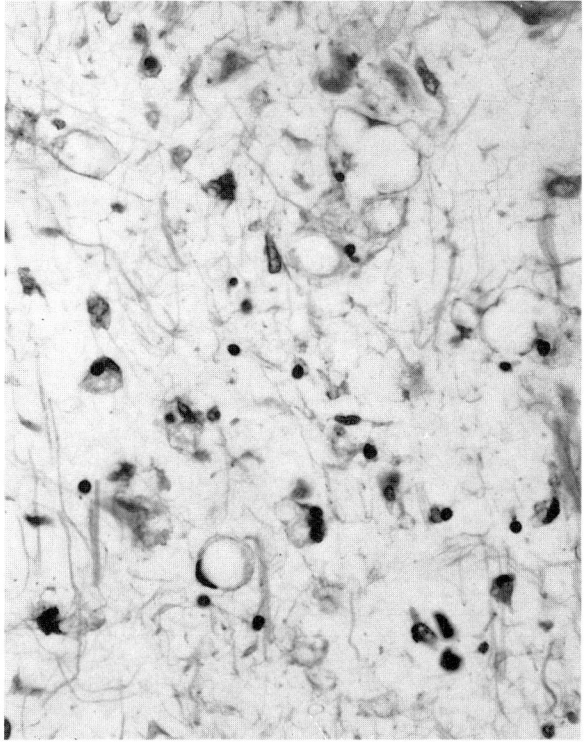

Figure 12-56
LIPOSARCOMA
A different area of the tumor shown in figure 12-55 shows
a signet ring lipoblast in a myxoid background.

myxoid background. In addition, interspersed hypertrophied myocytes are typically present, a feature lacking in liposarcoma.

Myxoid liposarcoma may resemble myxosarcoma or myxoid MFH. If there is a prominent capillary vascular background, the diagnosis of myxoid liposarcoma should be strongly considered and an extensive search for lipoblasts undertaken. In the absence of a plexiform capillary pattern, signet ring cell lipoblasts are easily identified if the tumor is a liposarcoma.

Lipid droplets that stain with oil red O may be present in MFH as well as liposarcoma. In at least one reported case of cardiac myxoid liposarcoma (130), neither a vascular pattern nor characteristic lipoblasts were identified, casting doubt on the diagnosis, which was based solely on the presence of cytoplasmic lipid.

Pleomorphic liposarcoma may resemble MFH or undifferentiated sarcoma. Lipoblasts are

present in liposarcoma, especially in myxoid, highly vascular areas. Cells of MFH may also contain vacuoles and lipid droplets within the cytoplasm, but these are Alcian blue positive, unlike the vacuoles of lipoblasts (126).

MALIGNANT SCHWANNOMA

Although malignant schwannomas (malignant peripheral nerve sheath tumor) metastatic to the heart have been reported (133), primary cardiac sarcomas with neurofibrosarcomatous differentiation are distinctly rare (131). McAllister and Fenoglio (134) reported four cases of cardiac neurofibrosarcoma, but did not demonstrate neurogenic differentiation by ultrastructural or immunohistochemical methods. Two recent cardiac sarcomas in the AFIP files are classified as malignant schwannomas, and in one there are also areas of rhabdomyosarcoma, indicating a so-called malignant Triton's tumor. One report of pericardial neurofibrosarcoma demonstrated ultrastructural features of neurogenic differentiation (135). Recently, a pericardial sarcoma positive for S-100 protein was described, but its precise taxonomy was elusive (132).

Histologically, malignant schwannomas are composed of tapered spindled cells with a plexiform pattern, a neural appearance (fig. 12-57), and irregular nuclear outlines (fig. 12-58). The diagnosis rests on the demonstration of neural antigens or origin within a epicardial nerve.

MALIGNANT MESENCHYMOMA

Because the putative cell of origin of cardiac sarcomas is the undifferentiated mesenchymal cell, it is not surprising that sarcomas with multiple forms of differentiation occur in the heart. By definition, malignant mesenchymoma contains two or more distinct types of cellular differentiation; these types of differentiation must be in addition to fibrosarcoma or MFH. Rhabdofibrosarcoma and neurofibrosarcoma occurring in the same tumor indicates a malignant Triton's tumor (see section on neurofibrosarcoma). Approximately 15 cases of cardiac malignant mesenchymoma have appeared in the literature, although in some cases divergent differentiation was not documented convincingly (138). The concomitant types of sarcoma were combinations of

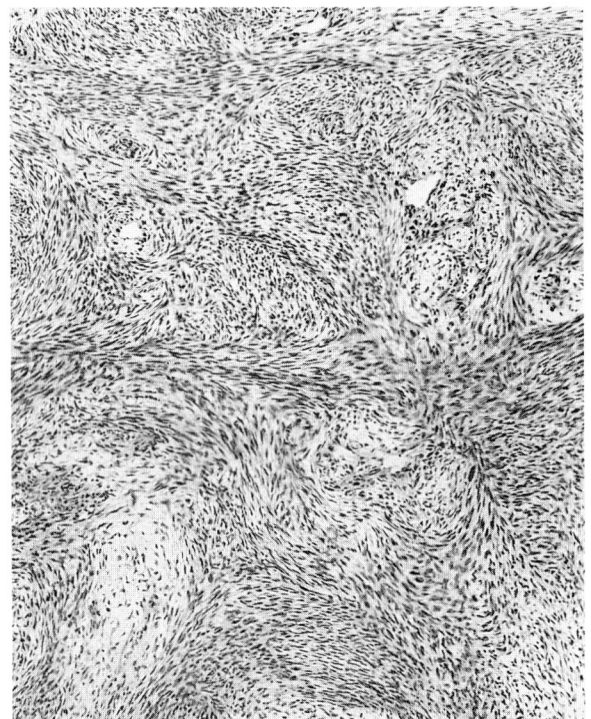

Figure 12-57
MALIGNANT SCHWANNOMA (MALIGNANT
PERIPHERAL NERVE SHEATH TUMOR)
This spindle cell neoplasm has a sweeping, plexiform growth pattern with a neural appearance.

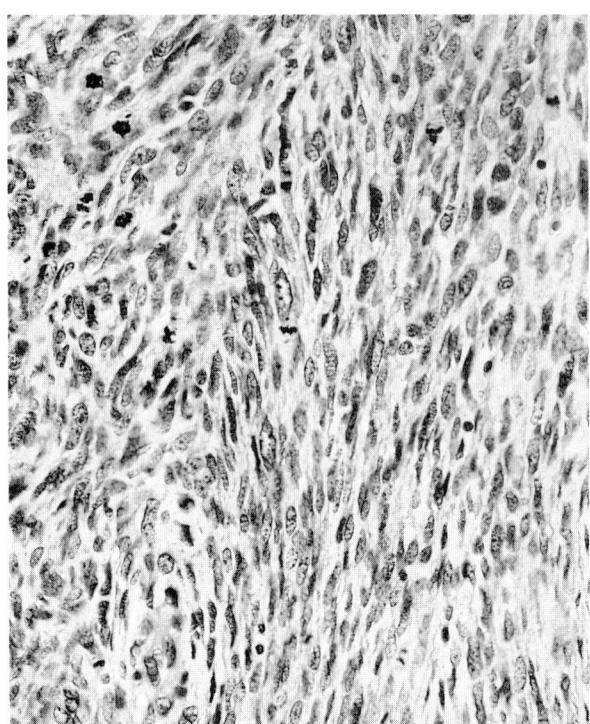

Figure 12-58
MALIGNANT SCHWANNOMA (MALIGNANT
PERIPHERAL NERVE SHEATH TUMOR)
The cellular features of this neoplasm, which is depicted at lower magnification in figure 12-57, are nonspecific. There are often irregularities in the nuclear contour. The diagnosis depends on the demonstration of neural markers or origin from a nerve. This tumor was a large epicardial nodule in a 59-year-old man. There was focal positivity for S-100 protein (not shown).

two or three of the following: osteosarcoma/chondrosarcoma, rhabdomyosarcoma, angiosarcoma, and liposarcoma (139). The mean age at presentation of patients with cardiac malignant mesenchymoma is 42 years (range, 26 to 60 years), and there is a 2 to 1 female predominance. Some of these tumors have been reported in patients with von Recklinghausen's neurofibromatosis (136). Cardiac mesenchymomas typically occur in the left atrium or mitral valve (137); those reported in the pulmonary trunk (136) are better considered intimal sarcoma (see chapter 16). The mean survival period of 12 patients was 20 months (136).

MALIGNANT RHABDOID TUMOR

Malignant rhabdoid tumor is a highly malignant, undifferentiated tumor of infants and children. Although originally described in the kidney, these tumors occur in many organs, including the heart (142). Although rhabdoid tumors superficially resemble embryonal

rhabdomyosarcoma, immunohistochemical studies fail to demonstrate myogenic differentiation. Ultrastructurally, there are masses of intermediate filaments; these give a rhabdomyoblastic appearance to the tumor cells when stained with hematoxylin and eosin. It is not certain whether these tumors are a distinct entity, since similar cells have been demonstrated in MFH and epithelial tumors (140). Recently, immunohistochemical and gene expression studies performed on cell cultures of two rhabdoid tumors have suggested a relationship between these unusual tumors and primitive neuroectodermal tumors (141). In one undifferentiated sarcoma in the AFIP files, ultrastructural features of rhabdoid cells were present; however, until these tumors are better characterized, we prefer to classify them in the undifferentiated category.

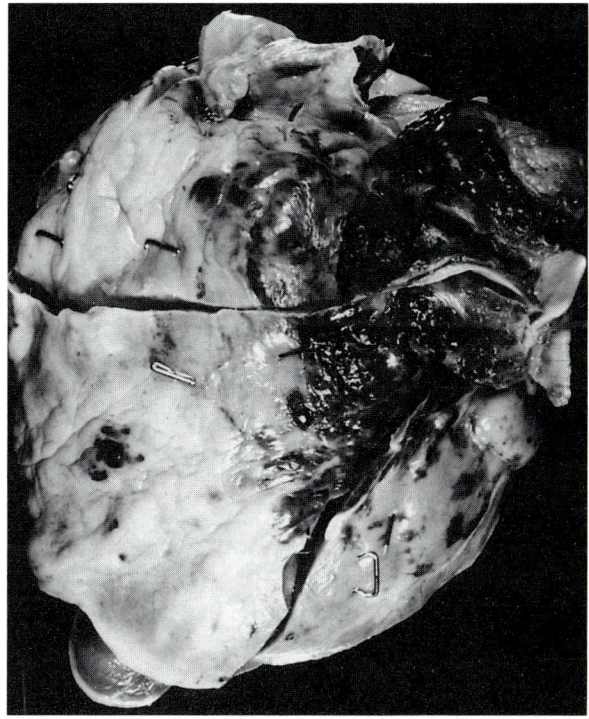

Figure 12-59
KAPOSI'S SARCOMA

The gross appearance of Kaposi's sarcoma is characterized by multiple, small epicardial nodules that are hemorrhagic and do not extensively infiltrate the heart. (Fig. 1 from Steigman CK, Anderson DW, Macher AM, Sennesh JD, Virmani R. Fatal cardiac tamponade in acquired immunodeficiency syndrome with epicardial Kaposi's sarcoma. Am Heart J 1988;116:1105–7.)

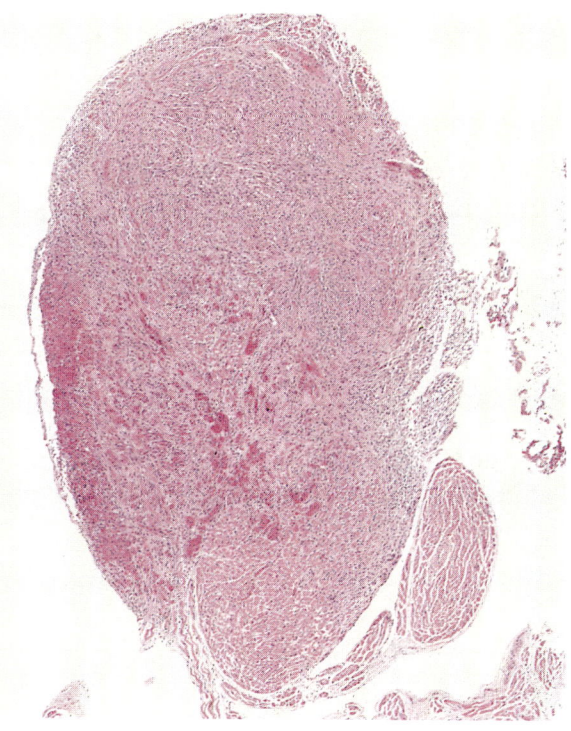

Figure 12-60
KAPOSI'S SARCOMA

Photomicrograph of tumor illustrated in figure 12-59 demonstrates hemorrhagic foci in papillary muscle. (Fig. 2 from Steigman CK, Anderson DW, Macher AM, Sennesh JD, Virmani R. Fatal cardiac tamponade in acquired immunodeficiency syndrome with epicardial Kaposi's sarcoma. Am Heart J 1988;116:1105–7.)

KAPOSI'S SARCOMA

Kaposi's sarcoma of the heart occurs in patients with skin and other visceral lesions in both the classic and epidemic forms of the disease (144). In patients with acquired immunodeficiency syndrome (AIDS), Kaposi's sarcoma of the heart occurs in about 5 percent of autopsy cases. Rarely, the heart is the sole site of involvement (143). The epicardium and pericardium are mainly involved, with minimal myocardial infiltration. In patients with cardiac involvement by Kaposi's sarcoma, significant clinical symptoms are rare. Fatal cardiac tamponade secondary to hemorrhagic effusion and heart failure without ventricular dilatation have been reported. Grossly, there are focal, small, firm, red-brown nodules that may coalesce (figs. 12-59–12-61). The histologic features are usually those of a late-stage lesion, because they are rarely diagnosed during life.

Seven reported cases of primary invasive Kaposi's sarcoma of the heart in immunocompetent individuals were reviewed by Janigan et al. (144). Because of their histologic and clinical similarities to angiosarcoma, these cases were probably spindled variants of angiosarcomas and not true Kaposi sarcomas (144). Spindled areas of angiosarcoma can mimic Kaposi's sarcoma, although typical PAS-positive eosinophilic hyaline globules are generally absent.

MALIGNANT HEMANGIOPERICYTOMA

Hemangiopericytomas are neoplasms of pericytes; benign and malignant examples have been described in the heart. This entity is described in chapter 7.

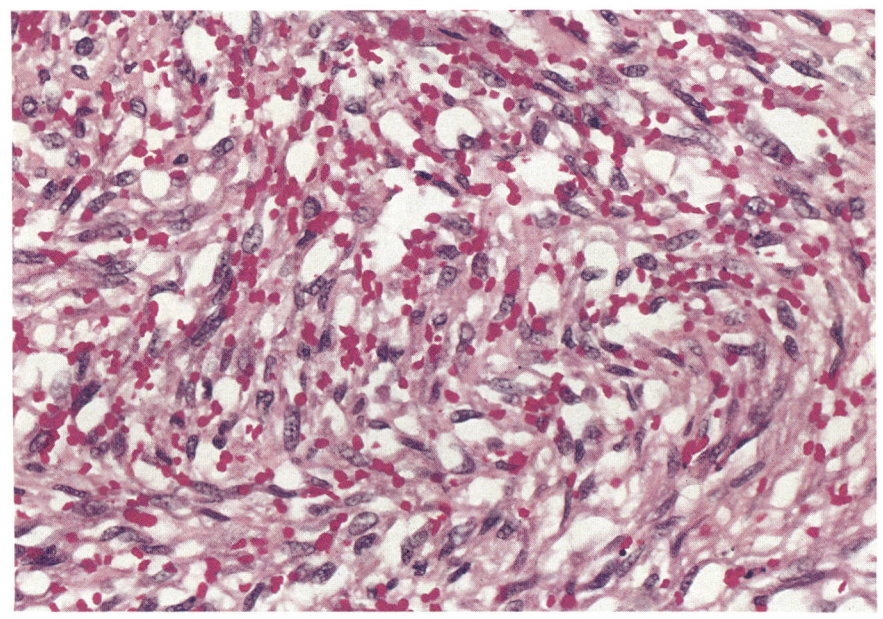

Figure 12-61
KAPOSI'S SARCOMA
Diagnostic area of tumor showing slit-like vascular spaces and atypical spindled and endothelial cells.

REFERENCES

Overview

1. Aravot DJ, Banner NR, Madden B, et al. Primary cardiac tumours—is there a place for cardiac transplantation? Eur J Cardiothorac Surg 1989;3:521–4.

2. Arcienegas E, Hakimi M, Farooki ZQ, Truccone NJ, Green EW. Primary cardiac tumors in children. J Thorac Cardiovasc Surg 1980;79:582–91.

3. Attum AA, Johnson GS, Masri Z, Girardet R, Lansing AM. Malignant clinical behaviour of cardiac mysomas and myxoid imitators. Ann Thorac Surg 1987;44:217–22.

4. Awad M, Dunn B, al Halees Z, Mercer E. Intracardiac rhabdomyosarcoma: transesophageal echocardiographic findings and diagnosis. J Am Soc Echocardiogr 1992;5:199–202.

5. Bear PA, Moodie DS. Malignant primary cardiac tumors. The Cleveland Clinic experience, 1956 to 1986. Chest 1987;92:860–2.

6. Blondeau P. Primary cardiac tumors—French studies of 533 cases. Thorac Cardiovasc Surg 1990;38:192–5.

7. Burke AP, Cowan D, Virmani R. Primary sarcomas of the heart. Cancer 1992;69:387–95.

8. Chan HS, Sonley MJ, Moes CA, Daneman A, Smith CR, Martin DJ. Primary and secondary tumors of childhood involving the heart, pericardium, and great vessels. A report of 75 cases and review of the literature. Cancer 1985;15:825–36.

9. Chomette G, Auriol M, Cabrol C, Tranbaloc P. Primary malignant tumors of the heart. Anatomo-clinical study of 12 cases. Ann Med Interne (Paris) 1985;136:301–5.

10. Dein JR, Frist WH, Stinson EB, et al. Primary cardiac neoplasms. Early and late results of surgical treatment in 42 patients. J Thorac Cardiovasc Surg 1987;93:502–11.

11. Enzinger FM, Weiss SW. General considerations. In: Enzinger FM, Weiss SW, eds. Soft tissue tumors. St. Louis: C.V. Mosby Co. 1988:1–18.

12. Faught PR, Waller BF, Hull MT. Spindle cell sarcoma of the heart in childhood: light microscopic, ultrastructural, and immunohistochemical evidence for smooth muscle, endothelial and fibroblastic differentiations. Pediatr Pathol 1988;8:649–56.

13. Flipse TR, Tazelaar HD, Holmes DR Jr. Diagnosis of malignant cardiac disease by endomyocardial biopsy. Mayo Clin Proc 1990;65:1415–22.

14. Hausheer FH, Josephson RA, Grochow LB, Weissman D, Brinker JA, Weisman HF. Intracardiac sarcoma diagnosed by left ventricular endomyocardial biopsy. Chest 1987;92:177–9.

15. Herhusky MJ, Gregg SB, Virmani R, Chun PK, Bender H, Gray GF Jr. Cardiac sarcomas presenting as metastatic disease. Arch Pathol Lab Med 1985;109:943–5.

16. Hui KS, Green LK, Schmidt WA. Primary cardiac rhabdomyosarcoma: definition of a rare entity. Am J Cardiovasc Pathol 1988;2:19–29.

17. Isner JM, Falcone MW, Virmani R, Roberts WC. Cardiac sarcoma causing ASH and simulating coronary heart disease. Am J Med 1979;66:1025–30.

18. Kim EE, Wallace S, Abello R, et al. Malignant cardiac fibrous histiocytomas and angiosarcomas: MR features. J Comput Assist Tomogr 1989;13:627–32.

19. Lazarus KH, D'Orsogna DE, Bloom KR, Rouse RH. Primary pericardial sarcoma in a neonate. Am J Pediatr Hematol Oncol 1989;11:343–7.

20. Loffler H, Grille W. Classification or malignant cardiac tumors with respect to oncological treatment. Thorac Cardiovasc Surgeon 1990;38:173–5.
21. Ludomirsky A, Vargo TA, Murphy DJ, Gresik MV, Ott DA, Mullins CE. Intracardiac undifferentiated sarcoma in infancy. J Am Coll Cardiol 1985;6:1362–4.
22. Mahar LJ, Lie JT, Groover RV, Sweard JB, Puga F, Feldt RH. Primary cardiac myxosarcoma in a child. Mayo Clin Proc 1979;54:261–6.
23. Miralles A, Bracamonte L, Soncul H, et al. Cardiac tumors: Clinical experience and surgical results in 74 patients. Ann Thorac Surg 1991;52:886–95.
24. Moriarty AT, Nelson WA, McGahey B. Fine needle aspiration of rhabdomyosarcoma of the heart. Light and electron microscopic findings and histologic correlation. Acta Cytol 1990;34:74–8.
25. Murphy MC, Sweeney MS, Putnam JB Jr, et al. Surgical treatment of cardiac tumors: a 25-year experience. Ann Thorac Surg 1990;49:612–7.
26. Prichard RW. Tumors of the heart. Review of the subject and report of one hundred and fifty cases. Arch Pathol 1951;51:98–128.
27. Putnam JB Jr, Sweeney MS, Colon R, Lanza LA, Frazier OH, Cooley DA. Primary cardiac sarcomas. Ann Thorac Surg 1991;5:906–10.
28. Reece IJ, Cooley DA, Frazier OH, Hallman GL, Powers PL, Montero GC. Cardiac tumors. Clinical spectrum and prognosis of lesions other than classical benign myxoma in 20 patients. J Thorac Cardiovasc Surg 1984;88:439–46.
29. Shah AA, Churg A, Sbarbaro JA, Sheppard JM, Lamberi J. Malignant fibrous histiocytoma of the heart presenting as an atrial myxoma. Cancer 1978;42:2466–71.
30. Shechter M, Glikson M, Agranat O, Motro M. Echocardiographic demonstration of mitral block caused by left atrial spindle cell sarcoma. Am Heart J 1992;1234:232–4.
31. Siebenmann R, Jenni R, Makek M, Oelz O, Turina M. Primary synovial sarcoma of the heart treated by heart transplantation [Letter]. J Thorac Cardiovasc Surg 1990;3:567–8.
32. Tazelaar HD, Locke TJ, McGregor CG. Pathology of surgically excised primary cardiac tumors. Mayo Clin Proc 1992;67:957–65.

Angiosarcoma

33. Blondeau P. Primary cardiac tumors—French studies of 533 cases. Thorac Cardiovasc Surg 1990;38:192–5.
34. Burke AP, Cowan D, Virmani R. Primary sarcomas of the heart. Cancer 1992;69:387–95.
35. Enzinger FM, Weiss SW. Malignant vascular tumors. In: Enzinger FM, Weiss SW, eds. Tumors of soft tissue. St. Louis: C.V. Mosby Co, 1988:545–80.
36. Glancy DL, Morales JB, Roberts WC. Angiosarcoma of the heart. Am J Cardiol 1968;21:413–9.
37. Herrmann MA, Shankerman RA, Edwards WD, Shub C, Schaff HV. Primary cardiac angiosarcoma: A clinicopathologic study of six cases. J Thorac Cardiovasc Surg 1992;103:655–64.
38. Janigan DT, Husain A, Robinson NA. Cardiac angiosarcomas. A review and a case report. Cancer 1986;57:852–9.
39. Kim EE, Wallace S, Abello R, et al. Malignant cardiac fibrous histiocytomas and angiosarcomas: MR features. J Comput Assist Tomogr 1989;13:627–32.
40. Marafioti T, Castorino F, Gula G. Cardiac angiosarcoma. Histological, immunohistochemical and ultrastructural study. Pathologica 1993;85:103–11.
41. Masauzi N, Ichikawa S, Nishimura F, et al. Primary angiosarcoma of the right atrium detected by magnetic resonance imaging. Intern Med 1992;31:1291–7.
42. McCaughey WT, Dardick I, Barr JR. Angiosarcoma of serous membranes. Arch Pathol Lab Med 1983;107:304–7.
43. Poole-Wilson PA, Farnsworth A, Braimbridge MV, Pambakian H. Angiosarcoma of pericardium. Problems in diagnosis and management. Br Heart J 1976;38:240–3.
44. Prichard RW. Tumors of the heart. Review of the subject and report of one hundred and fifty cases. Arch Pathol 1951;51:98–128.
45. Sanoudos G, Reed GE. Primary cardiac sarcomas. J Thorac Cardiovasc Surg 1972;3:482–5.
46. Tazelaar HD, Locke TJ, McGregor CG. Pathology of surgically excised primary cardiac tumors. Mayo Clin Proc 1992;67:957–65.

Unclassified and Undifferentiated Sarcomas

47. Aravot DJ, Banner NR, Madden B, et al. Primary cardiac tumours—is there a place for cardiac transplantation? Eur J Cardiothorac Surg 1989;3:521–4.
48. Arcienegas E, Hakimi M, Farooki ZQ, Truccone NJ, Green EW. Primary cardiac tumors in children. J Thorac Cardiovasc Surg 1980;79:582–91.
49. Bear PA, Moodie DS. Malignant primary cardiac tumors. The Cleveland Clinic experience, 1956 to 1986. Chest 1987;92:860–2.
50. Blondeau P. Primary cardiac tumors—French studies of 533 cases. Thorac Cardiovasc Surg 1990;38:192–5.
51. Burke AP, Cowan D, Virmani R. Primary sarcomas of the heart. Cancer 1992;69:387–95.
52. Dein JR, Frist WH, Stinson EB, et al. Primary cardiac neoplasms. Early and late results of surgical treatment in 42 patients. J Thorac Cardiovasc Surg 1987;93:502–11.
53. Domanski MJ, Delaney TF, Kleiner DE Jr, et al. Primary sarcoma of the heart causing mitral stenosis. Am J Cardiol 1990;66:893–5.
54. Faught PR, Waller BF, Hull MT. Spindle cell sarcoma of the heart in childhood: light microscopic, ultrastructural, and immunohistochemical evidence for smooth muscle, endothelial and fibroblastic differentiations. Pediatr Pathol 1988;8:649–56.
55. James CL, Leong AS. Epithelioid leiomyosarcoma of the left atrium: immunohistochemical and ultrastructural findings. Pathology 1989;21:308–13.
56. Lazoglu AH, DaSliva MM, Iwahara M, Marino N, Coplan NL. Primary pericardial sarcoma. Am Heart J 1994;127:453–8.
57. Molina JE, Edwards JE, Ward HB. Primary cardiac tumors: experience at the University of Minnesota. Thorac Cardiovasc Surg 1990;38:183–91.

58. Murphy MC, Sweeney MS, Putnam JB Jr, et al. Surgical treatment of cardiac tumors: a 25-year experience. Ann Thorac Surg 1990;49:612–7.
59. Rangdaeng S, Truong LD. Comparative immunohistochemical staining for desmin and muscle-specific actin. A study of 576 cases. Am J Clin Pathol 1991;96:32–45.

60. Tazelaar HD, Locke TJ, McGregor CG. Pathology of surgically excised primary cardiac tumors. Mayo Clin Proc 1992;67:957–65.
61. Whorton CM. Primary malignant tumors of the heart. Cancer 1949;2:245–60.

Malignant Fibrous Histiocytoma

62. Burke AP, Virmani R. Osteosarcomas of the Heart. Am J Surg Pathol 1991;15:289–95.
63. Enzinger FM, Weiss SW. Malignant fibrohistiocytic tumors. In: Enzinger FM, Weiss SW, eds. Soft tissue tumors. St. Louis: CV Mosby Co, 1988:269–300.
64. Harris GJ, Tio FO, Grover FL. Primary left atrial myxosarcoma. Ann Thorac Surg 1993;56:564–6.
65. Iwasaki H, Isayama T, Ohjimi Y, et al. Malignant fibrous histiocytoma. A tumor of facultative histiocytes showing mesenchymal differentiation in cultured cell lines. Cancer 1992;69:437–47.
66. Klima T, Milam JD, Bossart MI, Cooley DA. Rare primary sarcomas of the heart. Arch Pathol Lab Med 1986;110:1155–9.
67. Korbmacher B, Doering C, Schulte HD, Hort W. Malignant fibrous histiocytoma of the heart—case report of a rare left atrial tumor. Thorac Cardiovasc Surg 1992;40:303–7.
68. Lawson CW, Fisher C, Gatter KC. An immunohistochemical study of differentiation in malignant fibrous histiocytoma. Histopathol 1987;11:375–83.

69. Laya MB, Mailliard JA, Bewtra C, Levin HS. Malignant fibrous histiocytoma of the heart. A case report and review of the literature. Cancer 1987;59;1026–31.
70. Maruki C, Suzukawa K, Koike J, Sato K. Cardiac malignant fibrous histiocytoma metastasizing to the brain: development of multiple neoplastic cerebral aneurysms. Surg Neurol 1994;41:40–4.
71. Ovcak Z, Masera A, Lamovec J. Malignant fibrous histiocytoma of the heart. Arch Pathol Lab Med 1992;116:872–4.
72. Pasquale M, Katz NM, Caruso AC, Bearb ME, Bitterman P. Myxoid variant of malignant fibrous histiocytoma of the heart. Am Heart J 1991;122:248–50.
73. Rangdaeng S, Truong LD. Comparative immunohistochemical staining for desmin and muscle-specific actin. A study of 576 cases. Am J Clin Pathol 1991;96:32–45.
74. Tazelaar HD, Locke TJ, McGregor CG. Pathology of surgically excised primary cardiac tumors. Mayo Clin Proc 1992;67:957–65.
75. Terashima K, Aoyama K, Nihei K, et al. Malignant fibrous histiocytoma of the heart. Cancer 1983;52:1919–26.
76. Weiss SW, Enzinger FM. Myxoid variant of malignant fibrous histiocytoma. Cancer 1977;39:1672–85.

Osteosarcoma

77. Burke AP, Virmani R. Osteosarcomas of the Heart. Am J Surg Pathol 1991;15:289–95.
78. Dorney P. Osteoclastoma of the heart. Br Heart J 1967;29:276–8.
79. Hammond GL, Strong WW, Cohen LS, et al. Chondrosarcoma simulating malignant atrial myxoma. J Thorac Cardiovasc Surg 1976;72:575–80.
80. Heni HE, Bubenheimer P, Gornandt L, Birnbaum D, Roskamm H. Primary atrial heart tumors—a review of 21 cases. Z Kardiol 1988;787:425–31.
81. Johansson L, Kugelberg J, Thulin L. Myxofibrosarcoma in the left atrium originally presented as a cardiac myxoma with chondroid differentiation. A clinico-pathological report [clinical conference]. APMIS 1989;97:833–8.
82. Lowry WB, McKee EE. Primary osteosarcoma of the heart. Cancer 1972;30:1068–73.

83. Marvasti MA, Bove EL, Obeid AK, Bowser MA, Parker FB Jr. Primary osteosarcoma of the left atrium: complete surgical excision. Ann Thorac Surg 1985;40:402–4.
84. Reynard JS Jr, Gregoratos G, Gordon MJ, Bloor CM. Primary osteosarcoma of the heart. Am Heart J 1985;109:598–600.
85. Schneiderman H, Fordham EW, Goren CC, McCall AR, Rosenberg MS, Rozek S. Primary cardiac osteosarcoma: multidisciplinary aspects applicable to extraskeletal osteosarcoma generally. CA Cancer J Clin 1984;34:110–7.
86. Seidal T, Wandt B, Lundin SE. Primary chondroblastic osteogenic sarcoma of the left atrium. Case report. Scand J Thorac Cardiovasc Surg 1992;26:233–6.
87. Yashar J, Witoszka M, Savage DD, et al. Primary osteogenic sarcoma of the heart. Ann Thorac Surg 1979;28:594–600.

Leiomyosarcoma

87a. Antunes MJ, Vanderonck KM, Andrade CM, Rebelo LS. Primary cardiac leiomyosarcomas. Ann Thorac Surg 1991;51:999–1001.
88. Enzinger FM, Weiss SW. Leiomyosarcoma. In: Enzinger FM, Weiss SW, eds. Soft tissue tumors. St Louis: C.V. Mosby Co, 1988:402–21.
89. Fox JP, Freitas E, McGiffin DC, Firouz-Abadi AA, West MJ. Primary leiomyosarcoma of the heart: a rare cause of obstruction of the left ventricular outflow tract. Aust N Z J Med 1991;21:881–3.

90. Fyfe AI, Huckell VF, Burr LH, Stonier PM. Leiomyosarcoma of the left atrium: case report and review of the literature. Can J Cardiol 1991;7:193–6.
91. James CL, Leong AS. Epithelioid leiomyosarcoma of the left atrium: immunohistochemical and ultrastructural findings. Pathology 1989;21:308–13.
92. Takamizawa S, Sugimoto K, Tanaka H, Sakai O, Arai T, Saitoh A. A case of primary leiomyosarcoma of the heart. Intern Med 1992;31:265–8.

Fibrosarcoma

93. Knobel B, Rosman P, Kishon Y, Husar M. Intracardiac primary fibrosarcoma. Case report and literature review. Thorac Cardiovasc Surg 1992;40:227–30.
94. Nambiar CA, Tareif HE, Kishore KU, Ravindran J, Banderjee AK. Primary pericardial mesothelioma: one-year event-free survival. Am Heart J 1992;124:802–3.
95. Sethi KK, Nair M, Khanna SK. Primary fibrosarcoma of the heart presenting as obstruction at the tricuspid valve: diagnosis by cross-sectional echocardiography. Int J Cardiol 1989;24:228–30.
96. Witkin GB, Rosai J. Solitary fibrous tumor of the mediastinum. A report of 14 cases. Am J Surg Pathol 1989;13:547–57.

Myxosarcoma

97. Dein JR, Frist WH, Stinson EB, et al. Primary cardiac neoplasms. Early and late results of surgical treatment in 42 patients. J Thorac Cardiovasc Surg 1987;93:502–11.
98. Enzinger FM, Weiss SW. General considerations. In: Enzinger FM, Weiss SW, eds. Soft tissue tumors. St. Louis: CV Mosby Co, 1988:1–18.
99. Hammond GL, Strong WW, Cohen LS, et al. Chondrosarcoma simulating malignant atrial myxoma. J Thorac Cardiovasc Surg 1976;72:575–80.
100. Johansson L, Kugelberg J, Thulin L. Myxofibrosarcoma in the left atrium originally presented as a cardiac myxoma with chondroid differentiation. A clinico-pathological report [clinical conference]. APMIS 1989;97:833–8.
101. Molina JE, Edwards JE, Ward HB. Primary cardiac tumors: experience at the University of Minnesota. Thorac Cardiovasc Surg 1990;38:183–91.
102. Murphy MC, Sweeney MS, Putnam JB Jr, et al. Surgical treatment of cardiac tumors: a 25-year experience. Ann Thorac Surg 1990;49:612–7.
103. Okada M, Ohta T, Yasuoka S, et al. Surgical management of intracavitary tumors. A review of fifteen patients and current status in Japan. J Cardiovasc Surg 1986;27:641–9.
104. Putnam JB Jr, Sweeney MS, Colon R, Lanza LA, Frazier OH, Cooley DA. Primary cardiac sarcomas. Ann Thorac Surg 1991;5:906–10.
105. Reece IJ, Cooley DA, Frazier OH, Hallman GL, Powers PL, Montero GC. Cardiac tumors. Clinical spectrum and prognosis of lesions other than classical benign myxoma in 20 patients. J Thorac Cardiovasc Surg 1984;88:439–46.
106. Weiss SW, Enzinger FM. Myxoid variant of malignant fibrous histiocytoma. Cancer 1977;39:1672–85.

Rhabdomyosarcoma

107. Awad M, Dunn B, al Halees Z, Mercer E. Intracardiac rhabdomyosarcoma: transesophageal echocardiographic findings and diagnosis. J Am Soc Echocardiogr 1992;5:199–202.
108. Bear PA, Moodie DS. Malignant primary cardiac tumors. The Cleveland Clinic experience, 1956 to 1986. Chest 1987;92:860–2.
109. Hajar R, Roberts WC, Folger GM Jr. Embryonal botryoid rhabdomyosarcoma of the mitral valve. Am J Cardiol 1986;57:376.
110. Hui KS, Green LK, Schmidt WA. Primary cardiac rhabdomyosarcoma: definition of a rare entity. Am J Cardiovasc Pathol 1988;2:19–29.
111. McAllister HA, Fenoglio JJ Jr. Tumors of the cardiovascular system. Atlas of Tumor Pathology, 2nd Series, Fascicle 15. Washington, D.C.: Armed Forces Institute of Pathology, 1978:81–102.
112. Miralles A, Bracamonte L, Soncul H, et al. Cardiac tumors: Clinical experience and surgical results in 74 patients. Ann Thorac Surg 1991;52:886–95.
113. Putnam JB Jr, Sweeney MS, Colon R, Lanza LA, Frazier OH, Cooley DA. Primary cardiac sarcomas. Ann Thorac Surg 1991;5:906–10.
114. Moriarty AT, Nelson WA, McGahey B. Fine needle aspiration of rhabdomyosarcoma of the heart. Light and electron microscopic findings and histologic correlation. Acta Cytol 1990;34:74–8.
115. Orsmond GS, Knight L, Dehner LP, Micoloff FM, Nesbitt M, Bessinger FB. Alveolar rhabdomyosarcoma involving the heart. An echocardiographic, angiographic and pathologic study. Circulation 1976;54:837–43.
116. Satoh M, Horimoto M, Sakurai K, Funayama N, Igarashi K, Yamashiro K. Primary cardiac rhabdomyosarcoma exhibiting transient and pronounced regression with chemotherapy. Am Heart J 1990;120:1458–60.
117. Somers K, Lothe F. Primary lymphosarcoma of the heart. Review of the literature and report of 3 cases. Cancer 1960;13:449–57.
118. Tazelaar HD, Locke TJ, McGregor CG. Pathology of surgically excised primary cardiac tumors. Mayo Clin Proc 1992;67:957–65.
119. Whorton CM. Primary malignant tumors of the heart. Cancer 1949;2:245–60.

Synovial Sarcoma

120. Burke AP, Cowan D, Virmani R. Primary sarcomas of the heart. Cancer 1992;69:387–95.
121. Karn CM, Socinski MA, Fletcher JA, Corson JM, Craighead JE. Cardiac synovial sarcoma with translocation (X;18) associated with asbestos exposure. Cancer 1994;73:74–8.
122. Tak T, Goel S, Chandrasoma P, Colletti P, Rahimtoola SH. Synovial sarcoma of the right ventricle. Am Heart J 1991;121:933–6.
123. Witkin GB, Miettinen M, Rosai J. A biphasic tumor of the mediastinum with features of synovial sarcoma. A report of four cases. Am J Surg Pathol 1989;13:490–9.

Liposarcoma

124. Can C, Arpaci F, Celasun B, Gunham O, Finci R. Primary pericardial liposarcoma presenting with cardiac tamponade and multiple organ metastases [Letter]. Chest 1993;103:328.

125. Dreyer L, Marik PE, Potgieter AS. Myxoid liposarcoma of the right atrium. A case report. S Afr Med J 1986;69:572–4.

126. Enzinger FM, Weiss SW. Liposarcoma. In: Enzinger FM, Weiss SW, eds. Soft tissue tumors. St. Louis: CV Mosby Co, 1988:346–82.

127. Lionarons RJ, van Baarlen J, Hitchcock JF. Constrictive pericarditis caused by primary liposarcoma. Thorax 1990;45:566–7.

128. Macedo-Dias JA, Queiroz Machado F, Vouga L, Goncalves V, Gomes R. Liposarcoma of the heart. A case report. Am J Cardiovasc Pathol 1990;3:259–63.

129. Nzayinambaho K, Noel H, Cosyns J, Sonnet J, Chalant C. Primary cardiac liposarcoma simulating a left atrial myxoma. Thorac Cardiovasc Surg 1985;33:193–5.

130. Paraf F, Bruneval P, Balaton A, et al. Primary liposarcoma of the heart. Am J Cardiovasc Pathol 1990;3:175–80.

Malignant Schwannoma

131. Dammert K, Elfing G, Halonen PI. Neurogenic sarcoma in the heart. Am Heart J 1955;49:794–8.

132. Fukuda T, Ishikawa H, Ohnishi Y, et al. Malignant spindle cell tumor of the pericardium. Evidence of sarcomatous mesothelioma with aberrant antigen expression. Acta Pathol Jpn 1989;39:750–4.

133. Hussain R, Neligan MC. Metastatic malignant schwannoma in the heart. Ann Thorac Surg 1993;56:374–5.

134. McAllister HA, Fenoglio JJ Jr. Tumors of the cardiovascular system. Atlas of Tumor Pathology, 2nd Series, Fascicle 15. Washington, D.C.: Armed Forces Institute of Pathology, 1978:81–102.

135. Ursell PC, Albala A, Fenoglio JJ Jr. Malignant neurogenic tumor of the heart. Hum Pathol 1982;13:640–5.

Malignant Mesenchymoma

136. McKenney PA, Moroz K, Haudenschild CC, Shemin RJ, Davidoff R. Malignant mesenchymoma as a primary cardiac tumor. Am Heart J 1992;123:1071–5.

137. Muir CS, Seah CS. Primary chondrosarcomatous mesenchymoma of the mitral valve. Thorax 1966;21:254–62.

138. Peters P, Flachskampf FA, Hauptmann S, Lo HB, Schuster CJ. Bilocular atrial malignant mesenchymoma causing mitral and localized pulmonary vein flow obstruction: diagnosis by transoesophageal echocardiography. Eur Heart J 1992;13:1585–8.

139. Tanaka T, Bunai Y, Nishikawa A, Kawai T, Mori H, Takahashi M. Malignant mesenchymoma of the heart. Acta Pathol Jpn 1982;32:851–9.

Rhabdoid Tumor

140. Egawa S, Uchida T, Koshiba K, Kagata Y, Iwabuchi K. Malignant fibrous histiocytoma of the bladder with focal rhabdoid tumor differentiation. J Urol 1994;151:154–6.

141. Ota S, Crabbe DC, Tran TN, Triche TJ, Shimada H. Malignant rhabdoid tumor. A study with two established cell lines. Cancer 1993;71:2862–72.

142. Small EJ, Gordon GJ, Dahms BB. Malignant rhabdoid tumor of the heart in an infant. Cancer 1985;55:2850–3.

Kaposi's Sarcoma

143. Autran BR, Gorin I, Leibowitch M, et al. AIDS in a Haitian woman with cardiac Kaposi's sarcoma and Whipple's disease. Lancet 1983;1:767–8.

144. Janigan DT, Husain A, Robinson NA. Cardiac angiosarcomas. A review and a case report. Cancer 1986;57:852–9.

13
HEMATOLOGIC TUMORS OF THE HEART AND PERICARDIUM

PRIMARY CARDIAC LYMPHOMA

Definition. Lymphoma is a malignant proliferation of lymphoid cells that occasionally involves the heart and pericardium. There are two definitions of primary cardiac lymphoma: some observers require an absence of lymphoma outside the pericardial sac, demonstrated by a complete autopsy examination (9,17); others accept a lymphoma as primary to the heart if the bulk of tumor is within the pericardium or if there are cardiac symptoms from lymphomatous cardiac infiltration at the time of initial diagnosis (32). Currently, most cardiac lymphomas are diagnosed premortem, in contrast to those discussed in the previous Fascicle on cardiac tumors (17), which included only autopsy cases. It is clinically relevant and acceptable today to classify lymphomas presenting as cardiac disease as "primary cardiac lymphoma," especially if the bulk of tumor appears to be intrapericardial. In fact, the precise location of the lymphoid cell(s) at the time of incipient clonal expansion can never be stated with certainty (27).

Histogenesis. A discussion of the histogenesis of lymphoma in general will not be presented here; the reader is encouraged to read the Atlas of Tumors of the Hematopoietic System (16). Because many cardiac lymphomas diagnosed today occur in immunocompromised patients, their histogenesis is discussed briefly. Lymphomas in immunosuppressed patients often arise within potentially reversible benign lymphoid proliferations that have developed over years (16); the broad term "post-transplant lymphoproliferative disorder" has been used for such infiltrations (7,8,13,23). Most, but not all, lymphomas arising in immunocompromised patients contain episomal Ebstein-Barr virus DNA (13), which is believed to be oncogenic (7,8). Originally, it was thought that the lymphomas in these patients were polyclonal, based on immunohistochemical and flow cytometric studies (16,27); however, Southern blot analysis for gene rearrangements has shown monoclonality in the majority of lymphomas in immunosuppressed patients (8). Since multiple distinct immuno-globulin rearrangements may occur within a single patient if different lymph nodes are biopsied, either from the same site or from widely separated sites in the body (7), clonality of Ebstein-Barr viral DNA may be a better marker for tumor clonality than DNA rearrangements, which may theoretically occur after clonal expansion (13). In a recent series, one of eight post-transplant lymphomas had oligoclonal episomal Epstein-Barr viral DNA, suggesting that some lymphomas in immunosuppressed patients are oligoclonal (13).

Incidence. Although cardiac involvement in patients with disseminated lymphoma occurs in up to 24 percent of patients (24), primary cardiac lymphoma is rare. By strict criteria (documented absence of lymphoma outside the pericardium), fewer than 30 cases of primary cardiac lymphoma in immunocompetent patients have been reported in the English language literature (1,2,5, 6,9,12,14,17,19,20–22,25,28,30,31); at the Armed Forces Institute of Pathology (AFIP), seven new cases have been accessioned since the writing of the previous Fascicle (17). There are approximately 20 reports of cardiac lymphomas presenting as cardiac disease, with evidence of concomitant mediastinal, bone marrow, or subdiaphragmatic lymphoma at the time of diagnosis (3,4,10, 12,15,18,26,28,29,31,32); another 20 to 25 cases of primary cardiac lymphomas in immunosuppressed patients have been reported.

Clinical Features. Among 38 well-documented cases of primary cardiac lymphomas in immunocompetent patients, including 13 patients with regional lymph node involvement at autopsy or on mediastinal imaging, the mean age at presentation was 58 years (range, 13 to 80 years) (1–6,9–12,14,15,18–22,25,26,28–32). The male to female ratio was 1.3 to 1. The presenting symptoms were most commonly related to congestive heart failure, pleural effusions, and conduction system disturbances. Rarely, anginal pain was present, indicating infiltration of a coronary artery (5). Unusual clinical findings were related to pulmonary embolism secondary to tumor (1), complete heart block (4,6), valvular

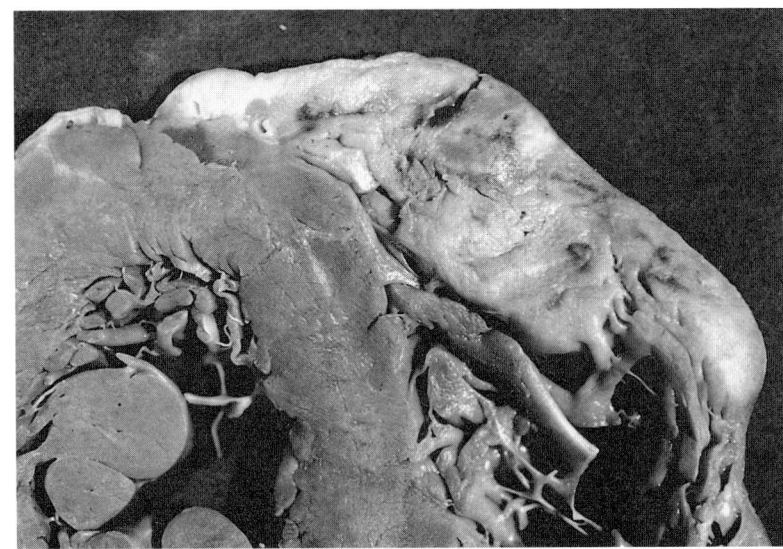

Figure 13-1
MALIGNANT LYMPHOMA
A 24-year-old drug addict was seropositive for HIV-1. There was widespread lymphoma that diffusely infiltrated the right ventricle. Histologically the tumor was large cell (not shown).

obstruction (28), and symptoms mimicking viral myocarditis (15). One patient died suddenly; cardiac lymphoma confined within the pericardium was the only significant finding at autopsy (25). Fourteen cases were diagnosed premortem either by biopsy, resection of tumor, or cytologic examination of pericardial fluid (5,12,21). Localization of tumor and assessment of response to treatment was facilitated by imaging techniques, including transesophageal echocardiography (19), magnetic resonance imaging (MRI) (18,20), and computed tomography (CT) (5). It may be difficult to detect extracardiac tumor in patients presenting with cardiac lymphoma: bone marrow biopsies, mediastinal CT, and MRI may confirm the presence of extracardiac lymphoma. However, mediastinal lymphadenopathy may, on histologic examination, be reactive hyperplasia (28,31), and imaging does not always detect mediastinal lymphoma (3).

Of the seven recent cases in the AFIP files, five patients were male (mean age 60 years). In only one case was the diagnosis made premortem. The initial clinical diagnoses were congestive failure (two patients), atypical chest pain, sudden death, cardiac "myxoma," and pericardial effusions; in one case, the tumor was an incidental finding.

Pathologic Findings. Grossly, primary cardiac lymphoma is characterized by multiple masses of the firm, white nodules characteristic of extracardiac lymphoma (figs. 13-1, 13-2) (2,3,9,11, 25,26,28,31). The heart is usually enlarged: autopsy weights range from 410 g (1) to 1,570 g (28),

with a mean weight of approximately 700 g in untreated cases (2,3,9,11,25,26,28,31). The gross appearance may suggest sarcoidosis. However, sarcoid granulomas do not form large nodules that extend into the pericardium or epicardium, as is typical for lymphoma, but form fine granules or irregular scars. Grossly, lymphomas may be impossible to distinguish from sarcomas. The latter, however, are more likely to demonstrate hemorrhage and necrosis on sections, and often extend into the ventricular or atrial cavities.

The right atrium is most often affected by lymphoma, followed by the right ventricle, left ventricle, left atrium, atrial septum, and ventricular septum (2,3,7,9,11,25,26,28,31). Extension of tumor onto valves is unusual (28), but extension onto the pericardial surfaces is typical. More than one cardiac chamber is involved in over 75 percent of cases, although tumors confined to the atria (1,2,12,14,19,22,28,31) or pericardium (12) and coronary artery infiltrates with aneurysm (11) have been reported. In one instance, there was no gross tumor and the diagnosis was made first at histologic evaluation (10). Of the seven cardiac lymphomas without extracardiac involvement in the AFIP files since 1975, three were localized to the left atrium, pericardium, and coronary artery, respectively; the remainder were multifocal tumors involving the ventricles, atria, and pericardium.

The microscopic features of many early cases of primary cardiac lymphoma were obscured by

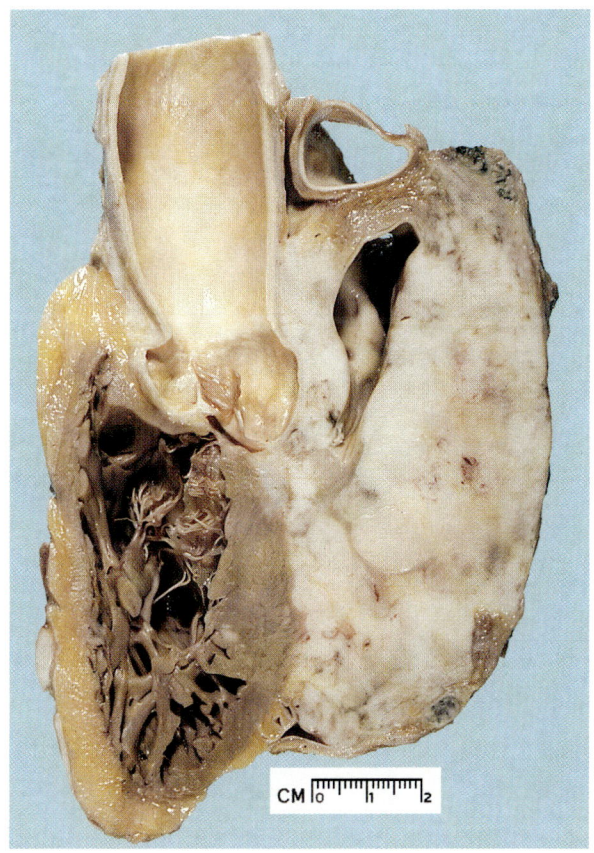

Figure 13-2
MALIGNANT LYMPHOMA
Note the fleshy white tumor infiltrating the left atrium.
The heart was the predominant organ involved.

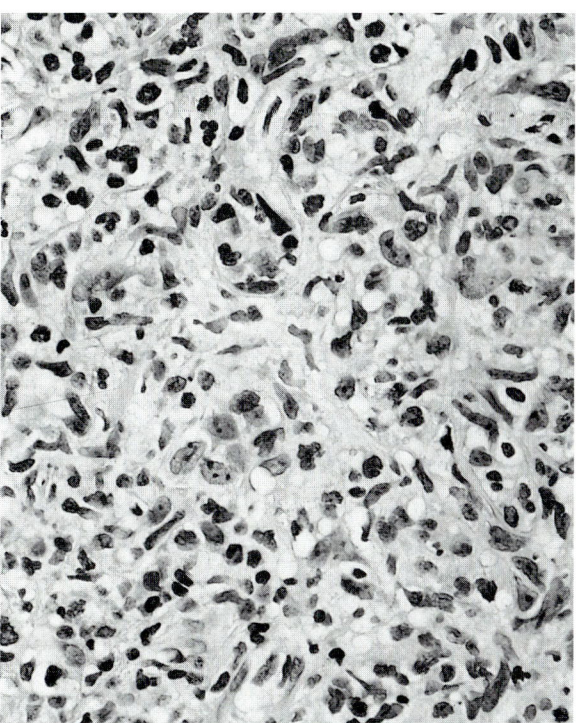

Figure 13-3
MALIGNANT LYMPHOMA, LARGE CELL TYPE
A middle-aged man had symptoms of coronary artery disease; at surgery for bypass grafting, a tumor was noted infiltrating the right ventricle. The tumor is composed of large cells that typed as B cells (not shown). No lymphoma was detected in regional lymph nodes or other extracardiac sites.

postmortem artifact. These tumors, diagnosed before the initiation of a functional classification system for lymphomas, bore designations such as lymphosarcoma, reticulum cell sarcoma, stem cell lymphoma, and histiocytic lymphoma. From the available photomicrographs, it appears that the majority of early cases were a form of large cell lymphoma (28,31). Recent cases have been designated small noncleaved follicular center cell (1,19), intermediate cell (19), B-immunoblastic (6,12), large cell undifferentiated (12), large cell noncleaved (12), and centroblastic/centrocytic (cleaved follicular center cell) lymphomas (11) (figs. 13-3–13-6). At the periphery of the tumor nodules, there is infiltration of the myocardium. In every case in which cell typing was performed, primary cardiac lymphomas have typed as B-cell proliferations (1,9,11,12,14,19,20,22).

Differential Diagnosis. The differential diagnosis of large cell lymphoma includes round cell sarcoma, undifferentiated carcinoma, malignant melanoma, and granulocytic sarcoma. Immunohistochemical stains for lymphoid markers, intermediate filaments, myoglobin, and epithelial markers such as cytokeratin and epithelial membrane antigen are helpful in distinguishing lymphoma, sarcoma, and carcinoma. Although we have not encountered a melanoma of the heart without a known primary, immunohistochemical studies for S-100 protein, HMB-45, and other melanoma-specific antigens are occasionally necessary for the complete evaluation of an undifferentiated malignancy. Rarely, chloromas (granulocytic sarcomas) occur within the heart (see below). For this reason, tumors with a histologic appearance of atypical high-grade lymphoma should be assessed with Leder's stain or another stain for myeloid granules.

173

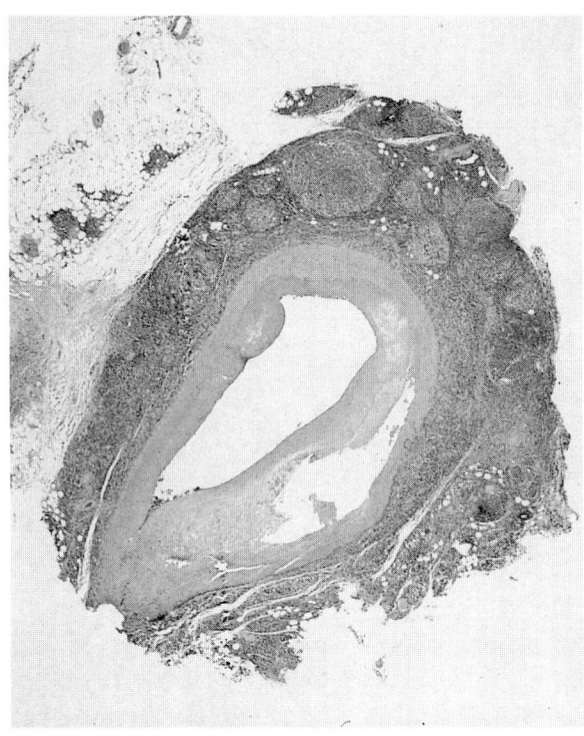

Figure 13-4
MALIGNANT LYMPHOMA, NODULAR
FOLLICULAR CENTER CELL TYPE

A 66-year-old man died suddenly and unexpectedly. At autopsy, the only significant finding was a mass surrounding the left anterior descending coronary artery. There is mild to moderate coronary atherosclerosis.

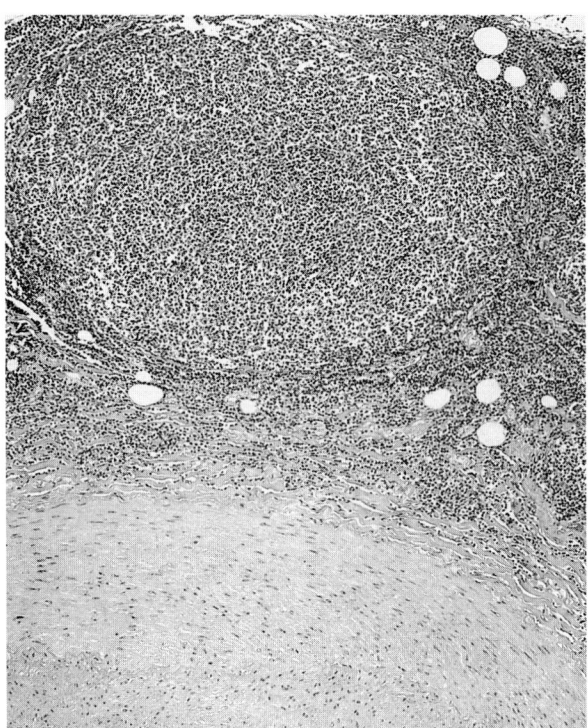

Figure 13-5
MALIGNANT LYMPHOMA,
FOLLICULAR CENTER CELL TYPE

A higher magnification of figure 13-4 shows a nodule of lymphoid cells adjacent to the coronary artery.

Cardiac Lymphomas in Immunosuppressed Patients. The incidence of cardiac lymphoma, and extranodal lymphoma in general, is on the rise. This trend reflects the increasing numbers of patients who are chronically immunosuppressed. As discussed above, these proliferations often evolve from a polymorphous, histologically benign lesion, which may result from activation of latent Epstein-Barr virus infection. These polymorphous proliferations may be difficult to distinguish from chronic rejection and have been designated *post-transplant lymphoproliferative disorder.* In patients with the acquired immunodeficiency syndrome (AIDS), benign proliferations that precede malignant lymphomas have also been identified, and may be termed *AIDS-associated lymphoproliferative disorder.*

There have been approximately 25 reports of cardiac lymphoma, generally associated with extracardiac lymphoma, in patients with AIDS or allografts (33–37,38–41,43,45,47). The heart is not a common site of lymphoma in immunosuppressed patients. In a series of 90 lymphomas developing prior to 1984 in homosexual men who were presumed infected with the AIDS virus, only 3 involved the heart or pericardium (48). The central nervous system, bone marrow, bowel, and mucocutaneous sites were the most common for extranodal lymphomas in these patients.

Clinically, cardiac lymphomas in patients with AIDS generally occur in 30- to 50-year-old men and cause cardiac symptoms (41). The occurrence of unexplained cardiac symptoms in patients with AIDS should alert the clinician to the possibility of cardiac lymphoma, which can be diagnosed by endomyocardial biopsy (34). In 5 of the 14 cases of cardiac lymphoma in AIDS patients reported before 1992, there was no apparent extracardiac involvement (39). Other extranodal sites, especially the gastrointestinal tract and lung, were involved in the remaining

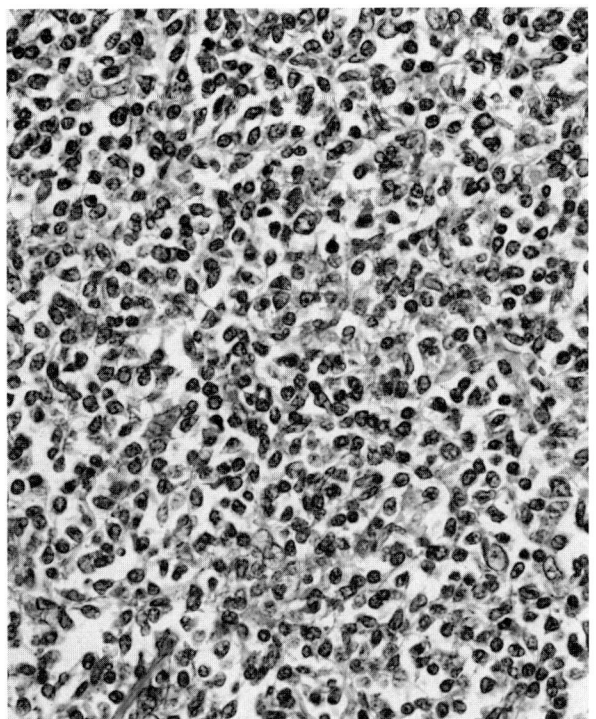

Figure 13-6
MALIGNANT LYMPHOMA,
FOLLICULAR CENTER CELL TYPE
The lymphoma cells within the follicle shown in figure 13-5 are generally small cleaved cells.

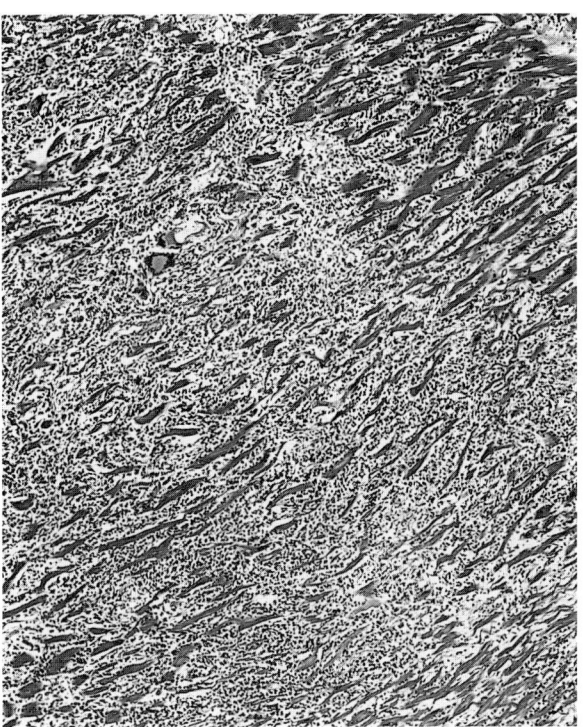

Figure 13-7
AIDS-RELATED LYMPHOPROLIFERATIVE DISORDER
A 22-year-old man was seropositive for HIV-1 and died suddenly. There was widespread inflammation of the myocardium with giant cells, resembling giant cell myocarditis, that may have represented a precursor to lymphoma.

cases. Virtually any site in the heart may be involved by cardiac lymphoma (39).

Cardiac and other extranodal lymphomas that arise in immunocompromised patients are usually high grade. Plasmacytoid immunoblastic lymphoma, small noncleaved cell lymphoma, and diffuse large cell lymphoma are the most common histologic types (39,41). Many other types of B-cell lymphomas have been described in extracardiac locations (48). T-cell lymphomas in immunocompromised patients are rare and have not been found in the heart (42,44).

We have seen a polymorphous lymphoid infiltrate associated with myocyte necrosis and giant cells (fig. 13-7) in a postmortem heart from a patient with AIDS. This infiltrate resembled the atypical lymphoid proliferations seen in lymph nodes of immunocompromised patients. In two cases of cardiac lymphoma in patients with AIDS, the apparent histologic progression from a polyclonal, polymorphous infiltrate to a monoclonal, monomorphous high-grade lymphoma was demonstrated (40).

Cardiac lymphomas in iatrogenically immunosuppressed patients with prior renal or heart transplants are usually part of disseminated disease (33,36,37,45,47), but are occasionally found confined to the heart at autopsy (45). They are generally high-grade B-cell lymphomas that arise within a polymorphous proliferation that is identified on biopsies for the evaluation of chronic rejection (figs. 13-8–13-10) (37,45). These proliferations rapidly progress to high-grade lymphoma, and may occur within months of the transplant (33).

Secondary Cardiac Involvement in Lymphoma. The incidence of secondary cardiac lymphoma in patients with malignant lymphoma ranges from 9 to 24 percent (see chapter 15) (50,53). In contrast to primary cardiac lymphomas and cardiac lymphomas arising in immunosuppressed patients, which are exclusively

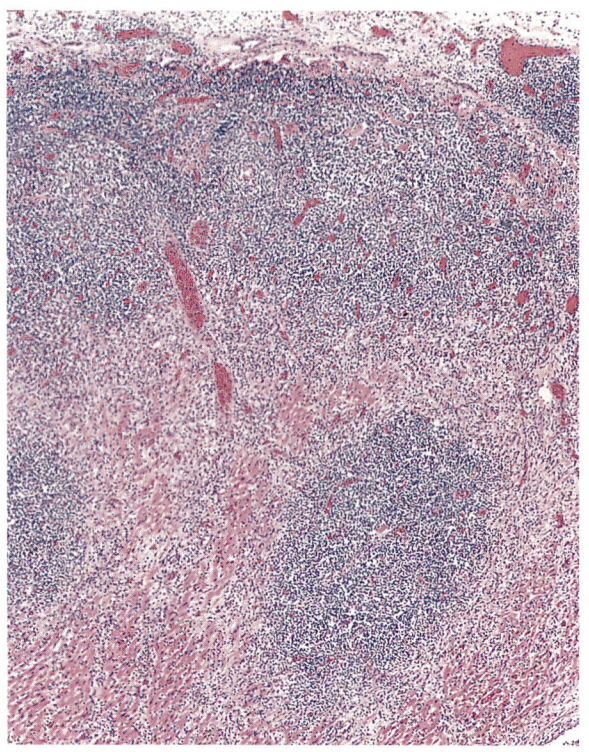

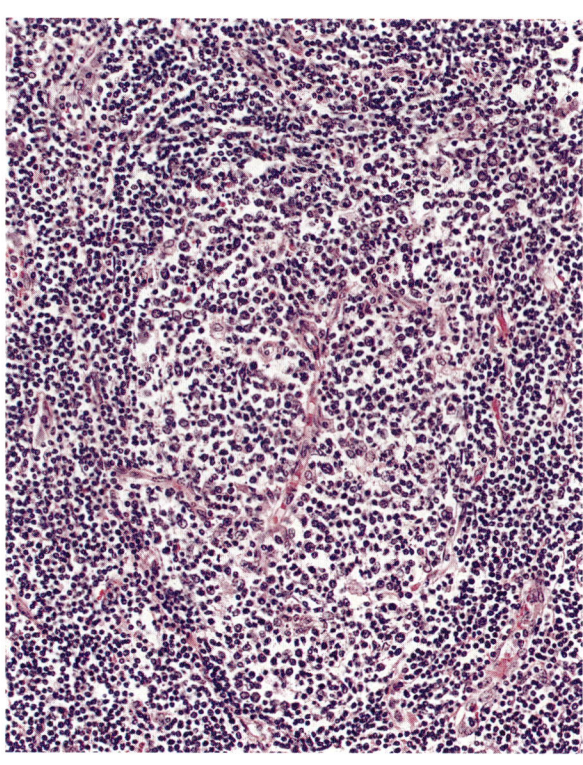

Figure 13-8
POST-TRANSPLANT
LYMPHOPROLIFERATIVE DISORDER

A 9-year-old boy died 13 months after receiving a heart transplant, with clinical evidence of rejection. In addition to severe rejection, there were widespread lymphoid infiltrates in the endocardium and epicardium.

Figure 13-9
POST-TRANSPLANT
LYMPHOPROLIFERATIVE DISORDER

In some areas of the case illustrated in figure 13-8, there were reactive germinal centers, indicating a benign process.

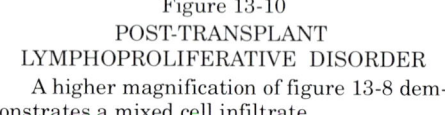

Figure 13-10
POST-TRANSPLANT
LYMPHOPROLIFERATIVE DISORDER

A higher magnification of figure 13-8 demonstrates a mixed cell infiltrate.

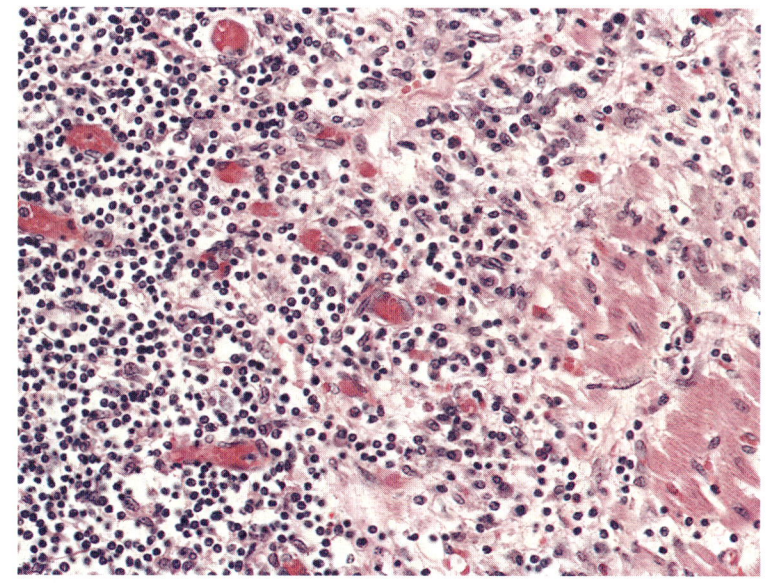

of B-cell origin, secondary cardiac lymphomas include Hodgkin's disease and T-cell lymphomas (49) as well as B-cell lymphomas. In early series, approximately 10 percent of patients with cardiac involvement had symptoms that were attributable to infiltration of the heart by lymphoma, but cardiac lymphoma was suspected only rarely before autopsy (50,53). Symptoms include chest pain and dyspnea, as well as others related to large pericardial effusions, left ventricular dysfunction (52), and congestive heart failure from intracavitary masses (54). Today, secondary cardiac involvement in patients with malignant lymphoma is diagnosed premortem in up to 40 percent of patients (51). MRI is very sensitive and superior to two-dimensional echocardiography for demonstrating cardiac infiltration in patients with mediastinal lymphoma (55), and may lead to early treatment. Because patients may respond to chemotherapy or combined radiation and chemotherapy, early diagnosis of cardiac involvement is essential (51).

Lymphomas spread to the heart by three pathways: direct extension from a mediastinal lymphoma, retrograde lymphatic spread in lymphatics along the coronary arteries and in the epicardium, and hematogenous spread. Hematogenous spread, which is characterized by interstitial and epicardial masses that resemble abscesses, is more typical of low-grade and intermediate follicular center cell lymphomas. Hodgkin's disease and high-grade non-Hodgkin's lymphomas are more likely to spread to the heart by direct extension or lymphatic routes (50).

Treatment. In patients with both primary and secondary cardiac lymphomas, remissions are possible with combination chemotherapy, with or without radiation therapy (56–61,63). Especially in immunocompetent individuals, treatment with chemotherapeutic regimens de-signed for nodal lymphomas can result in a reduction of tumor mass and a dramatic improvement of cardiac symptoms. Medical treatment may be combined with surgical debulking of tumor, which may necessitate synthetic grafts to repair surgical defects in the myocardium (62).

GRANULOCYTIC SARCOMA (LEUKEMIC INFILTRATION OF THE HEART)

Leukemic infiltrates are found at autopsy within the heart or pericardium in 37 percent of patients with acute leukemia (68). However, symptoms directly attributable to these deposits are uncommon (see chapter 15) (67,68).

There have been several reports of granulocytic sarcoma within the pericardium (64,65), adherent to the pericardium (66), and within the myocardium (69). In most of these cases, the granulocytic sarcoma occurred prior to the leukemic manifestations (64–66). In one patient, right ventricular failure resulted from leukemic infiltration (69).

GIANT LYMPH NODE HYPERPLASIA

Giant lymph node hyperplasia of the mediastinum was originally described by Castleman et al. (70) in 1956. Synonyms include *Castleman's disease, angiofollicular lymph node hyperplasia, angiomatous lymphoid hamartoma,* and *follicular lymphoreticuloma.* Rarely, giant lymph node hyperplasia can be entirely intrapericardial and result in a pericardial mass and cardiac symptoms (71). The histologic features include follicular hyperplasia, intrafollicular capillary proliferation and hyalinization, and perifollicular plasmacytosis.

REFERENCES

Primary Cardiac Lymphoma

1. Bestetti RB, Soares FA, Soares EG, Oliveira JS. Primary lymphoma of the right atrium with fatal neoplastic pulmonary embolism. Am Heart J 1992;124:1088–90.
2. Brucker EA, Glassy FJ. Primary reticulum cell sarcoma of the heart with review of the literature. Cancer 1955;8:921–31.
3. Cabin HS, Costello RM, Vasudevan G, Maron BJ, Roberts WC. Cardiac lymphoma mimicking hypertrophic cardiomyopathy. Am Heart J 1981;101:466–8.
4. Cairns P, Butany J, Fulop J, Rakowski H, Hassaram S. Cardiac presentation of non-Hodgkin's lymphoma. Arch Pathol Lab Med 1987;111:80–3.

5. Castelli MJ, Mihalov ML, Posniak HV, Gattuso P. Primary cardiac lymphoma initially diagnosed by routine cytology. Case report and literature review. Acta Cytol 1989;33:335–8.

6. Chou ST, Arkles LB, Gill GD, Pinkus N, Parkin A, Hicks JD. Primary lymphoma of the heart. A case report. Cancer 1983;52:744–7.

7. Cleary ML, Sklar J. Lymphoproliferative disorders in cardiac transplant recipients are multiclonal lymphomas. Lancet 1984;2:489–93.

8. _____, Warnke R, Sklar J. Monoclonality of lymphoproliferative lesions in cardiac transplant recipients: clonal analysis based on immunoglobulin-gene rearrangements. N Engl J Med 1984;310:477–82.

9. Curtsinger CR, Wilson MJ, Yoneda K. Primary cardiac lymphoma. Cancer 1989;64:521–5.

10. Fiester RF. Reticulum cell sarcoma of the heart. Arch Pathol 1975;99:60–1.

11. Gardiner DS, Lindop GB. Coronary artery aneurysm due to primary cardiac lymphoma. Histopathology 1989;15:537–40.

12. Gill PS, Chandraratna PA, Meyer PR, Levine AM. Malignant lymphoma: cardiac involvement at initial presentation. J Clin Oncol 1987;5:216–24.

13. Kaplan MA, Ferry JA, Harris NL, Jacobson JO. Clonal analysis of posttransplant lymphoproliferative disorders, using both episomal Epstein-Barr virus and immunoglobulin genes as markers. Am J Clin Pathol 1994;101:590–6.

14. Kasai K, Kuwao S, Sato Y, Murayama M, Harano Y, Kameya T. Case report of primary cardiac lymphoma. The applications of PCR to the diagnosis of primary cardiac lymphoma. Acta Pathol Jpn 1992;42:667–71.

15. Kissin M, Eisinger R. Reticulum cell sarcoma of the heart simulating viral pericarditis. Am Heart J 1961;62:549–52.

16. Lukes RJ, Collins RD. Tumors of the hematopoietic system. Atlas of Tumor Pathology, 2nd Series, Fascicle 28. Washington, D.C.: Armed Forces Institute of Pathology, 1992:378–9.

17. McAllister HA, Fenoglio JJ Jr. Tumors of the cardiovascular system. Atlas of Tumor Pathology. 2nd Series, Fascicle 15. Washington D.C.: Armed Forces Institute of Pathology, 1977:99–100.

18. Monsuez JJ, Frija J, Mertz-Pannier L, Miclea JM, Extra JM, Boiron M. Non-Hodgkin's lymphoma with cardiac presentation: evaluation and follow-up with echocardiography and MR imaging. Eur Heart J 1991;12:464–7.

19. Moore JA, DeRan BP, Minor R, Arthur J, Fraker TD. Transesophageal echocardiographic evaluation of intracardiac lymphoma. Am Heart J 1992;124:514–6.

20. Nand S, Mullen GM, Lonchyna VA, Moncada R. Primary lymphoma of the heart. Prolonged survival with early systemic therapy in a patient. Cancer 1991;68:2289–92.

21. Pozniak AL, Thomas RD, Hobbs CB, Lever JV. Primary malignant lymphoma of the heart. Antemortem cytologic diagnosis. Acta Cytol 1986;30:662–4.

22. Proctor MS, Tracy GP, Von Koch L. Primary cardiac B-cell lymphoma. Am Heart J 1989;118:179–81.

23. Purtilo DT, Strobach RS, Okano M, Davis JR. Epstein-Barr virus-associated lymphoproliferative disorders. Lab Invest 1992;67:5–23.

24. Roberts WC, Glancy DL, DeVita VT. Heart in malignant lymphoma (Hodgkin's disease, lymphosarcoma, reticulum cell sarcoma and mycosis fungoides). A study of 196 autopsy cases. Am J Cardiol 1968;22:85–107.

25. Roh LS, Papro GP. Primary malignant lymphoma of the heart in sudden unexpected death. J Forens Sci 1982;27:718–22.

26. Rucks WW, Russell HT, Motley RF. Primary reticulum cell sarcoma of the heart. Am Heart J 1963;66:97–102.

27. Scully RE, Mark EJ, McNeely BU. Case records of the Massachusetts General Hospital, Case 4-1985. N Engl J Med 1985;312:226–37.

28. Somers K, Lothe F. Primary lymphosarcoma of the heart. Review of the literature and report of 3 cases. Cancer 1960;13:449–60.

29. Stein M, Zyssman I, Kantor A, Spencer D, Lewis D, Bezwoda W. Malignant lymphoma with primary cardiac manifestations: a case report. Med Pediatr Oncol 1994;22:292–5.

30. Takagi M, Kugimiya T, Fujii T, et al. Extensive surgery for primary malignant lymphoma of the heart. J Cardiovasc Surg 1992;33:570–2.

31. Whorton CM. Primary malignant tumors of the heart. Report of a case. Cancer 1949;2:245–60.

32. Zaharia L, Gill PS. Primary cardiac lymphoma. Am J Clin Oncol 1991;14:142–5.

Cardiac Lymphoma in Immunosuppressed Patients

33. Abu-Farsakh H, Cagle PT, Buffone GJ, Bruner JM, Weilbaecher D, Greenberg SD. Heart allograft involvement with Epstein-Barr virus-associated posttransplant lymphoproliferative disorder. Arch Pathol Lab Med 1992;116:93–5.

34. Andress JD, Polish LB, Clark DM, Hossack KF. Transvenous biopsy diagnosis of cardiac lymphoma in an AIDS patient. Am Heart J 1989;118:421–3.

35. Balasubramanyam A, Waxman M, Kazal HL, Lee MH. Malignant lymphoma of the heart in acquired immune deficiency syndrome. Chest 1986;90:243–6.

36. Burtin P, Guerci A, Boman F, et al. Malignant lymphoma in the donor heart after heart transplantation. Eur Heart J 1993;14:1143–5.

37. Chang AC, Hruban RH, Levin HR, et al. Comparison of rejection in the atrioventricular node and bundles with the working myocardium in transplanted hearts. J Heart Lung Transplant 1991;10:915–20.

38. Gill PS, Chandraratna PA, Meyer PR, Levine AM. Malignant lymphoma: cardiac involvement at initial presentation. J Clin Oncol 1987;5:216–24.

39. Goldfarb A, King CL, Rosenzweig BP, et al. Cardiac lymphoma in the acquired immunodeficiency syndrome. Am Heart J 1989;118:1340–4.

40. Guarner J, Brynes RK, Chan WC, Birdsong G, Hertzler G. Primary non-Hodgkin's lymphoma of the heart in two patients with the acquired immunodeficiency syndrome. Arch Pathol Lab Med 1987;111:254–5.

41. Holladay AO, Siegel RJ, Schwartz DA. Cardiac malignant lymphoma in acquired immune deficiency syndrome. Cancer 1992;70:2203–7.

42. Kelsey RC, Saker A, Morgan M. Cardiac lymphoma in a patient with AIDS. Ann Intern Med 1991;115:370–1.

43. Kumar S, Kumar D, Kingma DW, Jaffe ES. Epstein-Barr virus-associated T-cell lymphoma in a renal transplant patient. Am J Surg Pathol 1993;17:1046–53.

44. Lukes RJ, Collins RD. Tumors of the hematopoietic system. Atlas of Tumor Pathology, 2nd Series, Fascicle 28. Washington, D.C.: Armed Forces Institute of Pathology, 1992:378–9.

45. Montone KT, Friedman H, Hodinka RL, Hicks DG, Kant JA, Tomaszewski JE. In situ hybridization for Epstein-Barr virus NotI repeats in posttransplant lymphoproliferative disorder. Mod Pathol 1992;5:292–302.

46. Rodenburg CJ, Kluin P, Maes A, Paul LC. Malignant lymphoma confined to the heart, 13 years after a cadaver kidney transplant. N Engl J Med 1985;313:122.

47. Scully RE, Mark EJ, McNeely BU. Case records of the Massachusetts General Hospital, Case 4-1985. N Engl J Med 1985;312:226–37.

48. Ziegler JL, Beckstead JA, Volberding PA, et al. Non-Hodgkin's lymphoma in 90 homosexual men. Relation to generalized lymphadenopathy and the acquired immunodeficiency syndrome. N Engl J Med 1984;311:565–70.

Cardiac Involvement in Lymphoma

49. Iemura A, Yano H, Kojiro M, Nouno R, Kouno K. Massive cardiac involvement of adult T-cell leukemia/lymphoma. An autopsy case. Arch Pathol Lab Med 1991;115:1052–4.

50. McDonnell PJ, Mann RB, Bulkley BH. Involvement of the heart by malignant lymphoma: a clinicopathologic study. Cancer 1982;49:944–51.

51. Peterson CD, Robinson WA, Klurnick JE. Involvement of the heart and pericardium in the malignant lymphomas. Am J Med Sci 1976;272:161–5.

52. Roberts WC, Glancy DL, DeVita VT. Heart in malignant lymphoma (Hodgkin's disease, lymphosarcoma, reticulum cell sarcoma and mycosis fungoides). A study of 196 autopsy cases. Am J Cardiol 1968;22:85–107.

53. Roistacher N, Preminger M, Macapinlac H, Pierre MK. Myocardial entrapment by lymphoma: a cause of reversible left ventricular dysfunction. Am Heart J 1992;124:516–21.

54. Sato H, Takahashi M. Non-Hodgkin's malignant lymphoma of the bone with intracavitary cardiac involvement. Intern Med 1993;32:502–7.

55. Tesoro-Tess JD, Biasi S, Balzarini L, et al. Heart involvement in lymphomas. The value of magnetic resonance imaging and two-dimensional echocardiography at disease presentation. Cancer 1993;72:2484–90.

Treatment

56. Castelli MJ, Mihalov ML, Posniak HV, Gattuso P. Primary cardiac lymphoma initially diagnosed by routine cytology. Case report and literature review. Acta Cytol 1989;33:335–8.

57. Gill PS, Chandraratna PA, Meyer PR, Levine AM. Malignant lymphoma: cardiac involvement at initial presentation. J Clin Oncol 1987;5:216–24.

58. Monsuez JJ, Frija J, Mertz-Pannier L, Miclea JM, Extra JM, Boiron M. Non-Hodgkin's lymphoma with cardiac presentation: evaluation and follow-up with echocardiography and MR imaging. Eur Heart J 1991;12:464–7.

59. Nand S, Mullen GM, Lonchyna VA, Moncada R. Primary lymphoma of the heart. Prolonged survival with early systemic therapy in a patient. Cancer 1991;68:2289–92.

60. Peterson CD, Robinson WA, Klurnick JE. Involvement of the heart and pericardium in the malignant lymphomas. Am J Med Sci 1976;272:161–5.

61. Roistacher N, Preminger M, Macapinlac H, Pierre MK. Myocardial entrapment by lymphoma: a cause of reversible left ventricular dysfunction. Am Heart J 1992;124:516–21.

62. Takagi M, Kugimiya T, Fujii T, et al. Extensive surgery for primary malignant lymphoma of the heart. J Cardiovasc Surg 1992;33:570–2.

63. Zaharia L, Gill PS. Primary cardiac lymphoma. Am J Clin Oncol 1991;14:142–5.

Granulocytic Sarcoma

64. Chu JY, Demello D, O'Connor DM, Chen SC, Gale GB. Pericarditis as presenting manifestation of acute nonlymphocytic leukemia in a young child. Cancer 1983;52:322–4.

65. Krause JR. Granulocytic sarcoma preceding acute leukemia: a report of six cases. Cancer 1979;44:1017–21.

66. Kubonishi I, Ohtsuki Y, Machida KI, et al. Granulocytic sarcoma presenting as a mediastinal tumor. Report of a case and cytochemical studies of tumor cells in vivo and in vitro. Am J Clin Pathol 1984;82:730–4.

67. Javier BV, Yount WJ, Crosby DJ, Hall TC. Cardiac metastasis in lymphoma and leukemia. Dis Chest 1967;52:481–4.

68. Roberts WC, Bodey GP, Wetlake PT. The heart in acute leukemia. A study of 420 autopsy cases. Am J Cardiol 1968;21:388–412.

69. Tillawi IS, Variokojis D. Refractory right ventricular failure due to granulocytic sarcoma. Arch Pathol Lab Med 1990;114:983–5.

Giant Lymph Node Hyperplasia

70. Castleman B, Iverson L, Menendez VP. Localized mediastinal lymph node hyperplasia resembling thymoma. Cancer 1956;9:822–30.

71. Virmani R, Bewtra C, McAllister HA, Schulte RD. Intrapericardial giant lymph node hyperplasia. Am J Surg Pathol 1982;6:475–81.

14
MALIGNANT MESOTHELIOMA OF THE PERICARDIUM

Definition. Malignant mesothelioma is a neoplasm that arises from mesothelial cells or possibly a more primitive precursor cell situated submesothelially (18). The definition of primary pericardial mesothelioma stipulates that there is no tumor present outside the pericardium, with the exception of lymph node metastases (2). Previously, a complete autopsy examination to exclude an occult primary tumor was also required to satisfy the criteria specified in the definition (2). Today, if an ultrastructural and immunohistochemical evaluation on adequate tissue is consistent with mesothelioma, the diagnosis of pericardial mesothelioma can be made on biopsy samples. Surgical evaluation of extent of tumor, with computed tomography (CT) or magnetic resonance imaging (MRI), is required to rule out extension of a pleural primary.

Pathogenesis. The pericardium consists of lining mesothelial cells and submesothelial mesenchymal cells that derive embryologically from coelomic epithelium. Cultures of normal mesothelium and mesothelial tumors demonstrate both epithelial and spindled cell types (19,42,53). It follows that the majority of malignant tumors of the pericardium demonstrate a biphasic growth pattern of spindled (sarcomatous) and epithelioid cells.

The association between malignant mesothelioma of the pleura and asbestosis was first described in 1954 (18), and subsequently established in 1960 (18). Because of the relative rarity of pericardial mesotheliomas, it has been difficult to establish a link between them and asbestos exposure (18). However, there have been increasing reports of pericardial mesothelioma arising in patients with known exposure to asbestos (3,7,13,21). It is currently believed that, like pleural mesotheliomas, at least some mesotheliomas of the pericardium are caused by asbestosis (21). One patient developed a pericardial mesothelioma 15 years after pericardial dusting with asbestos and fiber glass as a treatment for angina pectoris (7).

Exposure to various mineral fibers greatly increases the risk of developing mesothelioma (18). In general, those fibers with a high length-diameter ratio and good durability in biologic tissue are most likely to cause malignant mesothelioma. These include crocidolite asbestos and erionite, and nonasbestos fibrous zeolite. Types of asbestos with a moderate to high propensity to cause mesothelioma include amosite and tremolite asbestos. Chrysotile and anthophillite asbestos particles apparently cause a small increase in the incidence of mesothelioma in exposed populations (18).

Incidence. Mesothelioma of the pericardium is a rare tumor: using strict criteria, there were only 31 cases in the literature in 1974 (2); Hillerdal (6) compiled 33 cases from major Western journals in 1982; and approximately 25 cases have been reported since then (1,3,9,14,24,25,28, 30,32–34,37,41,44–47,52). Over 200 cases have been reported worldwide (46), including cases in which the histologic features and autopsy findings are poorly documented. Pericardial mesotheliomas represent approximately 0.7 percent of malignant mesotheliomas, while pleural and peritoneal tumors represent over 98 percent of the total (18). Of 240 thoracic mesotheliomas in the Armed Forces Institute of Pathology (AFIP) files from 1970 to the present, only 8 were limited to the heart and pericardium. In Canada, with a population of 40 million, approximately one case of pericardial mesothelioma occurs yearly, representing a yearly incidence of 0.0025 per 100,000 (27).

Clinical Features. *Patient Data and Role of Asbestos Exposure.* The mean age of patients at presentation of pericardial mesothelioma is 46 years, with an age range of 2 to 78 years. These figures are derived from the reports of 51 patients with primary pericardial mesothelioma (1,2,6,7,9,10,14,18,22,24,28,30,33,34,36,37,39, 41,44–47,52) and 8 additional cases in the AFIP files. Of these patients, 39 were men and 20 were women. The male to female ratio of nearly 2 to 1 is lower than the ratio of 3.5 to 1 for mesotheliomas of the pleura (18). The higher proportion of women suggests that the link with asbestos exposure is weaker for pericardial than for pleural mesothelioma, or that some pericardial mesotheliomas are pathogenetically distinct from their pleural counterparts.

In most cases of reported mesotheliomas of the pericardium, no history of asbestos exposure is mentioned; many of these reports, however, appeared before this link was established. Recently, several patients with a history of asbestos exposure developed pericardial mesothelioma (3,7, 13,21), as did four of eight patients in the AFIP files. A patient with tuberous sclerosis and pericardial mesothelioma has also been reported (32).

Signs and Symptoms. At the time of presentation, nearly 75 percent of patients with pericardial mesothelioma are dyspneic (43) and radiographically demonstrate cardiac enlargement (2). Pericardial effusions or solid tumor infiltrates are the cause of the cardiomegaly. Cardiac tamponade is unusual at the time of presentation (1,22,43), but often develops during the course of disease (10,43,46,52). Although effusions are the rule, the pericardial cavity may be obliterated by tumor, explaining the lack of fluid at pericardiocentesis in some cases (9).

Radiologic Evaluation. Two-dimensional echocardiography is effective in distinguishing pericardial mesothelioma from effusion (1,9,41), and MRI and CT help delineate mediastinal lymphadenopathy and the relationship of tumor to the great vessels (44,47). Gallium 67 and technetium 99 scintigraphy have also been used in the localization of pericardial mesothelioma (44). CT may guide transcutaneous needle biopsy for diagnostic tissue without sternotomy (47).

Tissue Sampling. Although the diagnosis may be made on the basis of ultrastructural and immunohistochemical evaluation of pericardial fluid (22), repeated pericardiocentesis may be necessary to diagnose the malignancy (9,10,22,46). Hyaluronic acid levels of greater than 800 mg/L are evidence of pleural mesothelioma (44); similarly, elevated levels of hyaluronic acid in pericardial fluid have been found in a patient with pericardial mesothelioma (44). Definitive diagnosis is based on the evaluation of tissue samples that demonstrate typical histologic, ultrastructural, and immunohistochemical findings.

Differential Diagnosis. Pericardial mesothelioma may occasionally mimic lupus erythematosus (28), rheumatic fever (36), tuberculous pericarditis (37), and cardiac myxoma (25). Cerebral ischemia may result from infiltration of the carotid vessels (14,28). Pericardial mesothelioma may compress mediastinal vessels, in-

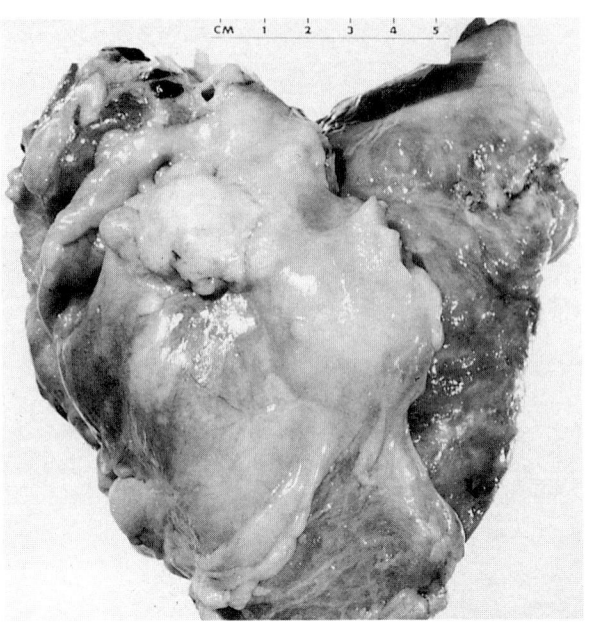

Figure 14-1
MALIGNANT MESOTHELIOMA: PERICARDIUM
Note the gross tumor studding the epicardial surface.

cluding the superior vena cava, resulting in superior vena cava syndrome (2,43). Rarely, extension into the epicardial coronary arteries may result in acute myocardial infarction (6).

Gross Pathologic Findings. Malignant mesotheliomas of the pericardium form bulky nodules that fill the pericardial cavity, often encircling the heart (figs. 14-1–14-3). Multiple satellite nodules are commonly found along the diaphragmatic and pleural surfaces. Pericardial mesotheliomas often encircle the great vessels (43,47), and may obstruct the vena cava (10). Deep infiltration of the myocardium is rare, although deep extension with infiltration of the tricuspid valve has been reported (48). The tumor itself is firm and white (fig. 14-1), although hemorrhagic, cystic, and necrotic areas may be present. One pericardial mesothclioma was grossly described as resembling placental tissue (46).

Microscopic Findings. Malignant mesotheliomas of the pericardium resemble pleural mesotheliomas. Mesotheliomas are divided into epithelial, mixed (biphasic), and sarcomatoid types on the basis of histologic growth patterns. The epithelial component forms tubules, papillary structures, and cords of infiltrating cells that can incite a desmoplastic response (figs. 14-4–14-12).

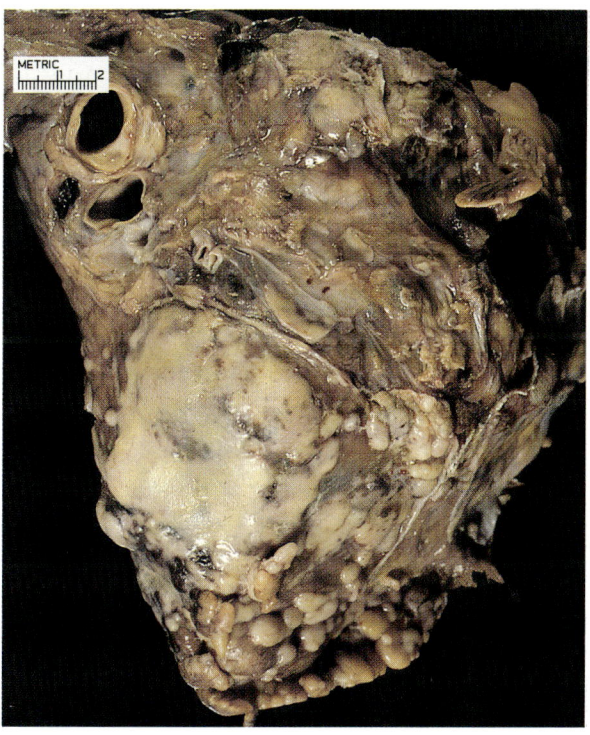

Figure 14-2
MALIGNANT MESOTHELIOMA: PERICARDIUM
There is studding of the pericardium with tumor deposits. The patient was a 50-year-old man with a 2-year history of pericarditis progressing to pericardial constriction.

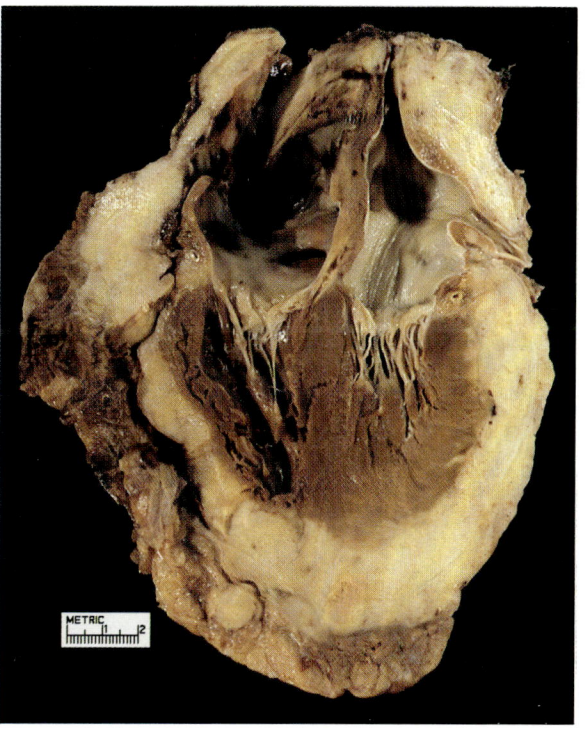

Figure 14-3
MALIGNANT MESOTHELIOMA: PERICARDIUM
There is total encasement of the atria and left ventricles by firm, white tumor.

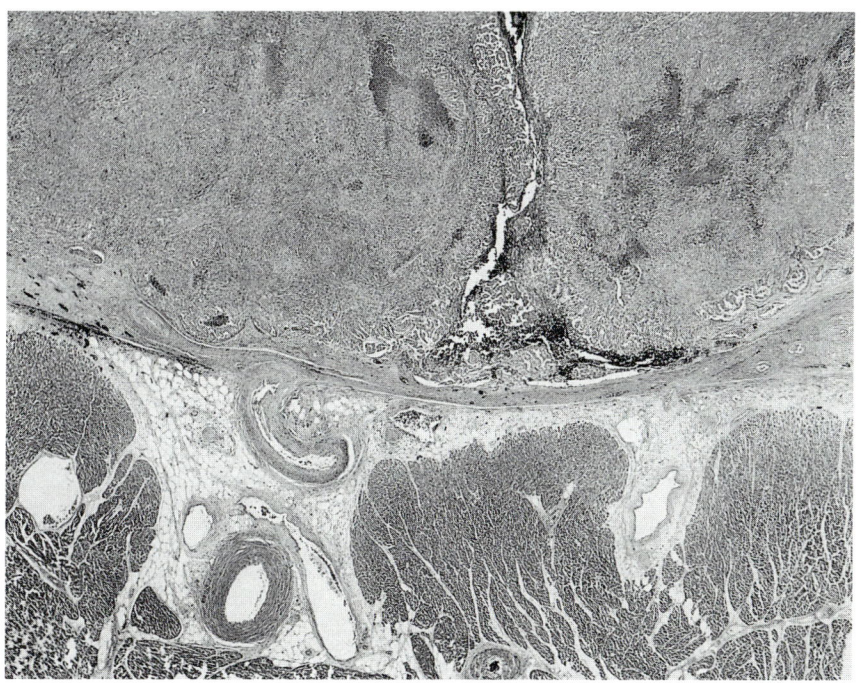

Figure 14-4
MALIGNANT
MESOTHELIOMA:
PERICARDIUM
There is a partly necrotic mass on the surface of the epicardium.

Figure 14-5
MALIGNANT
MESOTHELIOMA,
EPITHELIOID TYPE:
PERICARDIUM

A higher magnification of figure
14-4 demonstrates a predominantly
epithelioid tumor forming papillary
structures on the pericardial surface (left) and tubules infiltrating
stroma (right).

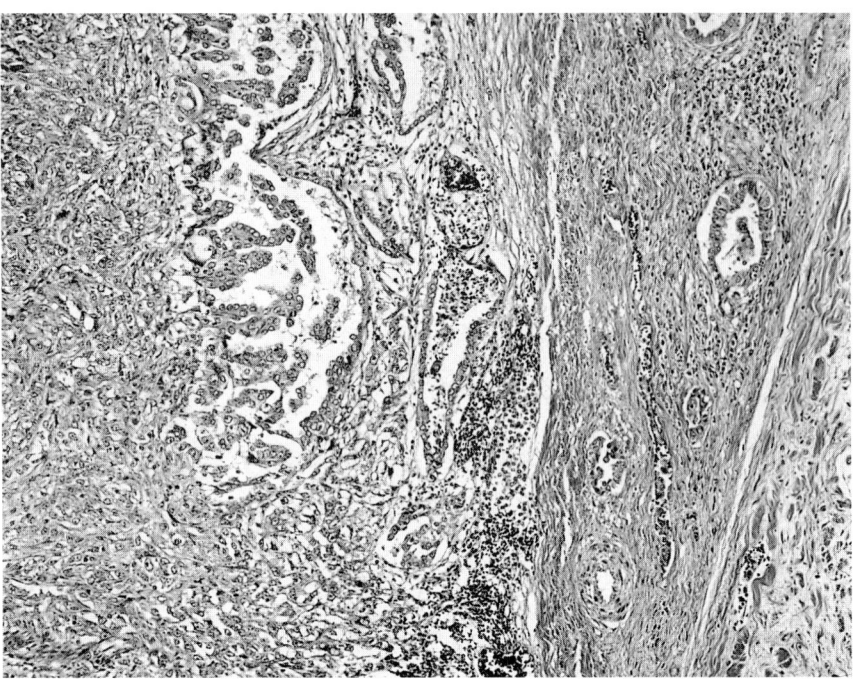

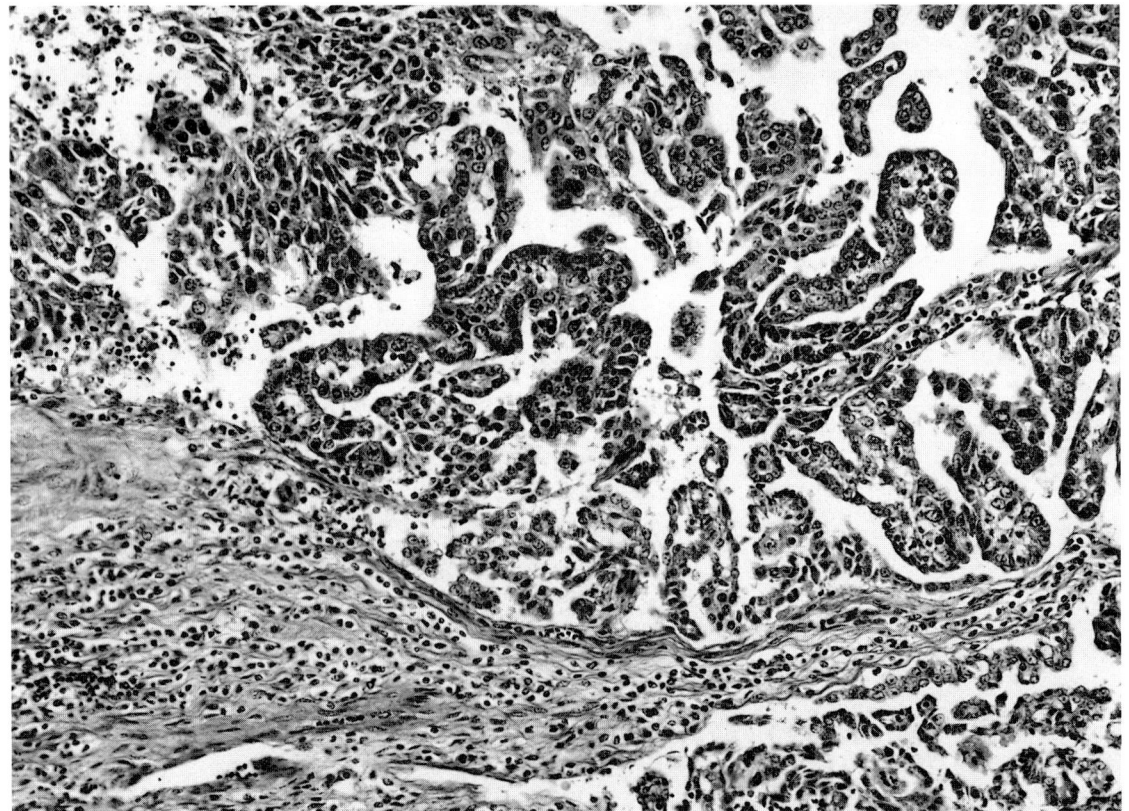

Figure 14-6
MALIGNANT MESOTHELIOMA, EPITHELIOID TYPE: PERICARDIUM
A higher magnification of figure 14-5 demonstrates papillary areas.

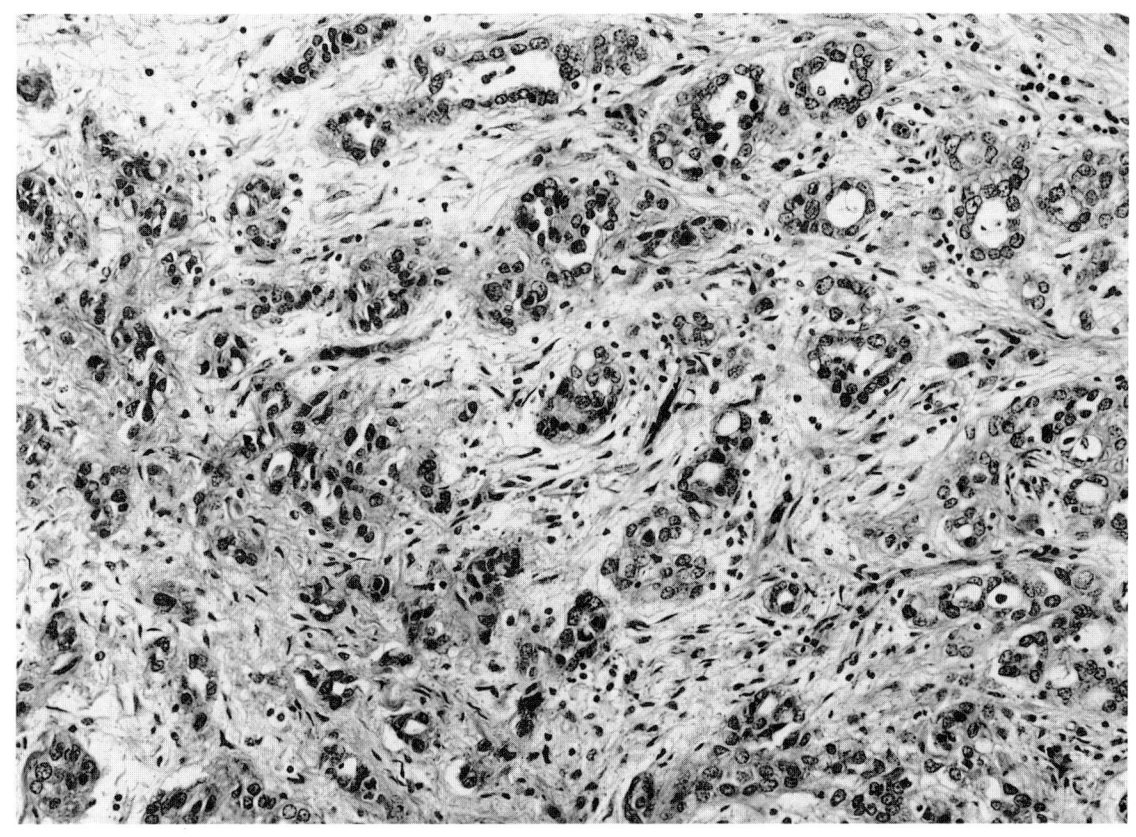

Figure 14-7
MALIGNANT MESOTHELIOMA, EPITHELIOID TYPE: PERICARDIUM
The tumor infiltrates as tubules which histologically mimic adenocarcinoma.

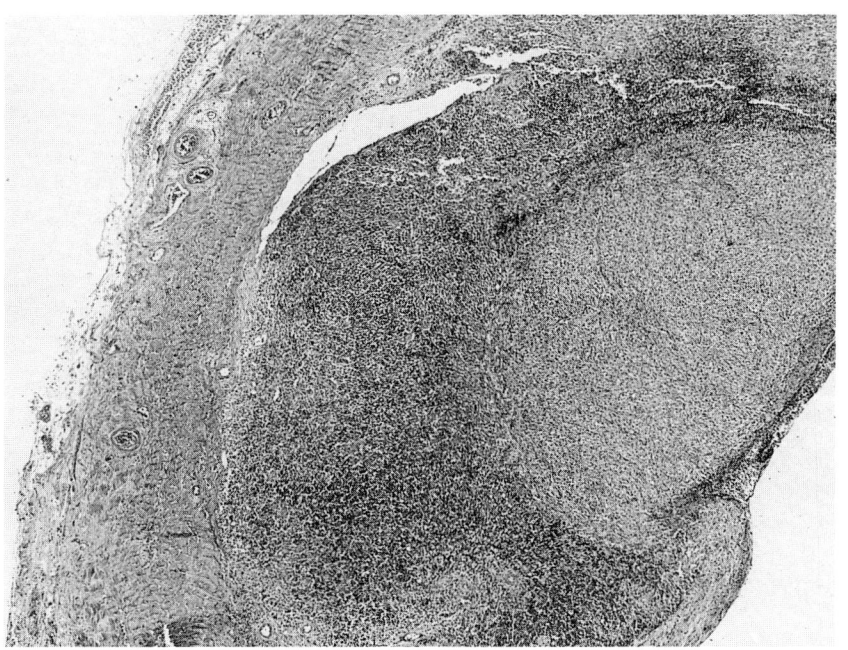

Figure 14-8
MALIGNANT MESOTHELIOMA,
EPITHELIOID TYPE:
PERICARDIUM
The patient was a 66-year-old male with a known history of asbestos exposure and pleural plaques who developed diffuse pericardial tumor. A low magnification view shows a section of pericardium that is markedly thickened.

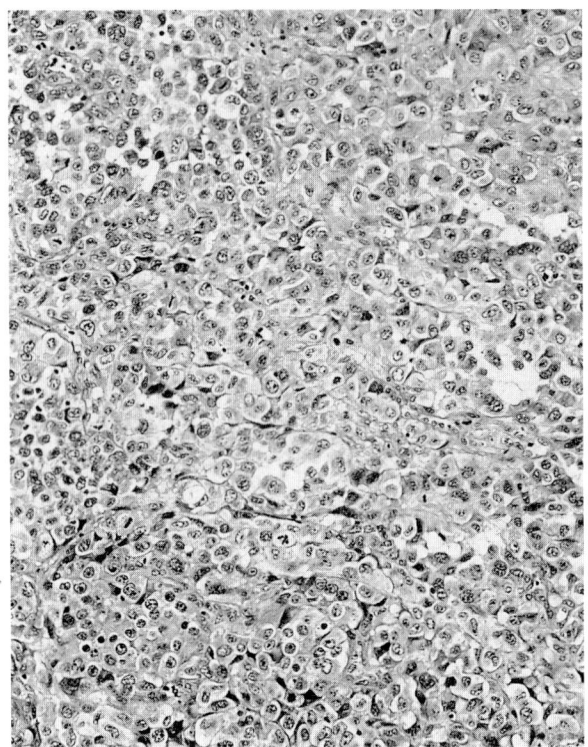

Figure 14-9
MALIGNANT MESOTHELIOMA,
EPITHELIOID TYPE: PERICARDIUM

A higher magnification of the tumor shown in figure 14-8 demonstrates an epithelioid neoplasm mimicking carcinoma. A primary carcinoma was ruled out at autopsy.

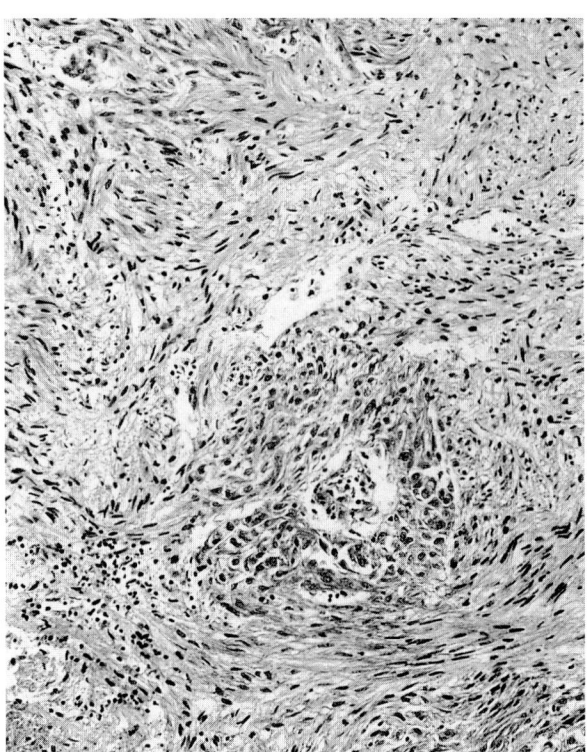

Figure 14-10
MALIGNANT MESOTHELIOMA,
BIPHASIC TYPE: PERICARDIUM

This tumor has epithelioid cells (lower half) surrounded by spindled cells. The patient was a 46-year-old woman with constrictive pericarditis; the pericardium was studded with coalescing tumor nodules.

In biphasic tumors, it may be difficult to separate reactive fibroblasts from the malignant spindle cell component of the tumor (figs. 14-10, 14-11). Sarcomatoid mesothelioma may focally resemble malignant fibrous histiocytoma or undifferentiated sarcoma (figs. 14-12, 14-13). The sarcomatoid cells have large oval nuclei, prominent nucleoli, and abundant cytoplasm, and there is usually a subpopulation of cells with a rounded contour. The epithelioid and spindle cell areas usually merge imperceptibly, and the nuclear features of the sarcomatoid cells are often similar to those of the epithelioid cells (7). Over 75 percent of pericardial mesotheliomas are of the biphasic variety (18,43): in the AFIP files, six pericardial mesothelial tumors had spindled and epithelial areas, one was predominantly sarcomatoid, and one was predominantly epithelial with a tubulopapillary pattern. Occasionally, a pattern reminiscent of adenomatoid tumor, a benign mesothelial tumor

found predominantly in the genital tract, may be present in malignant mesothelioma of the pericardium (figs. 14-14, 14-15).

The presence of hyaluronic acid in mesothelioma has been classically used as a criterion for diagnosis. Mesothelioma contains both intracellular and extracellular glycosaminoglycans. Cytoplasmic vacuoles containing hyaluronic acid and chondroitin sulfate are positive for colloidal iron and Alcian blue at pH 2.5. Staining disappears with pretreatment with hyaluronidase. Extracellular hyaluronic acid is generally plentiful in effusions, and is also detected in tissue sections by colloidal iron and Alcian blue stains. Unfortunately, fewer than 50 percent of pleural mesotheliomas reliably demonstrate hyaluronic acid–digestible colloidal iron or Alcian blue vacuoles (20,49). Mucicarmine rarely, if ever, stains cytoplasmic vacuoles of mesothelioma (26,49).

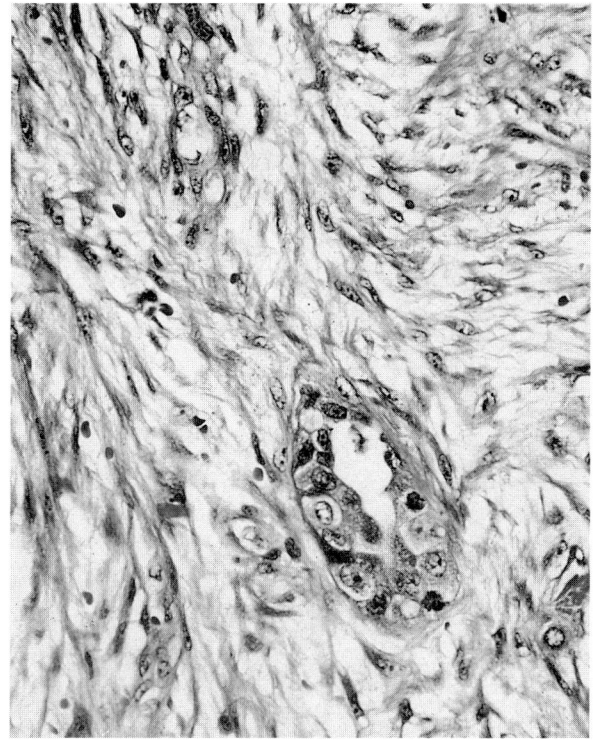

Figure 14-11
MALIGNANT MESOTHELIOMA: PERICARDIUM
A higher magnification of a different area of the tumor depicted in figure 14-10 shows biphasic tumor mimicking desmoplastic adenocarcinoma.

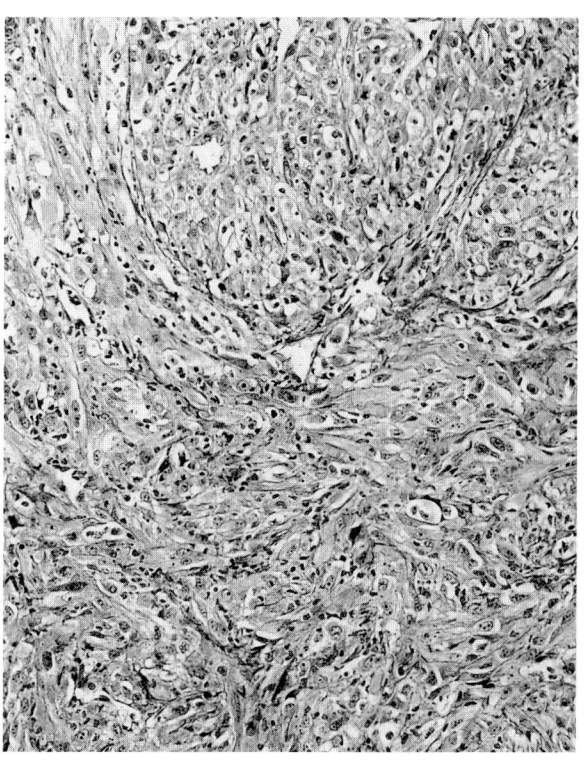

Figure 14-12
MALIGNANT MESOTHELIOMA: PERICARDIUM
The spindled and epithelioid areas may merge, imparting a sarcomatoid appearance. The patient was a 56-year-old woman with pericardial tamponade and diffuse pericardial tumor surrounding the root of the aorta.

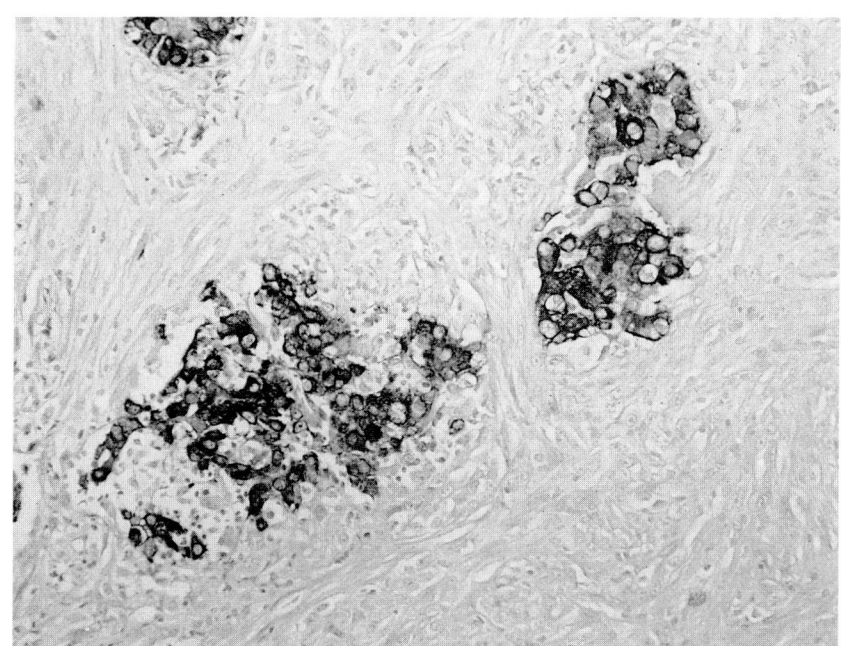

Figure 14-13
MALIGNANT MESOTHELIOMA:
PERICARDIUM
Immunohistochemical stain reveals epithelioid areas that strongly express cytokeratin; the spindled cells are often less strongly reactive for this antibody.

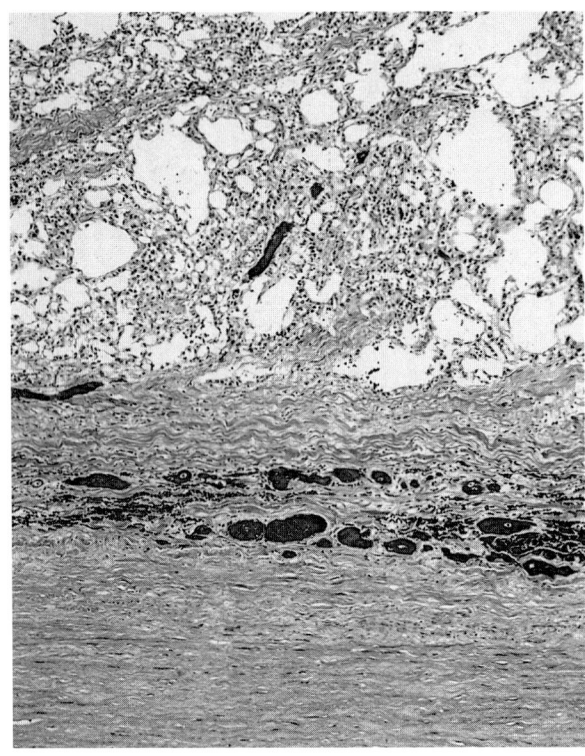

Figure 14-14
MALIGNANT MESOTHELIOMA: PERICARDIUM
The patient was a 69-year-old man who died shortly after open thoracotomy to relieve pericardial constriction. There were multiple tumor nodules on the epicardial surfaces of both atria, enveloping the aortic root. This tumor has a histologic appearance reminiscent of an adenomatoid tumor.

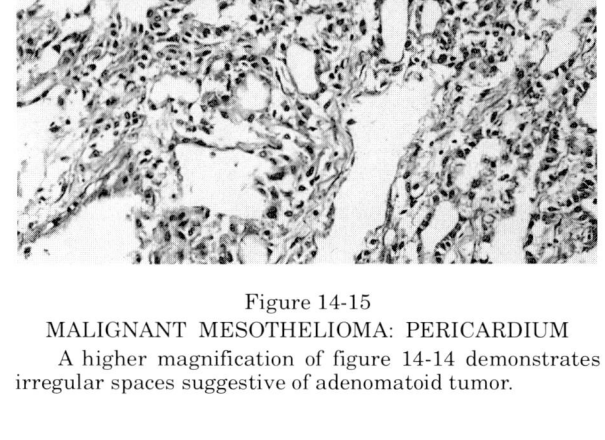

Figure 14-15
MALIGNANT MESOTHELIOMA: PERICARDIUM
A higher magnification of figure 14-14 demonstrates irregular spaces suggestive of adenomatoid tumor.

The incidence of intracytoplasmic and extracellular proteoglycans is difficult to determine from reports of pericardial mesothelioma. Most reports mention the presence of hyaluronidase-sensitive material within the tumor, but illustrations are generally lacking, as are specific methodologies in many cases.

Immunohistochemically, virtually 100 percent of pleural mesotheliomas express cytokeratin, primarily in its high molecular weight form, in epithelioid areas (fig. 14-13); sarcomatoid cells express cytokeratin in about 75 percent of cases, often focally. Vimentin is preferentially expressed in the spindle cell areas of mesothelioma, but less often than cytokeratin (49). Epithelial membrane antigen is frequently present in the epithelioid areas of mesothelioma (49), although expression of this antigen appears inconsistent (38). Mesotheliomas, in general, do not express car-cinoembryonic antigen, B72.3 antigen, and Leu-M1, although there are exceptions.

There is little reported immunohistochemical data regarding pericardial mesotheliomas (14). In our experience, epithelial membrane antigen and vimentin are present in fewer than 50 percent of pericardial cases. Cytokeratin is invariably present, diffusely within epithelioid areas and focally within the spindled or sarcomatous areas.

Ultrastructurally, mesothelioma cells from epithelioid areas contain branched, bushy microvilli in virtually all cases (fig. 14-16) (49). Cytoplasmic tonofibrils are present in approximately 50 percent of tumors. Again, there are few ultrastructural reports of pericardial mesotheliomas, but long microvilli are invariably mentioned (22). Asbestos bodies may be identified within pericardial mesothelioma, supporting an association with asbestos exposure (7,13).

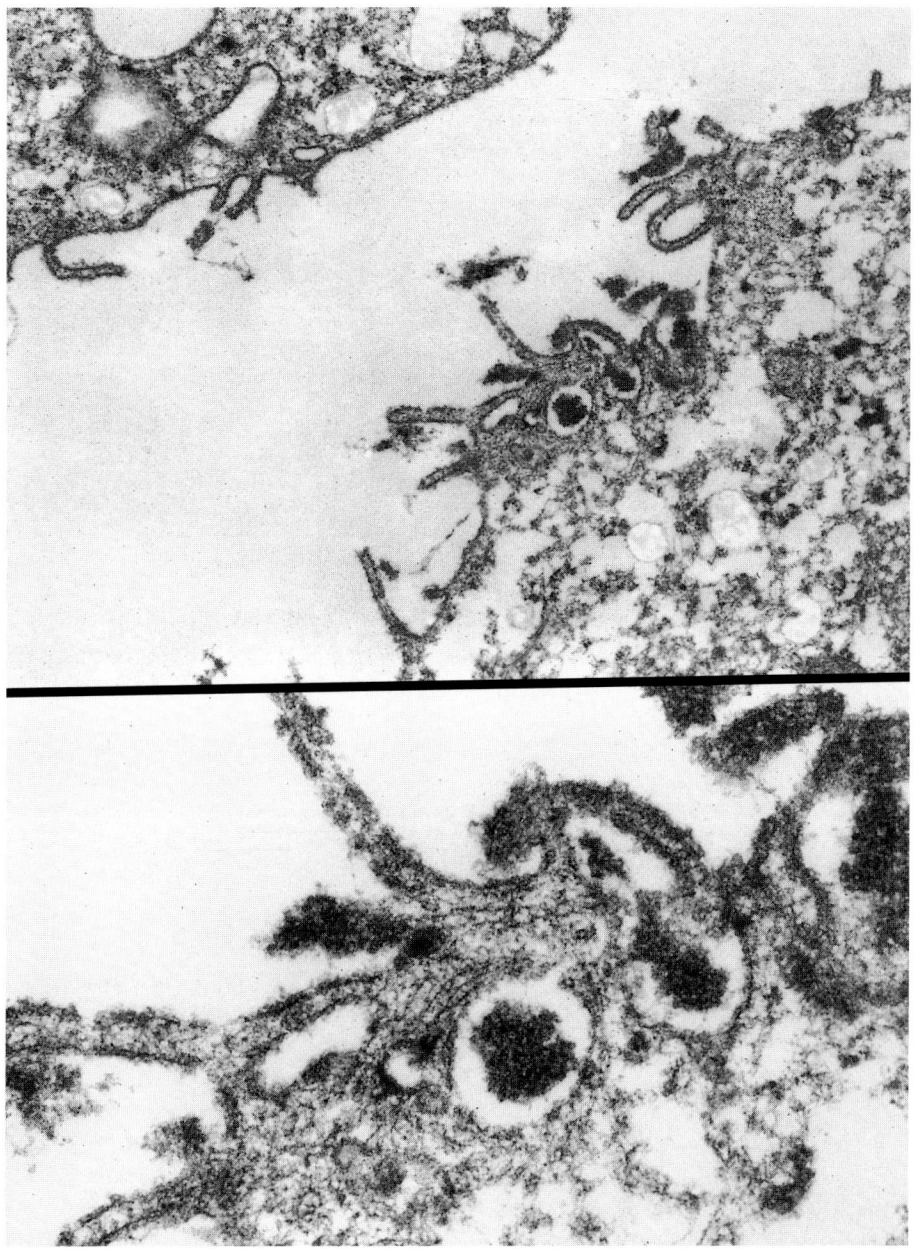

Figure 14-16
MALIGNANT MESOTHELIOMA: PERICARDIUM
Electron micrograph demonstrates elongated microvilli characteristic of mesothelial differentiation.

As with pleural mesothelioma, the diagnosis of pericardial mesothelioma may be made on the basis of cytologic smears of serous effusions (22, 40). While the presence of a biphasic cell population is suggestive of the diagnosis, immunohistochemical or ultrastructural studies on the exfoliated cells are necessary for a definitive diagnosis.

Differential Diagnosis. *Metastatic Adenocarcinoma.* The distinction between mesothelioma and pleural-based lung adenocarcinoma can be quite difficult (see chapter 15). Histologically, the same difficulties apply for pericardial mesothelioma and metastatic adenocarcinoma. If the tumor grossly encases the heart, and a primary tumor in the lung has been excluded, primary pericardial mesothelioma is likely. However, metastatic carcinoma to the pericardium may result in a bulky, infiltrating tumor, even if the primary tumor is small or occult (2).

Differentiating mesothelioma and adenocarcinoma is facilitated by histochemical, ultrastructural, and immunohistological studies. In general, a definitive diagnosis is rendered only after a panel of stains has been performed. The simplest histochemical stain that identifies adenocarcinoma is the periodic acid–Schiff (PAS) after diastase pretreatment. Intracytoplasmic PAS-positive vacuoles are rarely, if ever, present in mesotheliomas (26,49), but are present in 46 to 61 percent of adenocarcinomas of all types (20), and 52 percent of adenocarcinomas of the lung.

Acid mucins, as detected by colloidal iron or Alcian blue stains at pH 2.5, are present in approximately 40 percent of mesotheliomas and disappear when pretreated with hyaluronidase. Colloidal iron is positive in less than 25 percent of adenocarcinomas, and tends to disappear or diminish in intensity after hyaluronidase pretreatment (49).

Ultrastructurally, intracytoplasmic lumina and cytoplasmic mucin droplets are absent in virtually all mesotheliomas and are present in approximately 50 percent of adenocarcinomas of the lung (49). Branched, "bushy" microvilli are present in over 75 percent of mesotheliomas and absent in lung carcinomas (49). The length to diameter ratio of surface microvilli in mesothelioma ranges from 10–16 to 1, and in adenocarcinoma, from 4–7.5 to 1.

Many immunohistochemical markers have been used to distinguish adenocarcinoma from mesothelioma. The majority exclude mesothelioma if there is a positive reaction. Carcinoembryonic antigen is expressed in 77 to 95 percent of adenocarcinomas (8,20,29,31,50) and in 0 to 22 percent of mesotheliomas (4,11,29,31,49, 50). Polyclonal antisera should be absorbed against splenic tissues to remove antibodies that cross-react with nonspecific glycoproteins. Monoclonal antibodies are generally more specific than polyclonal antisera, and are less often positive in mesothelioma (11). Although those anticarcinoembryonic antigen reagents that react with neutrophils may react with some mesotheliomas, we believe that a positive reaction with carcinoembryonic antigen is very useful in excluding malignant mesothelioma (4).

Leu-M1, a cell membrane–associated glycoprotein, is present in 0 to 8 percent of mesotheliomas (8,38,49,50), but in 80 to 100 percent of adenocarcinomas of the lung (49,50), and 42 to 60 percent (8,31,38) of carcinomas of all types. B72.3 antigen, Ber-EP4, and MOC-31 are markers of adenocarcinoma that are also rarely, if ever, expressed by mesothelioma (15,38,49). Weak diffuse cytoplasmic staining may occur in mesothelioma (50), whereas the staining in adenocarcinoma is intense and membranous. More adenocarcinomas express MOC-31 than B72.3 antigen (38), although the reliability of this marker has yet to be thoroughly tested.

Blood group antigens, including Lewis^y, Lewis^x (stage-specific embryonic antigen), and blood group ABH, are preferentially expressed in adenocarcinoma (20). Of these, monoclonal antibody to blood group ABH is the most specific marker for adenocarcinoma when used to differentiate from mesothelioma (49).

Thrombomodulin has been used as a diagnostic marker in the differential diagnosis of adenocarcinoma and mesothelioma (8), but unlike other immunohistochemical tests, positivity with this reagent is indicative of mesothelioma. Although thrombomodulin is a sensitive marker for mesothelioma, it is also expressed in nearly 10 percent of adenocarcinomas (8). Other specific markers for mesothelioma have been developed, including MAb-45, anti-MS, OV632, and ME1 antibody; the specificity of these reagents and their lack of staining in adenocarcinomas has not been fully determined (53).

The published reports of vimentin reactivity in mesotheliomas are discrepant. Wirth et al. (50) found that vimentin positivity reliably identified mesotheliomas (80 percent positivity in epithelioid areas, 100 percent positivity in spindled areas) and was not expressed in lung adenocarcinomas. In contrast, other investigators have found vimentin positive in only 41 percent of epithelioid mesotheliomas (49), but in 17 to 100 percent of carcinomas (5,31,38,49). In our experience, vimentin antigenicity is especially susceptible to prolonged fixation, and staining is variable depending on the extent and type of digestion used.

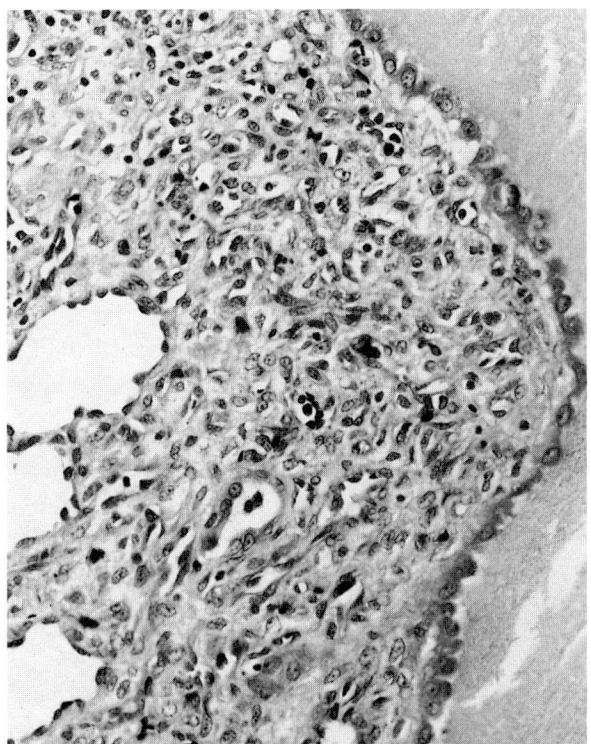

Figure 14-17
ANGIOSARCOMA: PERICARDIUM
A 43-year-old woman presented with pericardial tamponade. A hemorrhagic tumor was found infiltrating the pericardium and right atrium. Histologically, there is a layer of hyperplastic mesothelial cells (right) and a proliferation of atypical vessels (left). The patient died 6 months after surgery with multiple metastatic lesions of angiosarcoma.

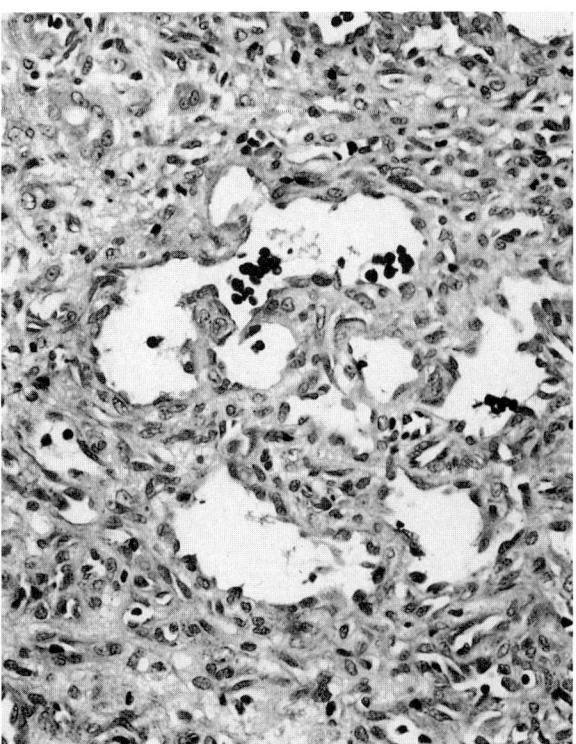

Figure 14-18
ANGIOSARCOMA: PERICARDIUM
A different area of the tumor shown in figure 14-17 demonstrates irregular vascular channels lined by atypical endothelial cells.

Reactive Mesothelial Hyperplasia. It is often difficult to distinguish reactive mesothelial proliferations from malignant mesotheliomas. Benign mesothelial proliferations occasionally result in recurrent pericardial effusions that suggest malignancy (17). In general, malignant mesotheliomas can form sheets of cells, infiltrate fibrous tissue or myocardium, and have spindle and sarcomatoid areas, all features lacking in reactive mesothelial processes. Immunohistochemical stains are of limited use in separating malignant from benign mesothelial reactions: vimentin may be expressed by both benign and malignant mesothelial cells (5,31,38,49); and epithelial membrane antigen has been described as prevalent (49) and rare (38) in both mesothelioma and reactive mesothelial hyperplasia and we have not noted any benefit in using this marker in this situation.

Angiosarcoma. The most common sarcoma that arises within the pericardium is angiosarcoma (see chapter 12). In 1979, 11 cases were reported (19). The relative propensity for angiosarcoma to develop within the pericardium has led to the idea that the cell of origin of mesothelioma may be the same as that of pericardial angiosarcoma. The term "angioblastic mesothelioma" has even been used for pericardial angiosarcomas in order to underscore the concept that these tumors are actually of mesothelial origin (19).

Grossly, angiosarcomas mimic mesothelioma, with diffuse infiltration of the pericardium (45). The diagnosis may be missed on repeated pericardial biopsy if adequate tissue is not retrieved (35), and reactive mesothelial hyperplasia may be present to confound the diagnosis (figs. 14-17, 14-18). Atypical endothelial-lined channels are identified within the tumor or metastases, which generally are restricted to the lungs and thorax (19). Immunohistochemical stains for factor

VIII–related antigen and cytokeratin may be helpful in differentiating angiosarcoma from spindled mesothelioma on biopsy samples.

Unclassifiable Pericardial Sarcomas. Rarely, a malignant spindle cell tumor of the pericardium diffusely infiltrates the pericardium, simulating mesothelioma. Like angiosarcomas of the pericardium, it is possible that these tumors arise from the same precursor cell as typical biphasic mesothelioma. Unlike mesothelioma, there are no epithelioid areas and the spindled areas do not express cytokeratin (23). Such tumors may represent sarcomatoid mesotheliomas which were not sampled sufficiently for identification of epithelioid or cytokeratin-expressing areas. Some spindle cell tumors of the pericardium have immunohistochemical features of both sarcoma and mesothelioma and are difficult to classify even after immunohistochemical and ultrastructural studies have been carried out (16).

Malignant Fibrous Tumor of the Pericardium. Solitary fibrous tumors of the pericardium are rare and are discussed in chapter 6. Although most are benign, some may have cellular areas with pleomorphism and mitotic figures (30,51). These malignant fibrous tumors may recur and infiltrate surrounding structures. In contrast to sarcomatoid mesotheliomas, solitary fibrous tumors are composed of relatively bland spindled cells similar to fibrosarcoma. There is no expression of neural or epithelial markers. Because these tumors immunohistochemically and ultrastructurally resemble fibrous tumors, they are believed to originate from submesothelial fibroblasts and are considered a type of fibrosarcoma (see chapter 12).

Synovial Sarcoma. Synovial sarcomas of the mediastinum have only recently been described (51). Both pericardial mesotheliomas and synovial sarcomas are extremely rare, and it may be very difficult to differentiate them. Although synovial sarcomas are often poorly demarcated, they do not diffusely infiltrate the pericardium, in contrast to mesotheliomas. Histologically, both are biphasic, possessing spindled and epithelioid areas. However, the glandular spaces of synovial sarcoma may be branched and elongated and contain PAS-positive, diastase-resistant material. Unlike typical mesothelioma cells, the spindled cells of synovial sarcoma tend to resemble fibrosarcoma, with finely stippled chromatin and inconspicuous nucleoli. Immunohistochemical studies are not particularly helpful in distinguishing synovial sarcoma and mesothelioma (51), and the differential diagnosis is largely made by the gross and histologic features mentioned above (51).

Malignant Thymoma. A thymoma that infiltrates its capsule or a nearby structure is by definition malignant. In most cases of pericardial infiltration, the bulk of thymoma is within the anterior mediastinum and there is no clinical consideration of mesothelioma, especially if there is a history of myasthenia gravis. Because thymoma and mesothelioma both have epithelioid or spindled growth patterns, and both strongly express cytokeratin, they may be difficult to differentiate on the basis of a small biopsy specimen. Diffuse infiltration of the pericardium, marked cellular atypia, prominent nucleoli, and the absence of a background infiltrate of lymphocytes are features of mesothelioma that help exclude thymoma from diagnostic consideration.

Treatment. There is no satisfactory treatment for pericardial mesothelioma. Pericardial resection is attempted both to prevent recurrent cardiac constriction and for surgical cure (12). Sclerotic agents may be instilled into the pericardium to prevent recurrent fluid accumulation (7). Radiation therapy (7) and combination chemotherapy (30,46) have been used with limited success.

Prognosis. The prognosis of pericardial mesothelioma is poor: 50 percent of patients are dead at 6 months; an exceptional patient may live as long as 48 months (18). The mean survival of patients with pericardial mesothelioma is shorter than that of patients with pleural and peritoneal mesotheliomas (18).

REFERENCES

1. Agatston AS, Robinson MJ, Trigo L, Machado R, Samet P. Echocardiographic findings in primary pericardial mesothelioma. Am Heart J 1986;111:986–8.

2. Andersen JA, Hamsen BF. Primary pericardial mesothelioma. Dan Med Bull 1974;21:195–200.

3. Beck B, Konetzke G, Ludwig V, Rothig W, Sturm W. Malignant pericardial mesotheliomas and asbestos exposure: a case report. Am J Ind Med 1982;3:149–59.

4. Burke AP, Anderson PG, Virmani R, James TN, Herrera GA, Ceballos R. Tumors of the atrioventricular node. Arch Pathol Lab Med 1990:114:1057–62.

5. Cagle PT, Truong LD, Roggli VL, Greenberg SD. Immunohistochemical differentiation of sarcomatoid mesotheliomas from other spindle cell neoplasms. Am J Clin Pathol 1989;92:566–71.

6. Chun PK, Leeburg WT, Coggin JT, Zajtchuk R. Primary pericardial malignant epithelioid mesothelioma causing acute myocardial infarction. Chest 1980;77:559–61.

7. Churg A, Warnock ML, Bensch KG. Malignant mesothelioma arising after direct application of asbestos and fiber glass to the pericardium. Am Rev Respir Dis 1978;118:419–24.

8. Collins CL, Ordonez NG, Schaefer R, et al. Thrombomodulin expression in malignant pleural mesothelioma and pulmonary adenocarcinoma. Am J Pathol 1992;141:827–33.

9. Coplan NL, Kennish AJ, Burgess NL, Deligdish L, Goldman ME. Pericardial mesothelioma masquerading as a benign pericardial effusion. J Am Coll Cardiol 1984;4:1307–10.

10. Dawe CJ, Wood DA, Mitchell S. Diffuse fibrous mesothelioma of the pericardium. Cancer 1953;6:794–800.

11. Dejmek A, Hjerpe A. Carcinoembryonic antigen-like reactivity in malignant mesothelioma. A comparison between different commercially available antibodies. Cancer 1994;73:464–9.

12. Dooley BN, Beckmann C, Hood RH. Primary mesothelioma of the pericardium. Successful surgical removal. J Thorac Cardiovasc Surg 1968;55:719–24.

13. Eck H, Berg-Schlosser V. Zur Pathogenese des malignen Mesotheliom des Perikards. Dtsch Med Wochenschr 1978;103:1751–3.

14. Fazekas T, Ungi I, Tiszlavicz L. Primary malignant mesothelioma of the pericardium. Am Heart J 1992;124:227–31.

15. Frisman DM, McCarthy WF, Schleiff P, Buckner SB, Nocito JD Jr, O'Leary TJ. Immunocytochemistry in the differential diagnosis of effusions: use of logistic regression to select a panel of antibodies to distinguish adenocarcinomas from mesothelial proliferation. Mod Pathol 1993;6:179–84.

16. Fukuda T, Ishikawa H, Ohnishi Y, et al. Malignant spindle cell tumor of the pericardium. Evidence of sarcomatous mesothelioma with aberrant antigen expression. Acta Pathol Jpn 1989;39:750–4.

17. Hansen RM, Caya JG, Clowry LJ Jr, Anderson T. Benign mesothelial proliferation with effusion. Clinicopathologic entity that may mimic malignancy. Am J Med 1984;77:887–92.

18. Hillerdal G. Malignant mesothelioma 1982: review of 4710 published cases. Br J Dis Chest 1983;77:321–43.

19. Hofler H, Schmid P, Tscheliessnigg KH. Malignes angioblastisches Mesotheliom des Perikards. Zentralbl Allg Pathol 1979;123:344–50.

20. Jordon D, Jagirdar J, Kaneko M. Blood group antigens, Lewis x and Lewis y in the diagnostic discrimination of malignant mesothelioma versus adenocarcinoma. Am J Pathol 1989;135:931–7.

21. Kahn EI, Rohl A, Barrett EW, Suzuki Y. Primary pericardial mesothelioma following exposure to asbestos. Environ Res 1980;23:270–81.

22. Kobayashi Y, Takeda S, Yamamoto T, Goi S. Cytologic detection of malignant mesotheliomas of the pericardium. Acta Cytol 1978;22:344–9.

23. Lazoglu AH, Da Silva MM, Iwahara M, et al. Primary pericardial sarcoma. Am Heart J 1994;127:453–8.

24. Llewellyn MJ, Atkinson MW, Fabri B. Pericardial constriction caused by primary mesothelioma. Br Heart J 1987;57:54–7.

25. Lund O, Hansen OK, Ardest S, Baandrup U. Primary malignant pericardial mesothelioma mimicking left atrial myxoma. Case Report. Scand J Thorac Cardiovasc Surg 1987;21:273–5.

26. MacDougall DB, Wang SE, Zidar B. Mucin-positive epithelial mesothelioma. Arch Pathol Lab Med 1992;116:874–80.

27. McDonald AD, Harper A, Jatter OA, McDonald JC. Epidemiology of primary malignant mesothelial tumors in Canada. Cancer 1970;26:94–113.

28. McGuigan L, Fleming A. Pericardial mesothelioma presenting as systemic lupus erythematosus. Ann Rheum Dis 1984;43:515–7.

29. Mezger J, Lamerz R, Permanetter W. Diagnostic significance of carcinoembryonic antigen in the differential diagnosis of malignant mesotheliomas. J Thorac Cardiovasc Surg 1990;100:860–6.

30. Nambiar CA, Tareif HE, Kishore KU, Ravindran J, Banerjee AK. Primary pericardial mesothelioma: one-year event-free survival. Am Heart J 1992;124:802–3.

31. Nance KV, Silverman JF. Immunocytochemical panel for the identification of malignant cells in serous effusions. Am J Clin Pathol 1991;95:867–74.

32. Naramoto A, Itoh N, Nakano M, Shigematsu H. An autopsy case of tuberous sclerosis associated with primary pericardial mesothelioma. Acta Pathol Jpn 1989;39:400–6.

33. Nishikimi T, Ochi H, Hirota K, et al. Primary pericardial mesothelioma detected by gallium-67 scintigraphy. J Nucl Med 1987;28:1210–2.

34. Nomori H, Shimosato Y, Tsuchiya R. Diffuse malignant pericardial mesothelioma. Acta Pathol Jpn 1985;35:1475–81.

35. Poole-Wilson PA, Farnsworth A, Braimbridge MV, Pambakian H. Angiosarcoma of pericardium. Problems in diagnosis and management. Br Heart J 1976;38:240–3.

36. Recant L, Lacy P. Clinical pathologic conference. Pericardial disease with effusion, systemic involvement and pulmonary edema. Am J Med 1962;33:442–9.

37. Rose DS, Vigneswaran WT, Bovill BA, Riordan JF, Sapsford RN, Stanbridge RD. Primary pericardial mesothelioma presenting as tuberculous pericarditis. Postgrad Med J 1992;68:137–9.

38. Ruitenbeek T, Gouw AS, Pappema S. Immunocytology of body cavity fluids. MOC-31, a monoclonal antibody discriminating between mesothelial and epithelial cells. Arch Pathol Lab Med 1994;118:265–9.

39. Sarrell WG. Primary pericardial mesothelioma. Am Heart J 1955;49:310–7.

40. Sherman ME, Mark EJ. Effusion cytology in the diagnosis of malignant epithelioid and biphasic pleural mesothelioma. Arch Pathol Lab Med 1990;114:845–51.

41. Spodick DH. Echography of pericardial mesothelioma. Am Heart J 1986;112:1347.

42. Stout AP, Murray MR. Localized pleural mesothelioma. Report of a case. Arch Pathol 1942;34:955–64.

43. Sytman AL, MacAlpin RN. Primary pericardial mesothelioma: report of two cases and review of the literature. Am Heart J 1971;81:760–9.

44. Takeda K, Ohba H, Hodo H, et al. Pericardial mesothelioma: hyaluronic acid in pericardial fluid. Am Heart J 1985;110:486–8.

45. Terada T, Nakanuma T, Matsubara T, Suematsu T. An autopsy case of primary angiosarcoma of the pericardium mimicking malignant mesothelioma. Acta Pathol Jpn 1988;38:1345–51.

46. Turk J, Kenda M, Kranjec I. Primary malignant pericardial mesothelioma. Klin Wochenschr 1991;69:674–8.

47. Vogel HJ, Wondergem JH, Falke TH. Mesotheliomas of the pericardium: CT and MR findings. J Comput Assist Tomogr 1989;13:543–4.

48. Walters LL, Taxy JB. Malignant mesotheliomas of the pleura with extensive cardiac invasion and tricuspid orifice occlusion. Cancer 1983;52:1736–8.

49. Wick MR, Mills SE, Swanson PE. Expression of myelomonocytic antigens in mesotheliomas and adenocarcinomas involving the serosal surfaces. Am J Clin Pathol 1990;94:18–26.

50. Wirth PR, Legier J, Wright GL. Immunohistochemical evaluation of seven monoclonal antibodies for differentiation of pleural mesothelioma from lung adenocarcinoma. Cancer 1991;67:655–62.

51. Witkin GB, Miettinen M, Rosai J. A biphasic tumor of the mediastinum with features of synovial sarcoma. Am J Surg Pathol 1989;13:490–9.

52. Yilling FP, Schlant RC, Hertzler GL, Krzyaniak R. Pericardial mesothelioma. Chest 1982;81:520–3.

53. Zeng L, Fleury-Feith J, Monnet I, Boutin C, Bignon J, Jaurand MC. Immunocytochemical characterization of cell lines from human malignant mesothelioma: characterization of human mesothelioma cell lines by immunocytochemistry with a panel of monoclonal antibodies. Human Pathol 1994;25:227–34.

✧✧✧

15

TUMORS METASTATIC TO THE HEART AND PERICARDIUM

Definition. The theoretical distinction between primary and metastatic tumors of the heart is straightforward. Carcinomas involving the heart are, by definition, metastatic. Sarcomas and mesotheliomas are considered metastatic if a primary extrapericardial site is identified at autopsy or upon clinical evaluation.

There are two tumors in which the definition of primary cardiac tumor is not always clear. The terms "primary" and "metastatic" lymphoma of the heart are not entirely meaningful, because the site of origin of multifocal or extranodal lymphoma is not generally possible to determine (see chapter 13). If the bulk of lymphoma is confined within the pericardium, and the patient presents with cardiac disease, the term primary lymphoma of the heart is often used. Similarly, there is some disagreement about the nomenclature of Kaposi's sarcoma when it involves the heart or pericardium. In almost every case of cardiac Kaposi's sarcoma, there is extracardiac involvement; whether the cardiac tumors are considered secondary lesions or new primary tumors is debated. Because the true nature of Kaposi's sarcoma is still unclear, we prefer the use of term "involvement" for cardiac Kaposi's sarcoma, rather than "metastasis."

Metastatic Pathways of Secondary Tumors of the Heart. Malignancies spread to the heart by four paths: direct extension, usually from mediastinal tumor; hematogenous spread; lymphatic spread; and intracavitary extension from the inferior vena cava, or rarely, the pulmonary veins. There may be a combination of more than one of these routes. Lymphatic spread is generally accompanied by tumor enlargement of pulmonary hilar or mediastinal lymph nodes (63), and there is histologic evidence of pericardial lymphatic infiltration (38). Hematogenous spread is characterized by myocardial metastatic tumors which, when small, resemble abscesses.

Although there are exceptions, epithelial malignancies typically spread to the heart by lymphatics. Melanoma, sarcomas, leukemia, and renal cell carcinoma metastasize to the heart by a hematogenous route. Lymphomas may involve the heart by virtually any path, including direct extension, hematogenous seeding, or lymphatic spread (48). Thymoma and esophageal carcinoma involve the heart by direct extension. Melanomas, renal tumors including Wilms' tumor and renal cell carcinoma, adrenal tumors, liver tumors, and uterine tumors are the most frequent intracavitary tumors (11,28,50). However, tumors of virtually any type may result in intracavitary metastasis.

Lymphatic dissemination in the heart is often the result of retrograde lymphatic spread secondary to blocked mediastinal or hilar lymphatics (63). The majority of lymph flow in the heart is efferent, which explains the low incidence of cardiac metastases (42). The mediastinal lymphatics include lymphatics of the superior vena cava, aortopulmonary artery, and pulmonary artery, and the left atrium-subcarinal lymph nodes (63). The lymphatic spread of metastasis is associated with a high incidence of malignant pericardial effusions, in contrast to hematogenous spread (63), which is associated with myocardial metastases.

Incidence. Tumor metastases to the heart are seen in approximately 15 percent of autopsies of patients with disseminated cancer (Table 15-1). The primary tumors can be divided into three categories of incidence (42): those that are uncommon primary tumors, but have a high rate of metastasis to the heart (malignant melanoma, malignant germ cell tumor, malignant thymoma); common tumors that have an intermediate rate of cardiac metastasis, but account for the greatest numbers of cardiac metastases (carcinoma of the lung and breast); and common tumors that have a low rate of cardiac metastasis (carcinoma of the stomach, liver, ovary, colon, and rectum). Table 15-1 lists, by relative incidence, rates of cardiac involvement by metastatic tumors as assessed by two large studies (37,42).

The frequency of cardiac metastasis in patients with metastatic epithelial malignancies ranges from 4.2 percent (35) to approximately 30 percent (1,2,36,37,60,63). The frequency depends in part on the primary neoplasm: lung, breast, thyroid, and kidney cancers have the

Table 15-1

TUMORS METASTATIC TO THE HEART AT AUTOPSY*

Primary Tumor	Total Autopsies	Heart Involvement**	Pericardial Involvement	Total (Heart and Pericardial Involvement)
Melanoma	69	32 (46%)	2 (3%)	34 (49%)
Malignant germ cell tumor	21	8 (38%)	1 (5%)	9 (42%)
Leukemia	202	66 (33%)	2 (1%)	68 (34%)
Carcinoma of lung	1037	180 (17%)	112 (11%)	292 (28%)
Sarcoma	159	24 (15%)	11 (7%)	35 (22%)
Lymphoma	392	67 (17%)	15 (4%)	82 (21%)
Carcinoma of breast	685	70 (10%)	69 (10%)	139 (20%)
Carcinoma of esophagus	294	37 (13%)	13 (4%)	50 (17%)
Carcinoma of kidney	114	12 (11%)	5 (4%)	17 (15%)
Carcinoma of oral cavity and tongue	235	22 (9%)	2 (1%)	24 (10%)
Carcinoma of larynx	100	9 (9%)	2 (2%)	11 (11%)
Carcinoma of thyroid	97	9 (9%)	3 (3%)	12 (12%)
Carcinoma of uterus	451	36 (8%)	5 (1%)	41 (9%)
Carcinoma of stomach	603	28 (5%)	16 (3%)	44 (7%)
Carcinoma of colon and rectum	440	22 (5%)	3 (1%)	25 (6%)
Carcinoma of pharynx	67	1	2	3 (4.5%)
Carcinoma of urinary bladder	128	8 (6%)	0	8 (6%)
Carcinoma of ovary	188	2 (1%)	6 (3%)	8 (4%)
Carcinoma of prostate	171	6 (4%)	0	6 (4%)
Carcinoma of nasal cavity	32	1	0	1 (3%)
Carcinoma of pancreas	185	6 (3%)	0	6 (3%)
Carcinoma of liver and biliary tract	325	7 (2%)	0	7 (2%)
TOTALS†	6240	654 (10%)	299 (5%)	953 (15%)

*From references 37, 42.
**Includes tumors with pericardial and myocardial involvement.
†Includes uncommon tumors not included in table.

highest rates of spread to the heart (35,37). Ovarian carcinoma involves the pericardium in 2.4 percent of patients, and 6 percent of those with stage IV disease (13). Cardiac metastases from the gastrointestinal and genitourinary tracts, especially prostate, are rare (1,35,37). In one series, a particular high rate of metastasis from the oral cavity was found (36). The rate of cardiac involvement by metastatic disease has not changed over a 14-year period (1), indicating that treatment may not have a significant effect on the rate of metastatic malignancy to the heart.

Hematologic malignancies are especially prone to involve the heart, especially the myocardium (37). Approximately 35 to 40 percent of patients with leukemia had cardiac involvement at autopsy (37,54). Lymphomatous cardiac infiltrates were found at autopsy in 7 (35) to 25 percent (55) of patients dying of lymphoma. Roberts et al. (55) reported a 16 percent incidence of cardiac metastases in Hodgkin's disease, a 33 percent incidence in mycosis fungoides, and a 27 percent incidence in other types of lymphoma.

Metastatic melanoma is the malignancy most likely to spread to the heart (18,37): up to 64 percent of patients who died of melanoma had cardiac involvement at autopsy. The heart is affected in 8 to 25 percent of patients with metastatic soft tissue or skeletal sarcoma (19).

In a series of childhood autopsies (10), only 1.6 percent of children with solid malignancies had evidence of cardiac involvement at autopsy. Tumors metastatic to the heart in children, in order of decreasing frequency, are non-Hodgkin's lymphoma, Wilms' tumor, neuroblastoma, rhabdomyosarcoma, undifferentiated sarcoma, hepatoma, and adrenal cortical carcinoma (10).

In patients with acquired immunodeficiency syndrome (AIDS), Kaposi's sarcoma is the most common neoplasm involving the heart (4), occurring in about 5 percent of autopsy cases (33). Of surgically resected cardiac tumors, metastatic lesions comprise 3 to 17 percent of all tumor resections and 22 to 61 percent of malignant tumors (40,43).

Clinical Features. *Symptoms.* Although cardiac metastases are relatively common at autopsy in patients with various malignancies, the clinical symptoms are often overlooked (38). Retrospectively, the incidence of cardiac symptoms presumed related to the cardiac metastases identified at autopsy ranges from 20 percent (10) to 43 percent (2), however, only half of these are ascribed clinically (10); at autopsy, it is often difficult to determine which cardiac symptoms were related to malignant cardiac infiltrates (18,54,55).

The signs and symptoms in patients with cardiac metastases documented at autopsy are widely variable. They include dyspnea on exertion, pleural effusions, echocardiographic low voltage effects, conduction block, supraventricular tachycardias, right ventricular outflow tract obstruction (28,45), and myocardial ischemia from coronary occlusion or tumor embolus (19, 35,42,45,63,65). In 8 to 32 percent of patients with metastatic cardiac disease the cause of death is related to the cardiac tumor (35, 42). In these cases, cardiac tamponade, cardiac rupture, congestive heart failure, compression of sino-

atrial node or coronary arteries, or coronary artery embolism have led to death (35,65).

Presenting symptoms in patients that undergo surgery for metastatic cardiac tumors are similar to those described in autopsy studies. A partial list follows, in order of decreasing frequency: dyspnea, cough, chest pain, hemiparesis, palpitations, fever, abdominal distension or pain, hemiparesis, pedal edema, and symptoms related to superior vena cava syndrome and right ventricular outflow obstruction (14).

Radiologic Diagnosis. Imaging studies, especially two-dimensional echocardiography (32), magnetic resonance scans (58,40), and gallium scans (31) are effective in localizing metastatic cardiac tumors. Because clinical recognition and treatment may increase patient survival (48), two-dimensional echocardiography (42) and computed tomography scans (10) have been recommended for early diagnosis of cardiac metastases. Imaging studies have resulted in diagnosis without pathologic documentation (9,24,26,48,49); in these cases, radiation or chemotherapy was given as an alternative treatment to surgery or the patient died before surgery could be accomplished.

Clinical Aspects of Pericardial Metastases. Pericardial involvement is suspected in patients with cancer if there is acute pericarditis, rapid enlargement of the heart shadow, low voltage changes on electrocardiography, serosanguinous or sanguinous effusions, or echocardiographic demonstration of echo-free spaces in pericardial effusions (59). Pericardial tamponade occasionally results from a variety of metastatic pericardial malignancies, including carcinomas of the lung, pancreas, kidney, breast, and ovary, as well as lymphoma, leukemia, and rhabdomyosarcoma (3,7,22,34,56). The diagnostic yield of pericardial biopsies may be enhanced by pericardioscopy, which allows the surgeon to endoscopically visualize the pericardial cavity, as compared to surgical subxiphoid biopsy, which is a relatively blind procedure (39). Recently, echocardiographically guided percutaneous biopsy has been successful in demonstrating metastatic malignancy (57). Occasionally, pericardial metastases are asymptomatic (67) and discovered incidentally at echocardiography.

Malignant infiltrates are not the only cause of pericardial effusions in cancer patients. In a series of patients with large pericardial effusions, metastatic tumor was the most common underlying cause, but accounted for only 23 percent of cases (12): effusions may be idiopathic or secondary to radiation or chemotherapy (20,27). In patients with breast cancer, small, asymptomatic effusions are likely benign; of those that are clinically apparent, only 50 percent are malignant (8).

Pericardial effusions in AIDS patients are generally secondary to infections, although lymphomas (53), and rarely, Kaposi's sarcoma (4) may cause effusions in AIDS patients. In patients with cardiac involvement by Kaposi's sarcoma, which rarely infiltrates deeply into the myocardium, significant clinical symptoms are rare. Fatal cardiac tamponade secondary to hemorrhagic effusion and heart failure without ventricular dilatation have been reported (61).

Distribution of Tumor Within the Heart.
In general, metastatic cardiac tumors affect the right side of the heart in 20 to 30 percent of cases (42,51), the left side in 10 to 33 percent of cases (42), bilaterally or diffusely in 30 to 35 percent of cases, and the endocardium or chamber cavities in 5 percent of cases. In a series of 407 autopsies in which metastatic tumors were present in the heart, Mukai et al. (42) found that 19 percent involved the pericardium only, 33 percent the epicardium predominantly, 42 percent the myocardium predominantly, and 6 percent the endocardium (intracavitary tumors). Metastatic deposits were not grossly evident in 6 of 407 hearts in this study (42). It is extremely uncommon for cardiac metastases to be isolated lesions (25,42,62). In only 1 of 30 cases of sarcoma metastatic to the heart was the heart the lone site of metastasis (19).

Carcinomas of the lung and breast commonly metastasize to the pericardium, while malignant thymomas directly invade the pericardium. In most (35,37), but not all (1,36) series, carcinomatous infiltration of the pericardium or epicardium was demonstrated more frequently than infiltration of the myocardium. However, superficial myocardial infiltration is present in over 90 percent of breast and lung carcinomas that metastasize to the pericardium (35). Pericardial metastases from other primary solid tumors are rare (Table 15-1) (37). The valves and endocardium are usually spared by metastatic carcinoma.

Leukemic infiltrates, when they occur in the heart, are typically widespread, involving the peri-

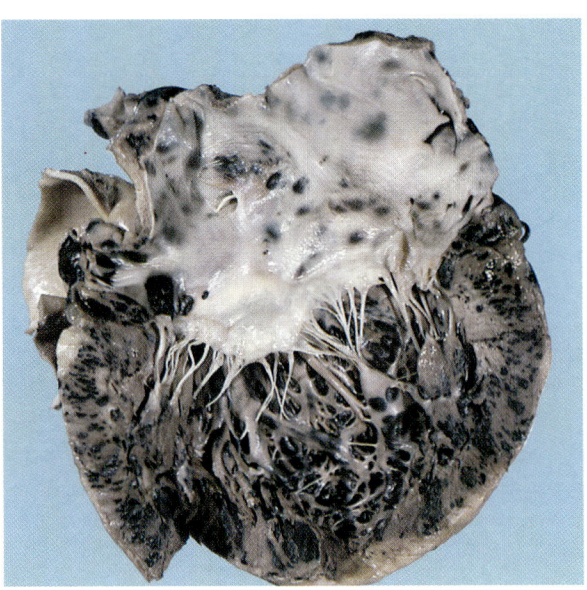

Figure 15-1
METASTATIC MALIGNANT MELANOMA: HEART
Note the pigmented masses throughout the heart.

cardium in 61 percent, left ventricle in 55 percent, and right atrium in 54 percent of cases (54). Pericardial involvement by lymphoma is considered unusual (37) to common (55); the reason for this discrepancy is unclear. McDonnell et al. (38) reported an equal distribution of lymphoma deposits in the myocardium and pericardium.

The myocardium is involved in virtually 100 percent of cases of melanoma metastatic to the heart; less frequently the epicardium and endocardium are infiltrated. The four chambers of the heart are involved with approximately equal frequency (18).

Sarcomatous deposits are found within the myocardium (50 percent), pericardium (33 percent), or both (17 percent). Valvular metastases are uncommon (19). Osteosarcoma (14,31), liposarcoma (6,29), leiomyosarcoma (19), unclassifiable sarcomas (19), rhabdomyosarcoma (19), neurofibrosarcoma (19), synovial sarcoma (19), and malignant fibrous histiocytoma (MFH) (19) have been reported to involve the heart secondarily. The type of soft tissue sarcoma does not appear to affect the incidence of metastases to the heart (37,42).

Gross Pathologic Findings. Metastatic deposits may be diffuse, multinodular, or consist of a single dominant mass greater than 2 cm (figs. 15-1, 15-2). There may be diffuse studding and

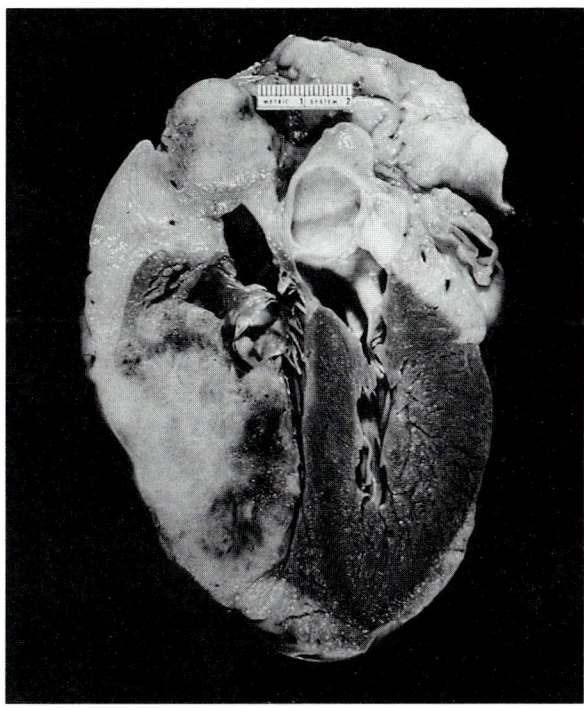

Figure 15-2
METASTATIC CARCINOMA: HEART
This elderly man had a primary colonic cancer with widespread metastases. Note massive infiltration of right ventricle and atrium.

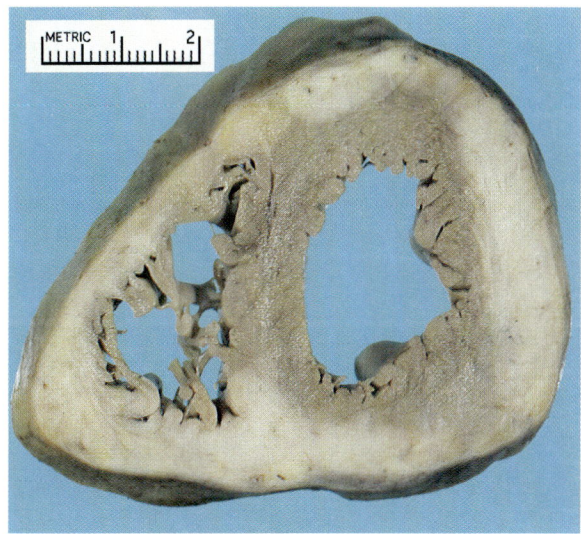

Figure 15-3
LEUKEMIA
Note the biventricular, predominantly subepicardial diffuse infiltrates. The patient was a 45-year-old man with acute myelogenous leukemia who died with disseminated disease.

thickening of the pericardial surfaces with little infiltration of the heart. This pattern generally occurs in carcinomatous metastases and can grossly be confused with mesothelioma or less commonly, benign fibrosing pericarditis. Mediastinal lymph nodes are involved in 80 percent of cases of cardiac metastases (42), especially if there is pericardial involvement.

It is not usually possible to determine tumor type by gross examination, although some generalizations may be made. Lymphoma nodules are epicardial or myocardial; merge imperceptibly with surrounding myocardium; and are large, homogeneous, white to tan, with little necrosis (figs. 15-3–15-5). Carcinomas are more variegated, gritty lesions that are usually epicardial- or pericardial-based tumors. The presence of melanotic pigment is suggestive of metastatic melanoma (fig. 15-1). The tumor burden in the heart is higher with melanoma than any other malignancy (66), although there may be massive involvement with lymphoma as well (23). Kaposi's sarcoma in-

volves the heart grossly as focal, small, firm, red-brown nodules that may coalesce, and only very rarely involves the heart in the absence of systemic disease (5,24); the epicardium and pericardium are usually involved and less frequently the myocardium and coronary arteries. Although metastatic transitional cell carcinoma to the bladder is rare (Table 15-1), it has been reported that metastatic bladder carcinoma may retain its papillary configuration within the pericardial space (17), thereby suggesting the diagnosis on gross inspection.

Primary sarcomas are impossible to distinguish from metastatic lesions without a complete autopsy, although they are generally larger, single tumors that extend into the cardiac cavities. Sarcoidosis may result in large, firm granulomas, but, unlike metastatic deposits, sarcoid granulomas rarely distort the endocardial or epicardial contours of the heart.

Microscopic Findings. The histologic features of cardiac metastases are identical to those of the primary tumor. In general, necrosis is not extensive. Hematologic malignancies infiltrate the surrounding myocardium, surrounding individual myocytes (figs. 15-6, 15-7). Hematogenous metastases of sarcomas and carcinomas form

199

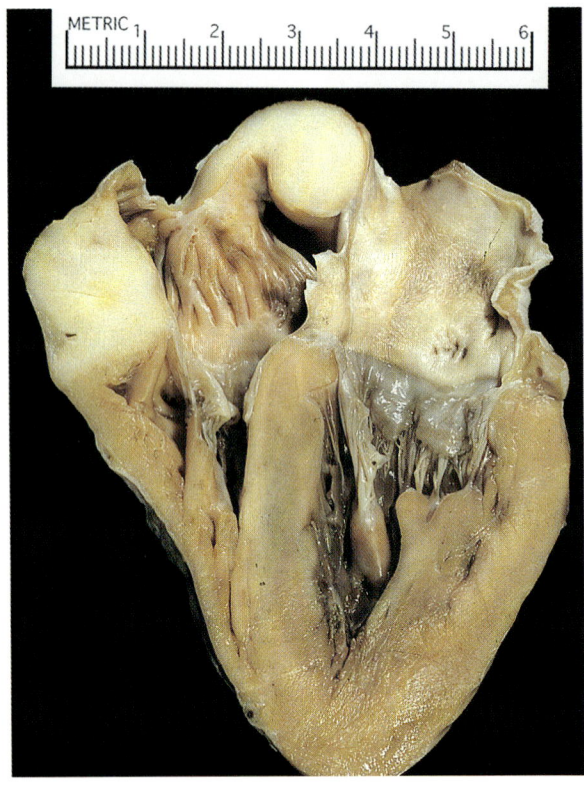

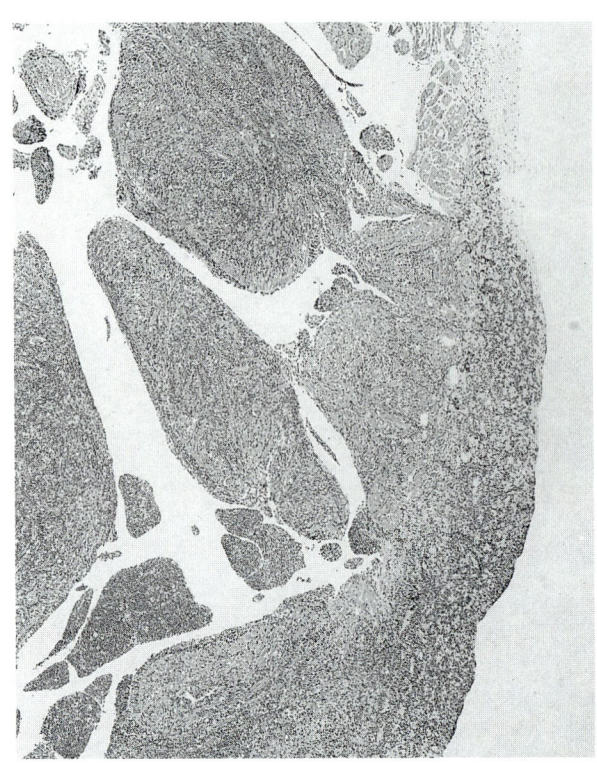

Figure 15-4
MALIGNANT LYMPHOMA

A 17-year-old female from Africa had widespread lymphoma involving ovaries, lymph nodes, and internal viscera, including the heart. Note infiltrates in atrial septum and right atrium.

Figure 15-5
MALIGNANT LYMPHOMA

Histologic section of the tumor depicted in figures 15-4 and 15-6 demonstrates infiltration by the lymphoma in the right atrial myocardium.

Figure 15-6
MALIGNANT LYMPHOMA

A closer view of the right atrium shown in figure 15-4 shows diffuse infiltration of the atrial wall by a homogeneous mass.

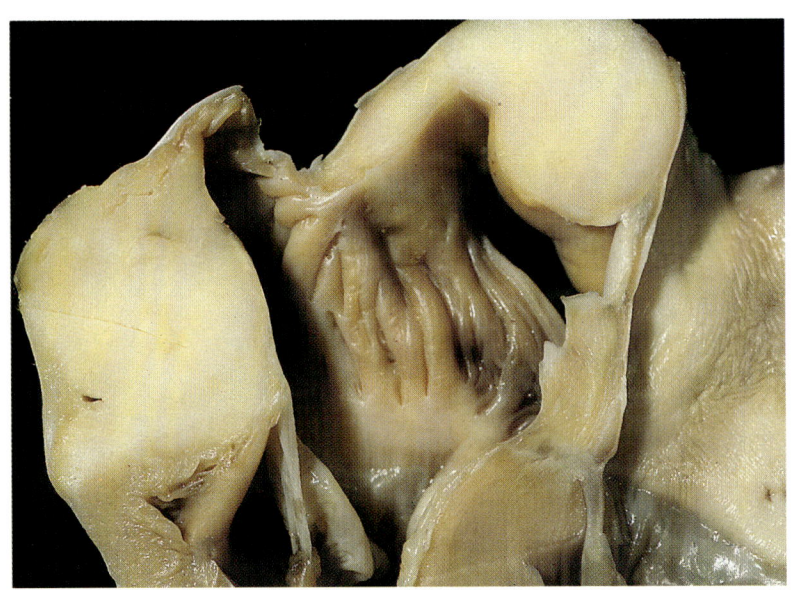

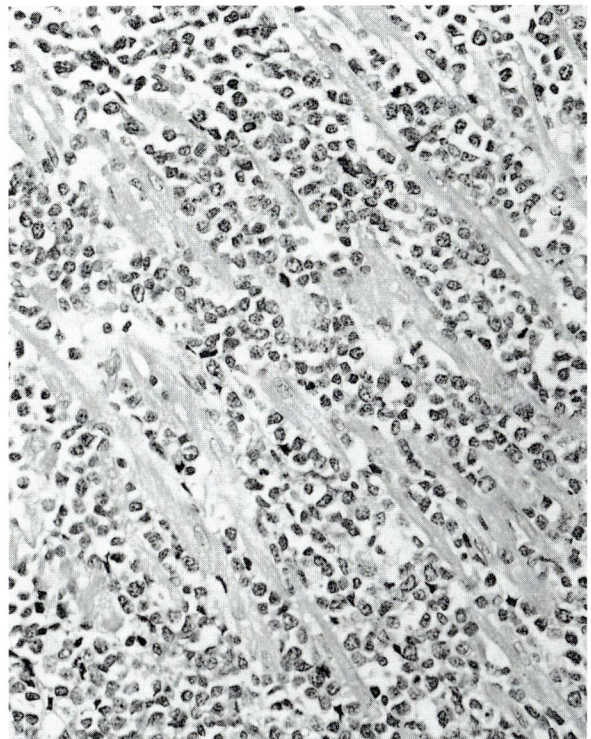

Figure 15-7
MALIGNANT LYMPHOMA: BURKITT'S TYPE
A higher magnification of figure 15-5 shows small cells infiltrating myocytes. The tumor was classified as small cell undifferentiated (Burkitt's type).

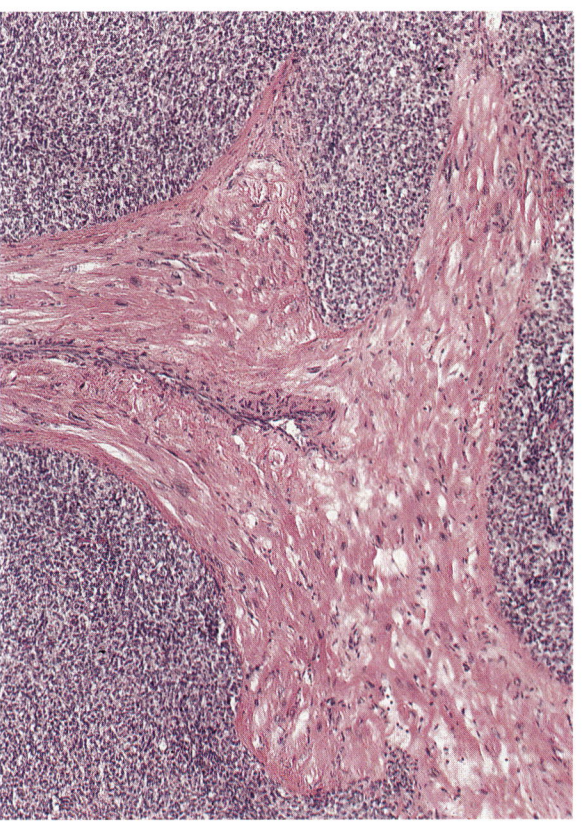

Figure 15-8
METASTATIC SARCOMA: RIGHT ATRIUM
The patient was a 21-year-old woman with a history of osteosarcoma of the humerus resected 9 years previously. Note the relatively sharp demarcation between tumor and cardiac muscle. The specimen was a surgical biopsy of a single cardiac metastasis.

more circumscribed masses (figs. 15-8–15-11). Although hematogenous deposits usually demonstrate little obvious relationship to blood vessels, there may be perivascular collections resembling microabscesses. Lymphatic spread is characterized by engorgement of pericardial and epicardial lymphatics with superficial infiltration of the myocardium (figs. 15-12, 15-13). Intracavitary metastases are often associated with tumor thrombi (42).

In addition to excisional biopsies, metastatic carcinomas to the heart can be detected in endomyocardial biopsies (15,21,58). Knowledge of the clinical history is crucial for histologic diagnosis on such limited material.

Pericardial Biopsies. The histologic features of metastatic pericardial tumors, most of which are carcinomas, are similar to their corresponding primaries. Carcinomas are classified as adenocarcinomas (figs. 15-14–15-17), squamous carcinomas (figs. 15-15–15-18), and undifferentiated large or small cell carcinomas (Table 15-2).

Undifferentiated carcinomas are usually of lung origin, but the small cell type rarely involves the pericardium. A surprisingly high percentage of malignant pericardial biopsies occur in patients in whom the diagnosis of malignancy has not yet been made clinically. Most adenocarcinomas presenting as pericardial metastases originate either in the lung or an undetermined primary site (34,63). Breast carcinoma, unlike lung carcinoma, usually manifests as pericardial disease only after the primary site is known (Table 15-3) (34).

Histologically, it is not possible to determine the primary site of adenocarcinoma unless there is expression of prostate-specific antigen or thyroglobulin in carcinomas of the prostate and thyroid, respectively. Although there is some site-specificity for carcinomas that express cytokeratins 7 and

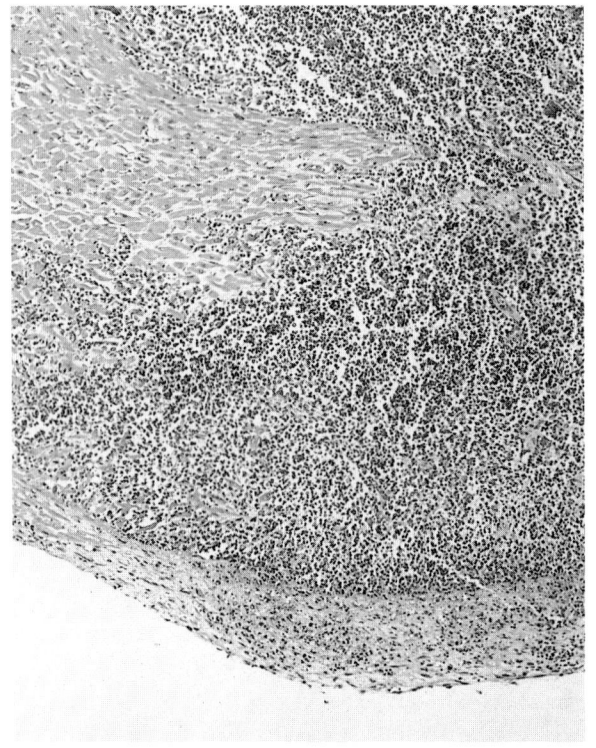

Figure 15-9
METASTATIC EMBRYONAL SARCOMA

The patient was a 13-year-old girl who died with disseminated embryonal rhabdomyosarcoma. The cardiac tumor was predominantly subendocardial.

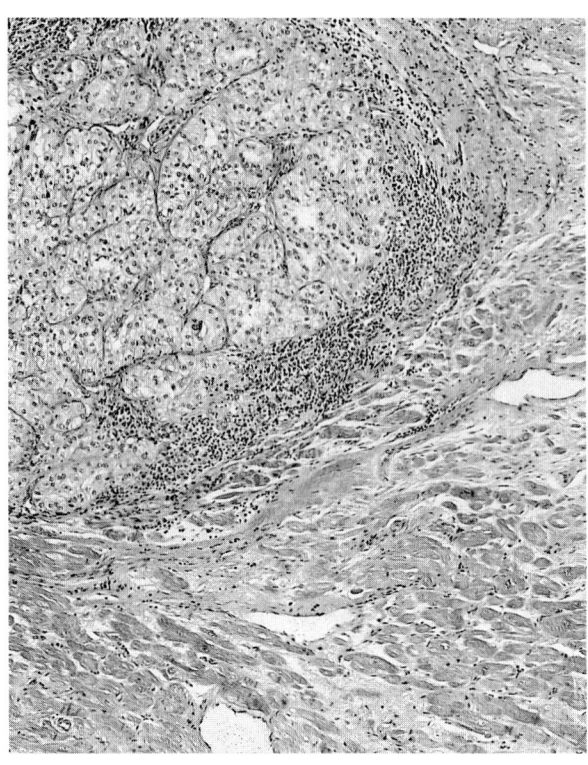

Figure 15-10
METASTATIC RENAL CELL CARCINOMA,
CLEAR CELL TYPE

The patient was a 65-year-old man with a remote history of nephrectomy for renal cell carcinoma. A tumor was demonstrated in the left ventricle after MRI and transesophageal echocardiography were performed for cyanosis and a cardiac murmur.

Figure 15-11
METASTATIC CARCINOID
TUMOR: MYOCARDIUM

An incidental mass in the right ventricle was removed at open heart surgery for coronary artery disease. Tumor cells are monotonous, with round to oval nuclei, stippled chromatin, and granular cytoplasm.

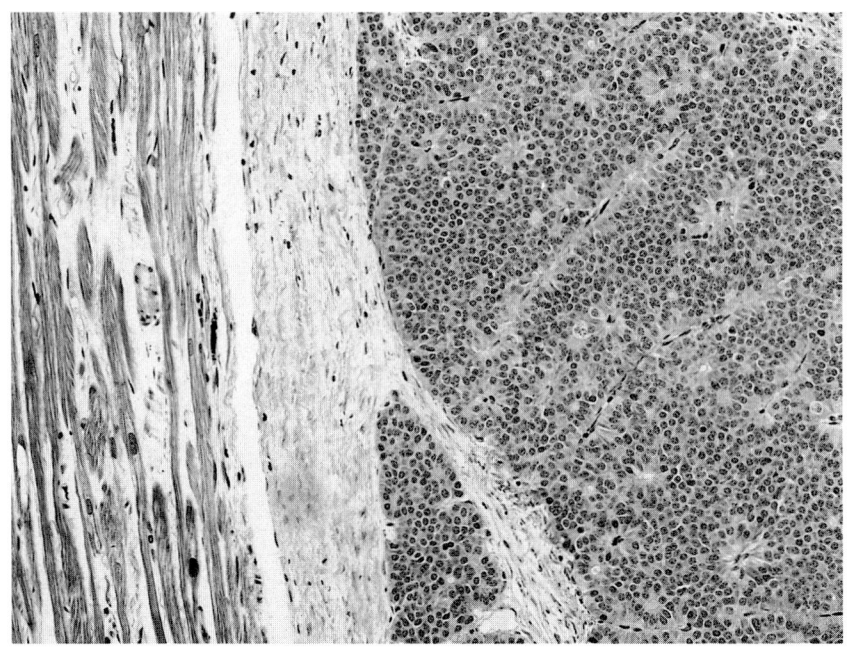

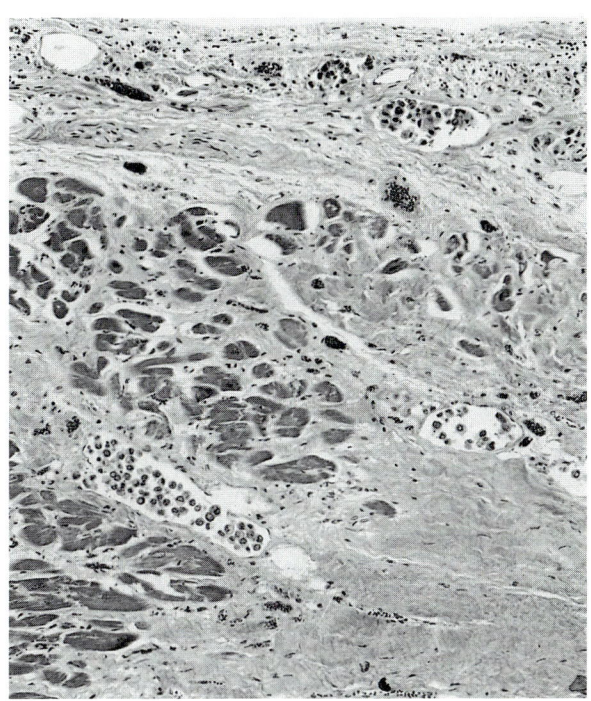

Figure 15-12
METASTATIC CARCINOMA OF THE LUNG:
EPICARDIUM
Nests of carcinoma cells are in the lymphatics at the junction of the myocardium and epicardium. Carcinomas of the lung and breast typically metastasize to the pericardium, epicardium, and superficial myocardium.

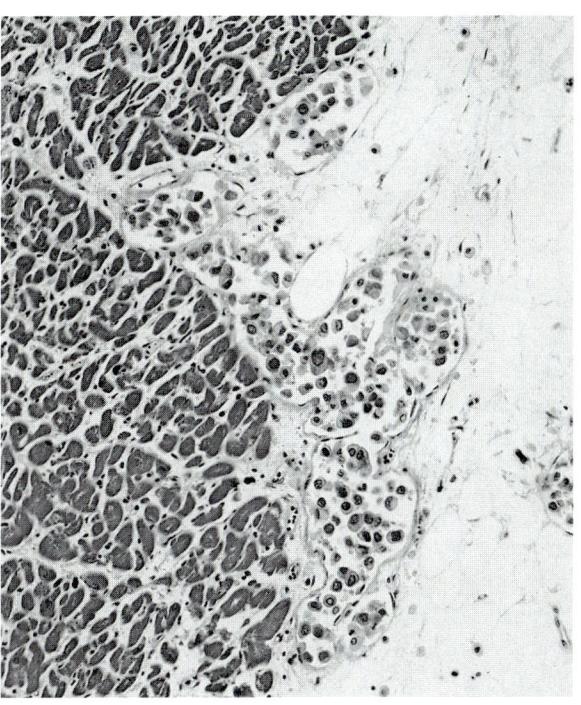

Figure 15-13
METASTATIC CARCINOMA OF THE LUNG
Higher magnification of a different area of the tumor seen in figure 15-12 demonstrates expansion of lymphatics by large cell carcinoma cells.

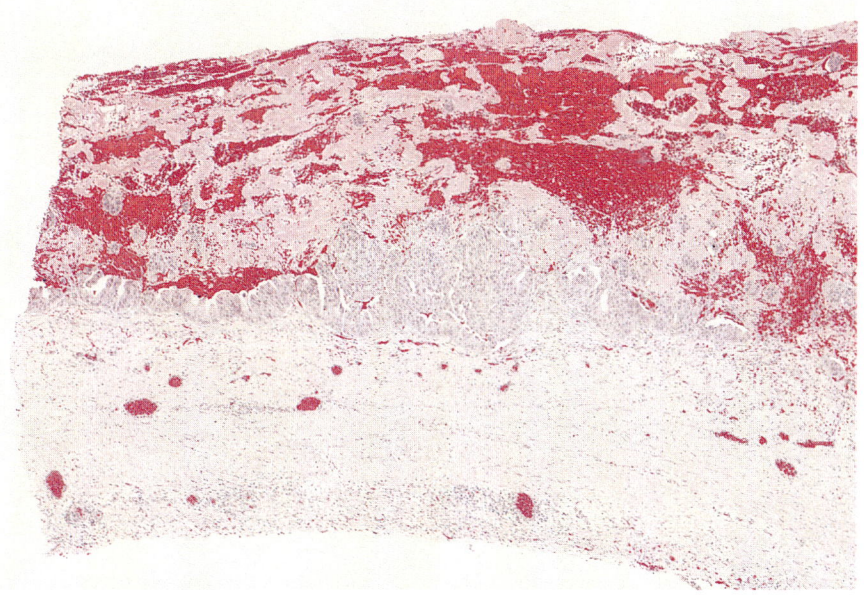

Figure 15-14
METASTATIC
ADENOCARCINOMA:
PERICARDIUM
A layer of tumor coats the parietal pericardium. There is abundant fibrin and blood, accounting for pericardial tamponade, which is typical in cases of metastatic pericardial tumor.

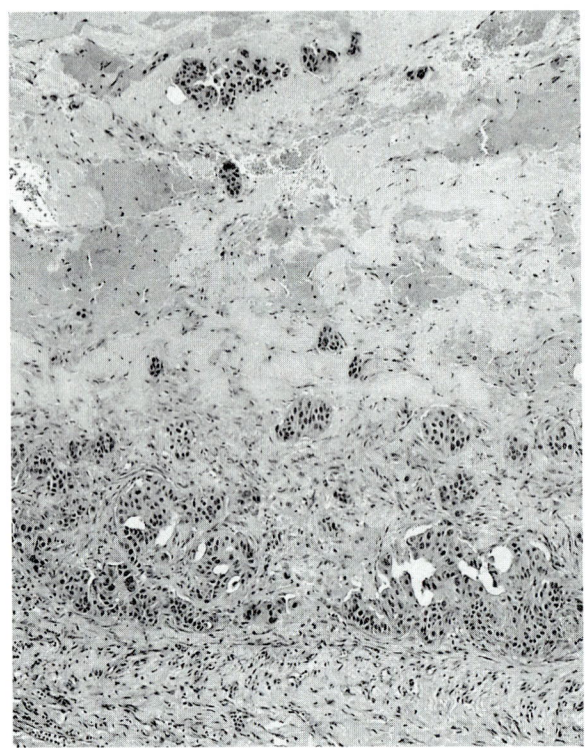

Figure 15-15
METASTATIC ADENOCARCINOMA: PERICARDIUM
This is a gland-forming neoplasm with organizing fibrin and blood on the surface of the pericardium. Numerous detached cell clusters are suggestive of malignancy.

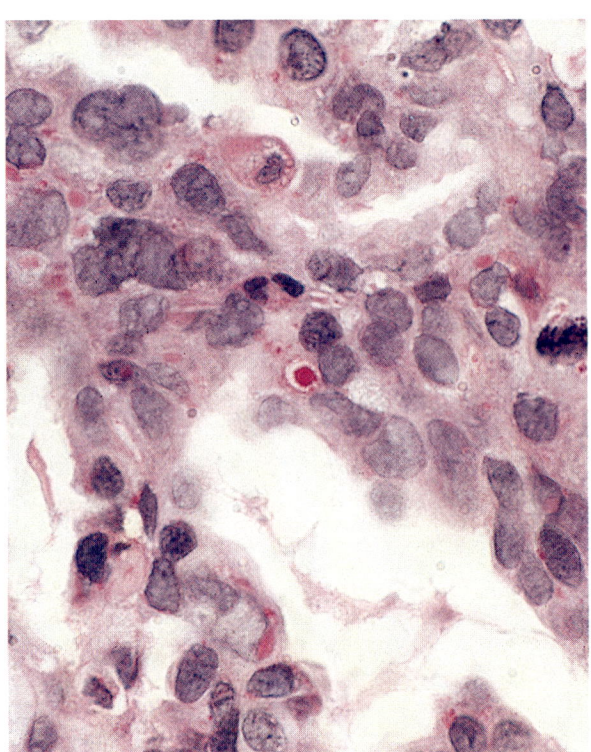

Figure 15-16
METASTATIC ADENOCARCINOMA: PERICARDIUM
Intracytoplasmic globules containing PAS-positive material are seen in adenocarcinoma and are absent in mesothelioma and reactive mesothelial cells. (Periodic acid–Schiff after diastase pretreatment. Oil immersion photomicrograph of tumor demonstrated in figure 15-15.)

Figure 15-17
METASTATIC
ADENOCARCINOMA:
PERICARDIUM
This intracytoplasmic globule was stained with mucicarmine. Although mucicarmine demonstrates cytoplasmic mucin vacuoles in most adenocarcinomas, it is not as sensitive as a PAS stain; for example, many gastric carcinomas are mucicarmine negative and PAS positive. (Oil immersion photomicrograph of tumor demonstrated in figure 15-15.)

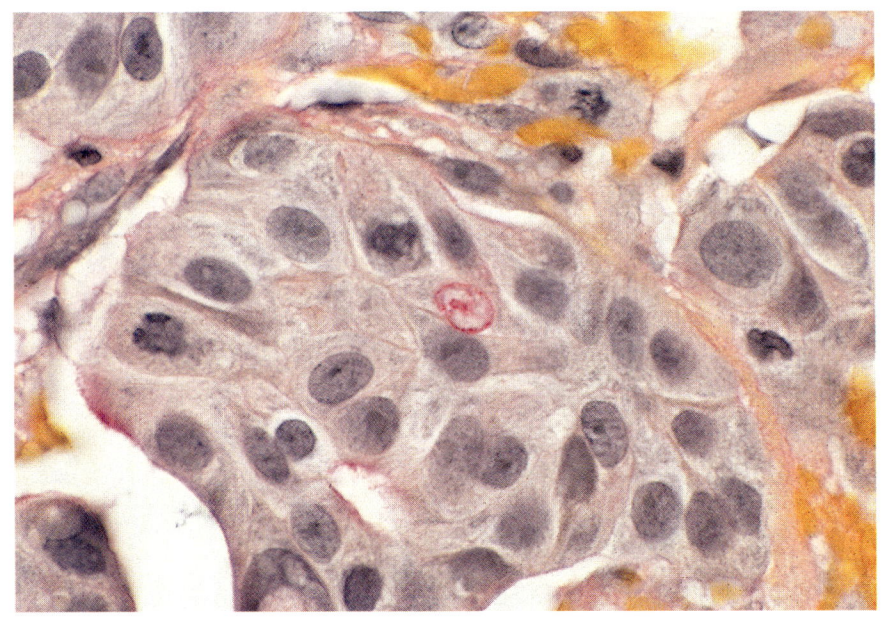

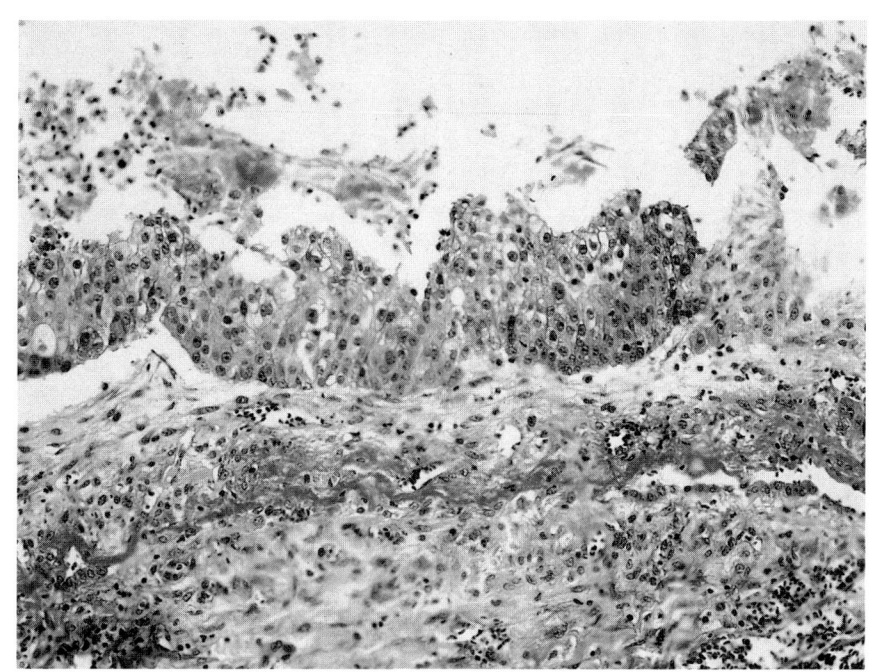

Figure 15-18
METASTATIC SQUAMOUS
CELL CARCINOMA:
PERICARDIUM
The patient was a 68-year-old
woman with a history of uterine cervical carcinoma and pericardial
tamponade.

Table 15-2

**MALIGNANT TUMORS DIAGNOSED
AT PERICARDIAL BIOPSY***

Tumor Type	Number	Percent
Carcinoma	**54**	**68**
Adenocarcinoma	32	40
Squamous cell	14	18
Large cell	7	9
Small cell	1	1
Lymphoma	**12**	**15**
Sarcoma	**7**	**9**
MFH**	3	3
Angiosarcoma	2	2
Leiomyosarcoma	1	1
Neurofibrosarcoma	1	1
Thymoma	**5**	**6**
Melanoma	**2**	**2**
Total	80	100

*From reference 34.
**MFH = malignant fibrous histiocytoma.

Table 15-3

**METASTATIC CARCINOMA DIAGNOSED
AT PERICARDIAL BIOPSY***

Histologic Type	Number (percent)	Primary Site, Number
Adenocarcinoma no previous diagnosis**	17 (31%)	Lung, 7 Unknown primary, 6[†] Thyroid, 1 Ovary ,1 Pancreas, 1 Kidney, 1
Adenocarcinoma with previous diagnosis	15 (28%)	Breast, 9 Prostate, 2 Kidney, 1 Stomach, 1 Parotid gland, 1 Lung, 1
Squamous cell carcinoma with previous diagnosis	8 (15%)	Esophagus, 4 Lung, 2 Uterine cervix, 2
Squamous cell carcinoma with no previous diagnosis**	6 (11%)	Lung, 4 Unknown primary, 2
Large cell	7 (13%)	Lung, 7
Small cell	1 (2%)	Lung, 1

*From reference 34.
**Indicates that the presenting symptom of carcinoma was related to pericardial disease.
†No primary tumor discovered during follow-up period or to death of the patient.

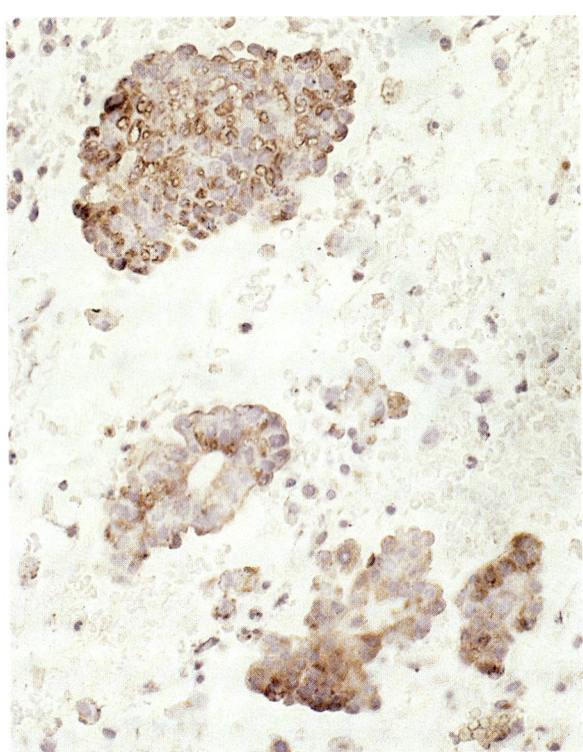

Figure 15-19
METASTATIC ADENOCARCINOMA: PERICARDIUM
Immunohistochemical stain for monoclonal car-cinoembryonic antigen demonstrates diffuse membrane pos-itivity, excluding a mesothelial proliferation.

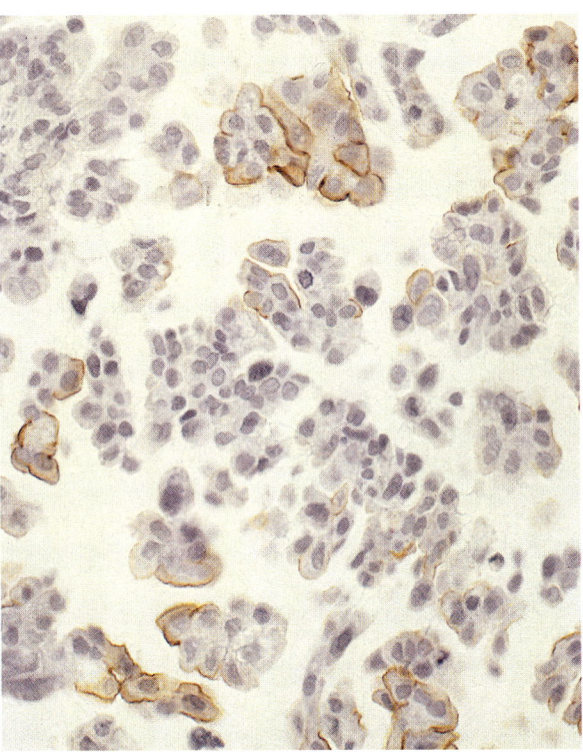

Figure 15-20
METASTATIC ADENOCARCINOMA: PERICARDIUM
A 65-year-old man had pericardial constriction and tam-ponade; malignant cells were noted in the pericardial fluid. A biopsy showed carcinoma without mucin vacuoles. This figure demonstrates B72.3 antigen positivity by immunohis-tochemical stain; expression of this antigen virtually ex-cludes a mesothelial proliferation.

18 (52), these markers do not differentiate be-tween carcinomas of the breast and lung, which commonly metastasize to the pericardium. Many "breast-specific antigens" have been pro-posed, although none has been a reliable marker for mammary carcinoma (68). Recently, gross cystic disease fluid protein-15 has been shown to be relatively specific for breast carcinoma (68), but this remains to be established.

The differential diagnosis of metastatic carci-noma to the pericardium includes reactive and malignant conditions (see chapter 14). The dis-tinction between reactive mesothelial hyperpla-sia and metastatic carcinoma can be difficult. Diastase-pretreated PAS and mucicarmine stains are helpful in identifying intracytoplas-mic glandular lumens of metastatic adenocarci-noma (figs. 15-16, 15-17), which are absent in reactive mesothelial proliferations. The pres-ence of carcinoembryonic antigen, Ber-EP4, B72.3 antigen, and Leu-M1 favors carcinoma

over mesothelial hyperplasia (figs. 15-19, 15-20). In reactive mesothelial cells there is usually a diffuse expression of vimentin, which is only weakly expressed in adenocarcinoma (16,44).

Other tumors found in pericardial biopsies include lymphoma (34), melanoma (34), multiple myeloma (56), thymoma (34), testicular seminoma (67), primary sarcomas of the pericardium, pri-mary malignant pericardial mesotheliomas, angiosarcomas (30), and undifferentiated sarcomas. Malignant thymoma is diagnosed on the basis of its typical histologic appearance and the presence of a mediastinal tumor; the characteristics of the other tumors are described in chapter 14.

Treatment. *Surgical Resection of Myocardial Metastases.* The aim of cardiac surgery in pa-tients with metastatic disease is usually pallia-tion (64). Only rarely are isolated metastases resected for possible cure (24,29,47,62).

In a recent series of 133 surgically resected cardiac tumors, 19 were metastatic to the heart, and in most cases surgery was performed for palliative, rather than diagnostic, purposes (43). Metastases from lung carcinomas, renal cell carcinomas, hepatocellular carcinomas, and cervical carcinomas (50) have all been removed at surgery. Metastatic sarcomas (chondrosarcomas, osteosarcomas, uterine leiometrial and endometrial stromal sarcomas, and rhabdosarcomas and liposarcomas of the extremity) (50) and a variety of miscellaneous metastatic tumors (paragangliomas, non-Hodgkin's lymphoma, testicular teratoma, and choriocarcinoma) (28,40,43,46,47, 64) have also been resected under cardiac bypass. In the AFIP files, there are 15 cases of surgically removed cardiac metastases: carcinomas (4 cases), malignant melanomas (4 cases); uterine adenosarcoma (1 case); anaplastic thyroid carcinoma (1 case); osteosarcoma (1 case); alveolar soft part sarcoma (1 case); metastatic endocrine tumor, not otherwise specified (1 case); incidental metastatic carcinoid tumor (1 case); and metastatic renal cell carcinoma (1 case).

From a surgical standpoint, metastatic tumors to the heart are divided into invasive tumors and intracavitary, noninfiltrating tumors (50). Metastases that invade the myocardium and are surgically removed are often sarcomas and nonepithelial neoplasms (6,29,50). Noninvasive intracavitary cardiac tumors that are surgically resected are often renal cell carcinomas that extend into the right atrium; other neoplasms that grow into the right atrium without myocardial infiltration and that are amenable to surgical excision are Wilms' tumor, hepatic embryonal rhabdomyosarcoma, hepatocellular carcinoma, adrenal pheochromocytoma, and uterine leiomyosarcoma (50). Rarely, lung carcinomas are resected after invading the pulmonary veins (50).

Unfortunately, results of follow-up in early cases of surgical treatment of cardiac metastases were not entirely encouraging (50): all of 10 patients with invasive metastases were dead at follow-up, with a mean survival of 7.5 months. Patients with intracavitary disease had a better prognosis: the mean survival was 17 months and 3 of 12 patients were alive at last follow-up. In 27 more recent cases of surgically resected cardiac metastases selected from the literature (28,40,43,46,47,64), survival was still poor, typically less than 10 months. However, some patients, especially those with unusual tumor types, live for extended periods, validating the use of surgery for treatment of cardiac metastases. Tumors that do better with resection include metastatic teratoma (46), breast carcinoma (28), choriocarcinoma (47), pelvic leiomyosarcoma (41), and alveolar rhabdomyosarcoma (45): postoperative survival ranges from 1 to 5 years.

Treatment of Pericardial Tamponade. The treatment of malignant pericardial disease includes establishing a pericardial window, sclerosis with tetracycline or other agents (27), and radiation therapy (50). Malignant pericardial effusions are generally a sign of rapidly progressive disease (8,12,27), necessitating emergency treatment.

Radiation Therapy and Chemotherapy for Myocardial Metastases. Radiation therapy often results in relentless congestive failure due to myocardial replacement by tumor (50). Chemotherapy or radiation therapy is generally reserved for cardiac involvement by lymphoma (48), which may regress dramatically with such treatment. The use of chemotherapy for metastatic cardiac soft tissue tumors is limited because cardiotoxic anthracyclines are often a component of chemotherapeutic regimens for these neoplasms.

REFERENCES

1. Abraham DP, Reddy V, Gattusa P. Neoplasms metastatic to the heart: review of 3314 consecutive autopsies. Am J Cardiovasc Pathol 1990;3:195–8.

2. Adenle AD, Edwards JE. Clinical and pathologic features of metastatic neoplasms of the pericardium. Chest 1982;81:166–9.

3. Almagro UA, Caya JG, Remeniuk E. Cardiac tamponade due to malignant pericardial effusion in breast cancer: a case report. Cancer 1982;49:1929–33.

4. Anderson DW, Virmani R. Cardiac pathology of HIV disease. In: Joshi VV, ed. Pathology of AIDS and other manifestations of HIV infection. New York: Igaku-Shoin 1990:165–85.

5. Autran B, Gorin I, Leibowitch M, et al. AIDS in a Haitian woman with cardiac Kaposi's sarcoma and Whipple's disease. Lancet 1983;1:767–8.

6. Bartels P, O'Callaghan WG, Peyton R. Metastatic liposarcoma of the right ventricle with outflow tract obstruction: restrictive pathophysiology predicts poor surgical outcome. Am Heart J 1988;114:696–8.

7. Bird DJ, Semple JP, Seiler MW. Sarcomatoid renal cell carcinoma metastatic to the heart: report of a case. Ultrastruct Pathol 1991;15:361–6.

8. Buck M, Ingle JN, Giuliani ER, Gordon JR, Therneau TM. Pericardial effusion in women with breast cancer. Cancer 1987;60:263–9.

9. Catton C, Shulman H, Rusthoven J, Wilk A. Gated magnetic resonance imaging of metastatic intracardiac malignant fibrous histiocytoma. Can Assoc Radiol J 1990;41:96–7.

10. Chan HS, Sonley MJ, Moes CA, Daneman A, Smith CR, Martin DJ. Primary and secondary tumors of childhood involving the heart, pericardium, and great vessels. A report of 75 cases and review of the literature. Cancer 1985;56:825–36.

11. Cleveland DC, Westaby S, Karp RB. Treatment of intra-atrial cardiac tumors. J Amer Med Assoc 1983;249:2799–802.

12. Corey GR, Campbell PT, Van Trigt P, et al. Etiology of large pericardial effusions. Am J Med 1993;95:209–13.

13. Dauplat J, Hacker NF, Nieberg RK, Berek JS, Rose TP, Sagae S. Distant metastases in epithelial ovarian carcinoma. Cancer 1987;60:1561–6.

14. Fiorentini G, Spinolo L, Bosi S, Cavallini B. Osteogenic sarcoma symptomatic metastases presenting as obstruction to the right heart. Pathologica 1987;79:367–76.

15. Flipse TR, Tazelaar HD, Holmes DR. Diagnosis of malignant cardiac disease by endomyocardial biopsy. Mayo Clin Proc 1990;65:1415–22.

16. Frisman DM, McCarthy WF, Schleiff P, Buckner SB, Nocito JD, O'Leary T. Immunocytochemistry in the differential diagnosis of effusions: use of logistic regression to select a panel of antibodies to distinguish adenocarcinomas from mesothelial proliferation. Mod Pathol 1993;6:179–84.

17. Gibbs JL, Rao RS, Williams GJ. Polypoid tumour of the pericardium—a previously unrecognised macroscopic appearance of metastatic bladder carcinoma. Int J Cardiol 1985;8:205–8.

18. Glancy DL, Roberts WC. The heart in malignant melanoma. A study of 70 autopsy cases. Am J Cardiol 1968;21:555–71.

19. Hallahan DE, Vogelzang NJ, Borow KM, Bostwick DG, Simon MA. Cardiac metastases from soft-tissue sarcomas. J Clin Oncol 1986;4:1662–9.

20. Hancock EW. Neoplastic pericardial disease. Cardiol Clin 1990;8:673–82.

21. Hanley PC, Shub C, Seward JB, Wold LE. Intracavitary cardiac melanoma diagnosed by endomyocardial left ventricular biopsy. Chest 1983;84:195–8.

22. Haskell RJ, French WJ. Cardiac tamponade as the initial presentation of malignancy. Chest 1985;88:70–3.

23. Iemura A, Yano H, Kojira M, Nouno R, Kouno K. Massive cardiac involvement of adult T-cell leukemia/lymphoma. Arch Pathol Lab Med 1991;115:1052–4.

24. James CL, Byard RW, Knight WB, Rice MS. Metastatic osteogenic sarcoma to the heart presenting as bacterial endocarditis. Pathology 1993;25:190–2.

25. Janssen DP, Van de Kaa CA, Moyez L, Van Haelst UJ, Lacquet LK. A solitary metastasis in the heart from Ewing's sarcoma. Eur J Cardiothorac Surg 1994;8:51–3.

26. Kamlow FJ, Padaria SF, Wainwright RJ. Metastatic cardiac malignant fibrous histiocytoma presenting as right ventricular outflow tract obstruction. Clin Cardiol 1991;134:173–5.

27. Kralstein J, Frishman W. Malignant pericardial diseases: diagnosis and treatment. Am Heart J 1987;113:785–80.

28. Labib SB, Schick EC Jr, Isner JM. Obstruction of right ventricular outflow tract caused by intracavitary metastatic disease: analysis of 14 cases. J Am Coll Cardiol 1992;19:1664–8.

29. Lagrange JL, Despins P, Spielman M et al. Cardiac metastases. Case report of an isolated cardiac metastasis of a myxoid liposarcoma. Cancer 1986;58:2333–7.

30. Lazoglu AH, Da Silva MM, Iwahara M, et al. Primary pericardial sarcoma. Am Heart J 1994;127:453–8.

31. Leonard JC, Raftery RG. Metastatic osteogenic sarcoma involving the left ventricle. Identification with gallium-67 citrate. Clin Nucl Med 1985;10:440.

32. Lestuzzi C, Biasi S, Nicolosi GL, et al. Secondary neoplastic infiltration of the myocardium diagnosed by two-dimensional echocardiography in seven cases with anatomic confirmation. J Am Coll Cardiol 1987;9:439–45.

33. Lewis W. AIDS: cardiac findings from 115 autopsies. Prog Cardiovascul Dis 1989;32:207–15.

34. Loire R, Hellal H. Neoplastic pericarditis. Study by thoracotomy and biopsy in 80 cases. Presse Med 1993;22:244–8.

35. MacGee W. Metastatic and invasive tumours involving the heart in a geriatric population: a necropsy study. Virchows Arch [A] 1991;419:183–9.

36. Manojlovic S. Metastatic carcinomas involving the heart. Review of postmortem examination. Zentralbl Allg Pathol 1990;136:657–61.

37. McAllister HA, Fenoglio JJ Jr. Tumors of the cardiovascular system. Atlas of Tumor Pathology. 2nd Series, Fascicle 15. Washington, D.C.: Armed Forces Institute of Pathology, 1977:111–9.

38. McDonnell PJ, Mann RB, Bulkley BH. Involvement of the heart by malignant lymphoma: a clinicopathologic study. Cancer 1982;49:944–51.

39. Millaire A, Wurtz A, de Groote P, Saudemont A, Chambon A, Ducloux G. Malignant pericardial effusions: usefulness of pericardioscopy. Am Heart J 1992;124:1030–4.

40. Miralles A, Bracamonte L, Soncul H, et al. Cardiac tumors: clinical experience and surgical results in 74 patients. Ann Thorac Surg 1991;52:886–95.

41. Mitchell D, Mitchell D, Davidson M, et al. Nongenital pelvic leiomyosarcoma metastatic to the heart. Gynecol Oncol 1991;43:84–7.

42. Mukai K, Shinkai T, Tominaga K, Shimosato Y. The incidence of secondary tumors of the heart and pericardium: a 10-year study. Jpn J Clin Oncol 1988;18:195–201.

43. Murphy MC, Sweeney MS, Putnam JB, et al. Surgical treatment of cardiac tumors: a 25-year experience. Ann Thorac Surg 1990;49:612–7.

44. Nance KV, Silverman JF. Immunocytochemical panel for the identification of malignant cells in serous effusions. Am J Clin Pathol 1991;95:867–74.

45. Orsmond GS, Knight L, Dehner LP, Micoloff FM, Nesbitt M, Bessinger FB. Alveolar rhabdomyosarcoma involving the heart: an echocardiographic, angiographic and pathologic study. Circulation 1976;54:837–43.

46. Parker M, Russo P, Reuter V, Bosl G, Keefe D. Intracardiac teratoma 15 years after treatment of a nonseminomatous germ cell tumor. J Urol 1993;150:478–80.

47. Perroni D, Grecchi GL, LaCiura P, Landoni F. Right ventricular metastasis from choriocarcinoma: report of a rare case and review of the literature. Eur J Surg Oncol 1993;19:378–81.

48. Peterson CD, Robinson WA, Klurnick JE. Involvement of the heart and pericardium in the malignant lymphomas. Am J Med Sci 1976;272:161–5.

49. Pizzarello RA, Goldberg SM, Goldman MA, et al. Tumor of the heart diagnosed by magnetic resonance imaging. J Am Coll Cardiol 1985;5:989–91.

50. Poole GV Jr, Meredith JW, Breyer RH, Mills SA. Surgical implications in malignant cardiac disease. Ann Thorac Surg 1983;36:484–91.

51. Prichard RW. Tumors of the heart. Review of the subject and report of one hundred and fifty cases. Arch Pathol 1951;51:98–128.

52. Ramaekers F, van Niekerk C, Poels L, Schaafsma G, Huijsmans A, Vooijs P. Use of monoclonal antibodies to keratin 7 in the differential diagnosis of adenocarcinomas. Am J Pathol 1990;136:641–5.

53. Reynolds MM, Hecht SR, Berger M, Kolokathis A, Horowitz SF. Large pericardial effusions in the acquired immunodeficiency syndrome. Chest 1992;102:1746–7.

54. Roberts WC, Bodey GP, Wertlake PT. The heart in acute leukemia. A study of 420 autopsy cases. Am J Cardiol 1968;21:388–412.

55. _____, Glancy DL, DeVita VT. Heart in malignant lymphoma (Hodgkin's disease, lymphosarcoma, reticulum cell sarcoma and mycosis fungoides). A study of 196 autopsy cases. Am J Cardiol 1968;22:85–107.

56. Santana O, Vivas PH, Ramos A, Safirstein S, Agatston AS. Multiple myeloma involving the pericardium associated with cardiac tamponade and constrictive pericarditis. Am Heart J 1993;126:737–40.

57. Selig MB. Percutaneous pericardial biopsy under echocardiographic guidance. Am Heart J 1991;122:879–82.

58. Shyu KG, Chiang FT, Kuan PL, Lien WP, Chen CL, How SW. Cardiac metastasis of hepatocellular carcinoma mimicking pericardial effusion on radionuclide angiocardiography. Chest 1992;101:261–2.

59. Skhvatsabaja LV. Secondary malignant lesions of the heart and pericardium in neoplastic disease. Oncology 1986;43:103–6.

60. Sokolova IN, Shkhvatsabaia LV. Secondary tumors of the heart (based on autopsy materials in the Oncology Research Center of the Academy of Medical Sciences of the USSR over the period of 1960-1977). Arkh Patol 1980;42:38–41.

61. Steigman CK, Anderson DW, Macher AM, Sennesh JD, Virmani R. Fatal cardiac tamponade in acquired immunodeficiency syndrome with epicardial Kaposi's sarcoma. Am Heart J 1988;116:1105–17.

62. Steinherz LJ, Rosen G, Steinherz PG, Robins J, Huvos A, Exelby PR. Isolated cardiac metastatic recurrence of epithelioid sarcoma after two and a half disease-free years. NY State J Med 1987;87:231–3.

63. Tamura A, Matsubara O, Yoshimura NH, Kasuga T, Akagawa A, Aoki N. Cardiac metastasis of lung cancer. A study of metastatic pathways and clinical manifestations. Cancer 1992;70:437–42.

64. Vargas-Barron J, Keirns C, Barragan-Garcia R, et al. Intracardiac extension of malignant uterine tumors. Echocardiographic detection and successful surgical resection. J Thorac Cardiovasc Surg 1990;99:1099–103.

65. Virmani R, Khedekar RR, Robinowitz M, McAllister HA Jr. Tumor embolization in coronary artery causing myocardial infarction Arch Pathol Lab Med 1983;107:243–5.

66. Waller BF, Gottdiener JS, Virmani R, Roberts WC. The charcoal heart; melanoma to the cor. Chest 1980;77:671–6.

67. White JE, Fincher RM, D'Cruz IA. Pericardial metastasis from testicular seminoma: appearance and disappearance by echocardiography. Am J Med Sci 1991;301:182–5.

68. Wick MR, Lillemoe TJ, Copland GT, Swanson PE, Manivel JC, Kiang DT. Gross cystic disease fluid protein-15 as a marker for breast cancer: immunohistochemical analysis of 690 human neoplasms and comparison with alpha-lactalbumin. Hum Pathol 1989;94:18–26.

16
TUMORS OF THE GREAT VESSELS

Primary tumors of the great vessels are rare lesions: between 300 and 400 have been reported in the world literature (1–5). The first description of a primary tumor of a large blood vessel was recorded by Perl (4), who reported a leiomyosarcoma of the inferior vena cava in 1891.

Most tumors of the great vessels are sarcomas. The sarcomas of great arteries are generally luminal, myofibroblastic tumors with divergent types of cellular differentiation. In contrast, those of the inferior vena cava are usually mural, well-differentiated leiomyosarcomas.

Paragangliomas of the aortic arch and organ of Zuckerkandl are briefly mentioned in this chapter because they occasionally present as an aortic mass.

SARCOMAS OF THE AORTA

Definition. By definition, a sarcoma that arises in the aorta must be predominantly intraluminal or be firmly attached to the aortic wall, so that part of the aorta must be removed to excise the tumor.

Incidence. Primary tumors of the aorta are exceptionally rare: there are 50-100 cases reported in the English language literature (6–18).

Classification. The majority of aortic sarcomas are found predominantly within the lumen, and are of putative intimal derivation. For this reason, they have been termed "intimal" sarcomas, similar to those of the pulmonary artery (see below). Most luminal sarcomas of the aorta are myofibroblastic sarcomas that are probably derived from subendothelial intimal mesenchymal cells. Angiosarcomas are less commonly luminal sarcomas of the aorta and express endothelial-specific antigens (7,10); the cellular origin of these tumors is likely the intimal endothelial cell.

Sarcomas that arise from the wall or adventitia are classified as are their soft tissue, extra-aortic counterparts. Intimal sarcomas differ both clinically and prognostically from mural sarcomas of the aorta. Therefore, we prefer to primarily classify them by site: those that are predominantly luminal are designated intimal sarcomas. They can then be subclassified by tissue type, such as undifferentiated, malignant fibrous histiocytoma (MFH), angiosarcoma, etc.

Clinical Features. Most patients with sarcomas of the aorta are middle-aged: in a recent series the mean age was 62 years (7). There appears to be no sex predilection (7,8). Because most tumors are intraluminal, the most common manifestations are related to embolic phenomena: claudication and absent pulses, usually of the lower extremities, are common. Other symptoms include back pain, abdominal angina from mesenteric artery occlusion, shock from rupture of aneurysm formed by the tumor, and symptoms related to malignant hypertension (13). Treatment consists of surgical removal of the affected aortic segment with repair by synthetic graft. Occasionally, the surgical diagnosis is atherosclerotic aneurysm, and the diagnosis of malignancy is first made at histologic examination of the aortic aneurysm.

The prognosis for patients with intimal sarcomas of the aorta is generally poor. Distant metastases are frequent, presumably due to arterial dissemination. The most common sites of metastases are bone, peritoneum, liver, and mesenteric lymph nodes. There are exceptional patients, especially those with mural tumors, who live years without symptoms after surgery. In our series, the mean survival of patients with luminal aortic sarcoma was 5.5 months. In contrast, two patients with mural sarcomas survived for 5 and 14 years.

Gross Findings. By definition, intimal sarcomas are either entirely intraluminal, in which case they grossly resemble thrombi (fig. 16-1), or are predominantly luminal with focal extension into the wall or adventitia. Occasionally, intimal sarcomas cause thinning and aneurysmal dilatation of the aortic wall. When they occur in the abdominal aorta, they can be mistaken for an atherosclerotic aneurysm (figs. 16-2, 16-3).

Unlike sarcomas of the venae cavae, aortic sarcomas rarely arise in the vessel wall. Those rare examples that have little luminal component and are predominantly mural are histologically more likely to be differentiated leimyosarcomas or angiosarcomas (7,8).

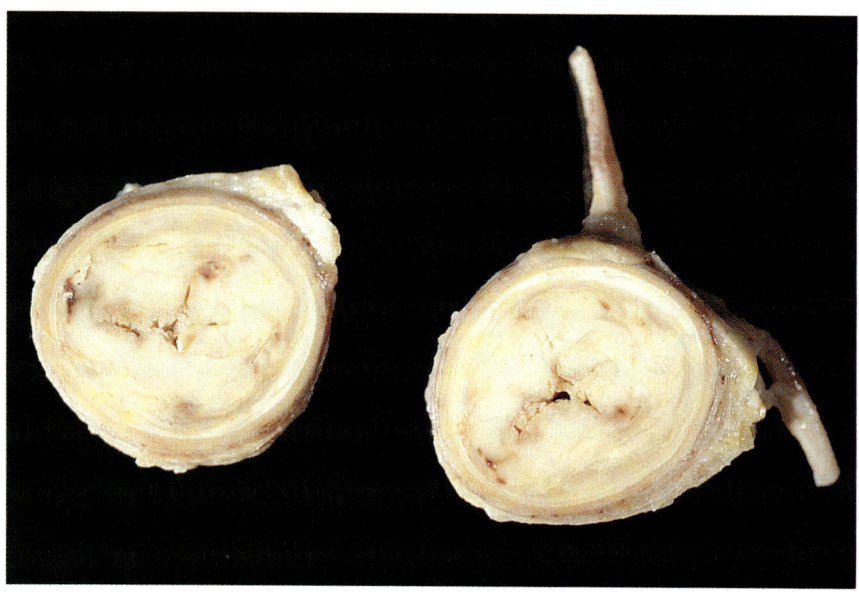

Figure 16-1
AORTIC INTIMAL SARCOMA
The tumor fills the aortic lumen without gross infiltration of the aortic wall.

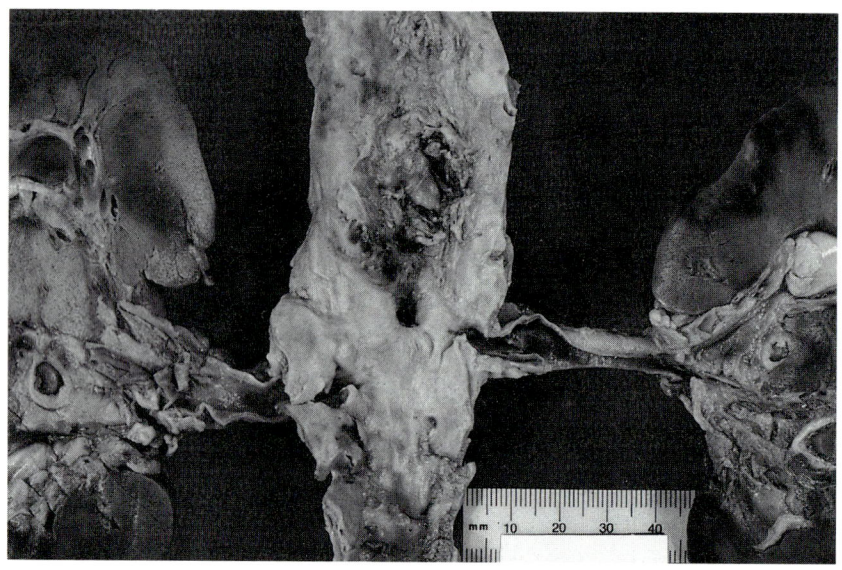

Figure 16-2
AORTIC INTIMAL SARCOMA
Gross photograph of aorta opened longitudinally at postmortem demonstrates an irregular area proximal to the renal arteries resembling an ulcerated atherosclerotic plaque. (Fig. 1 from Wright EP, Glick AD, Virmani R, Page DL. Aortic intimal sarcoma with embolic metastases. Am J Surg Pathol 1985;9:890-7.)

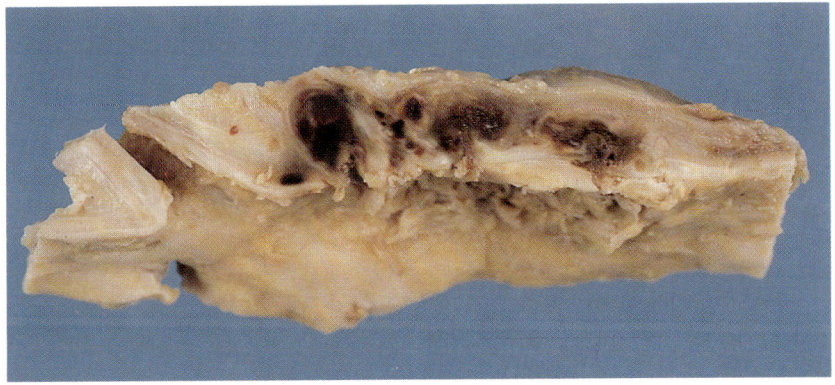

Figure 16-3
AORTIC INTIMAL SARCOMA
Cut section of aorta seen in figure 16-2 shows a hemorrhagic tumor extending from the intima into the adventitia. (Fig. 2 from Wright EP, Glick AD, Virmani R, Page DL. Aortic intimal sarcoma with embolic metastases. Am J Surg Pathol 1985;9:890–7.)

Most aortic sarcomas occur in the abdominal aorta between the celiac artery and the iliac bifurcation; approximately 30 percent occur in the descending thoracic aorta. There have been several reported cases of aortic sarcomas arising at the site of a synthetic aortic graft anastomosis (7,17). It is not unusual for the initial diagnosis to be made on the basis of embolectomy material, grossly considered by the surgeon to be a thrombus (7,8).

Histologic Findings. Intimal aortic sarcomas are usually poorly differentiated sarcomas of fibroblastic or myofibroblastic differentiation. They are composed of mitotically active spindle cells with varying degrees of atypia, necrosis, and pleomorphism. The luminal surface is often stratified into a layer of cellular neoplasm overlying a second layer of dense fibrous tissue or organizing thrombus. The tumor cells show mild to severe atypia (figs. 16-4–16-6). There may be an epithelioid appearance to tumor cells (fig. 16-7), and a mixture of pleomorphic fibrocytic and histiocytic cells resembling malignant fibrous histiocytoma; some intimal aortic sarcomas have, for this reason, been classified as such (16).

Unlike pulmonary intimal sarcomas, those of the aorta uncommonly contain areas of specific differentiation other than myofibroblastic cells. Intimal sarcomas may demonstrate histologic angiosarcomatous differentiation (7); we have recently encountered several epithelioid angiosarcomas arising in the aortic lumen. The intimal surface of the aorta adjacent to the gross tumor may have a lining of atypical cells that has been

termed "dysplasia." These cells may demonstrate endothelial differentiation (10). We have seen one case of aortic intimal sarcoma with chondrosarcomatous and osteosarcomatous differentiation (figs. 16-8, 16-9), but this is an unusual finding. Leiomyosarcomas with characteristic fascicular growth, intracytoplasmic glycogen, and ultrastructural characteristics of smooth muscle cells are rare as luminal (intimal) aortic sarcomas.

Sarcomas of the aorta that have only a minor luminal component are, in contrast to intimal sarcomas, generally better differentiated. The few examples that we have encountered are leiomyosarcomas similar to sarcomas of the venae cavae, and angiosarcomas (figs. 16-10–16-12).

NONSARCOMATOUS AORTIC NEOPLASMS

Benign Soft Tissue Tumors

Benign tumors of the aorta are exceedingly rare. We have seen a few benign fibrous histiocytomas and inflammatory pseudotumors of the aorta in young adults and children. These tumors are attached to the aortic adventitia, usually occur in the proximal aorta, and are cured by resection.

Paragangliomas

The soft tissue adjacent to the aortic adventitia contains dispersed paraganglia that function similarly to the carotid body. These paraganglia

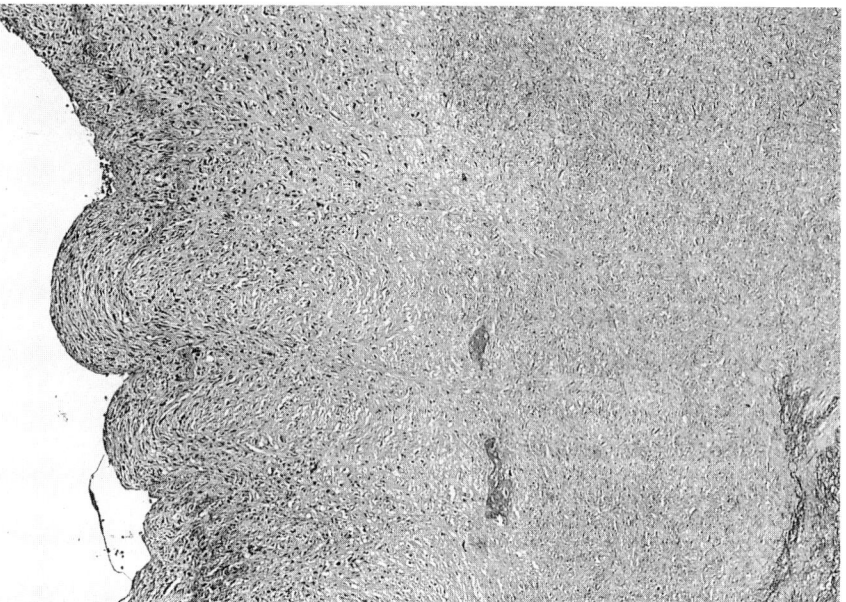

Figure 16-4
AORTIC INTIMAL SARCOMA
The luminal surface (left side of field) is composed of cellular tumor overlying a hypocellular area. (Figures 16-4–16-6 are from the same tumor.)

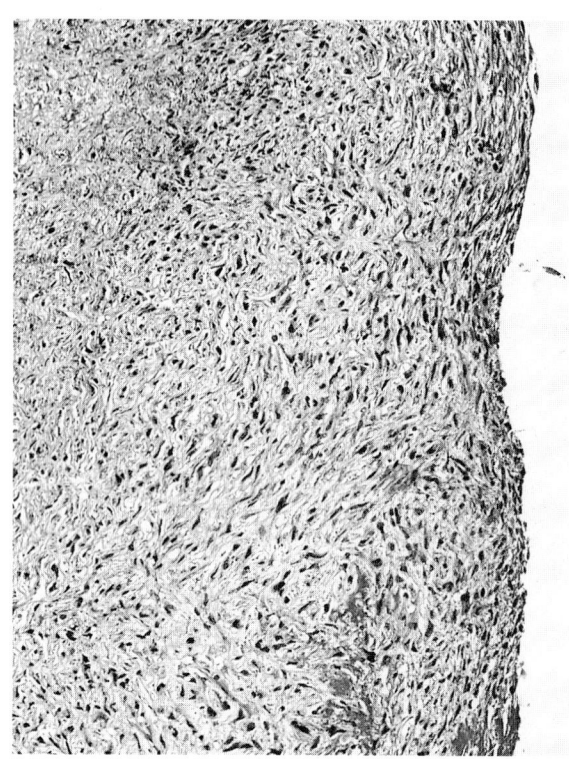

Figure 16-5
AORTIC INTIMAL SARCOMA
Higher magnification of figure 16-4 shows features of sarcoma, including cellular pleomorphism and atypia.

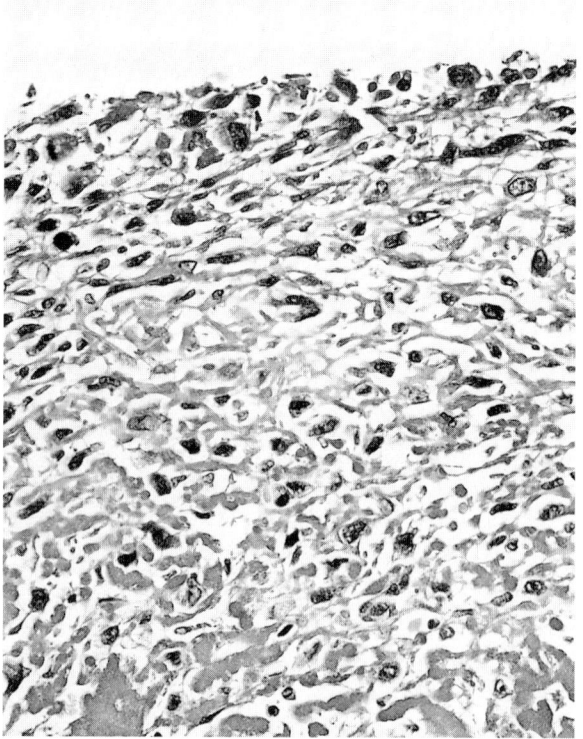

Figure 16-6
AORTIC INTIMAL SARCOMA
High magnification of tumor shown in figure 16-4 demonstrates atypical cells overlying a fibrin thrombus.

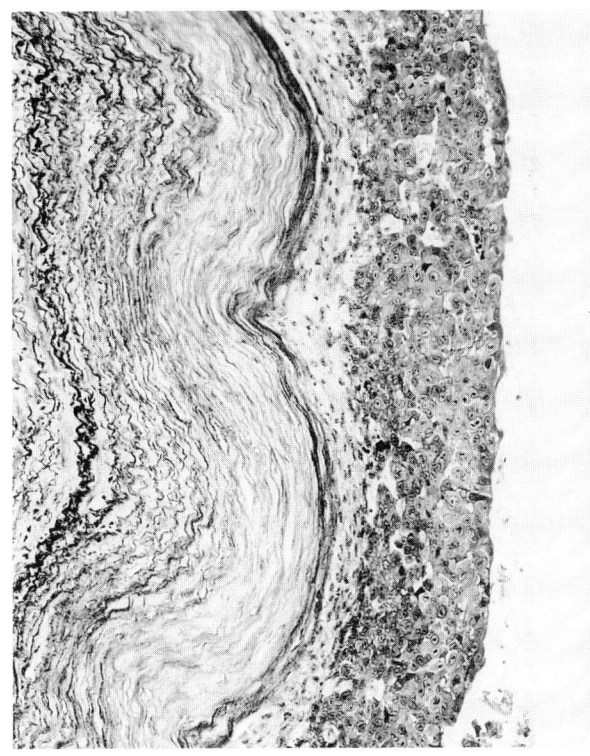

Figure 16-7
AORTIC INTIMAL SARCOMA
These tumors may have an epithelioid appearance and line the intimal surface of the internal elastic lamina, especially at the margins of the tumor. (Fig. 3 from Burke AP, Virmani R. Sarcomas of the great vessels. Cancer 1993;71:1761-73.)

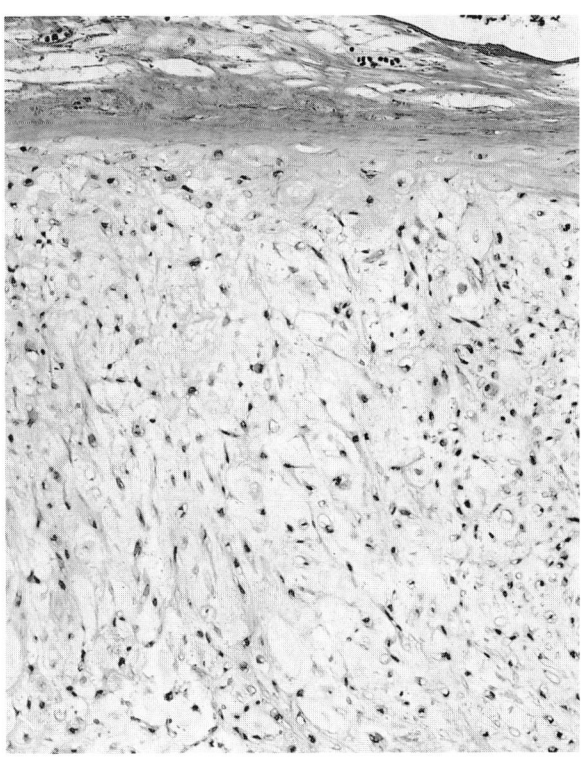

Figure 16-8
AORTIC INTIMAL SARCOMA:
CHONDROSARCOMATOUS DIFFERENTIATION
Rarely, chondrosarcomatous areas may be present. The patient was an elderly man with recurrent emboli to kidneys, gastrointestinal tract, and lower extremities. Imaging studies revealed a mass in the thoracic aorta. Note the myxoid tumor with chondroid features.

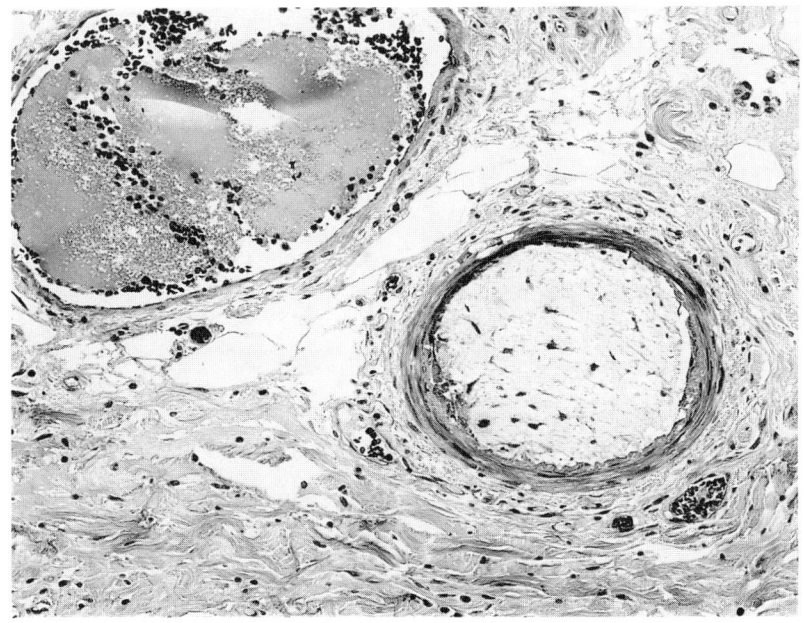

Figure 16-9
AORTIC INTIMAL SARCOMA:
EMBOLIC
The microscopic tumor resembled myxoma. Unlike myxoma, cords and ring structures were absent.

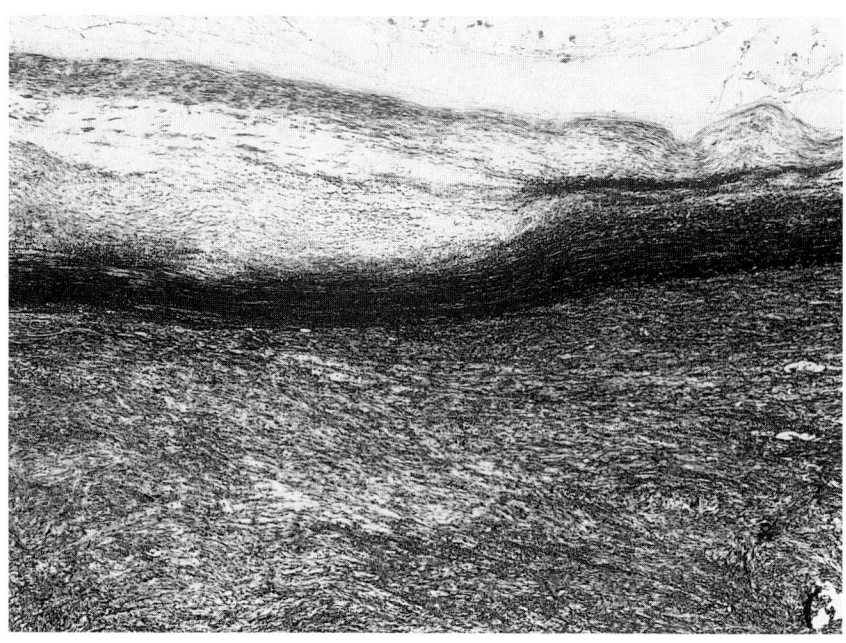

Figure 16-10
AORTIC MURAL SARCOMA

At repair of an abdominal aortic aneurysm in a 67-year-old woman, surgeons unexpectedly found a mass attached to the wall of the dilated aorta. The tumor is at the lower half of the field; the aortic wall shows an atherosclerotic plaque. (Movat pentachrome stain)

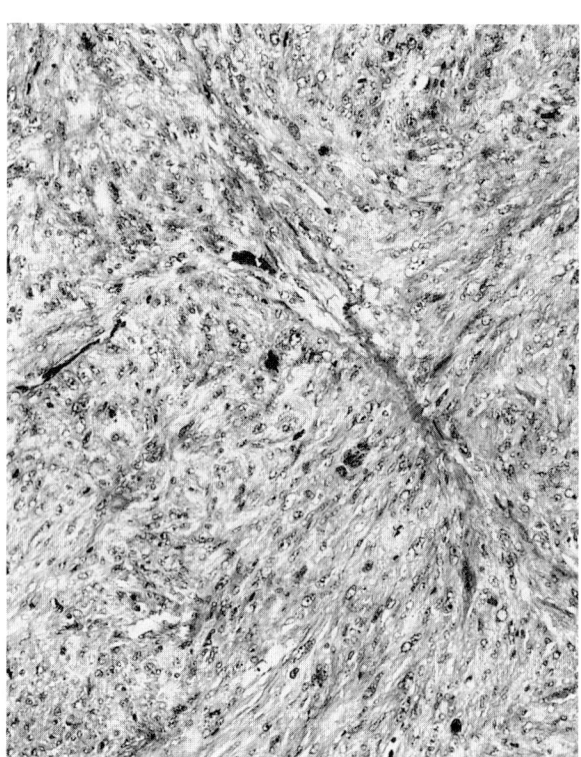

Figure 16-11
AORTIC MURAL SARCOMA

A higher magnification of figure 16-10 shows a pleomorphic spindle cell neoplasm. The patient survived nearly 5 years postoperatively.

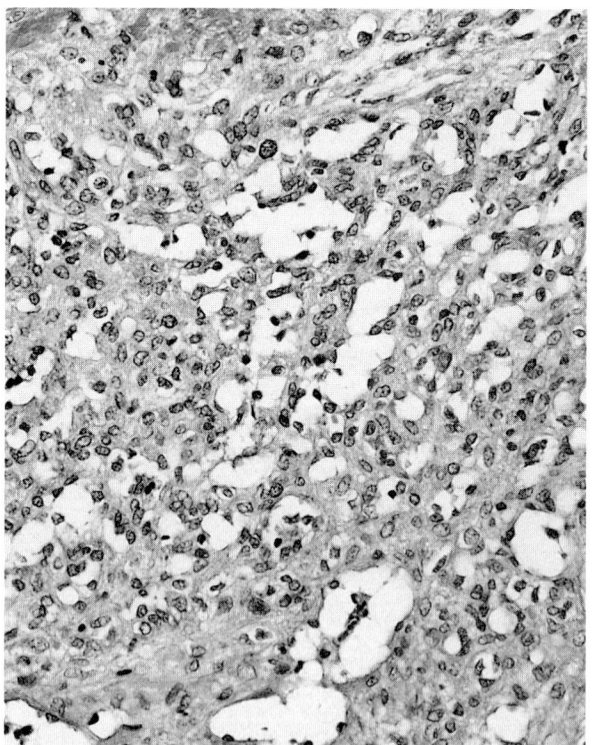

Figure 16-12
AORTIC MURAL ANGIOSARCOMA

The patient was a 49-year-old woman with a mass attached to the wall of the ascending thoracic aorta. Microscopically, there are irregular vascular channels lined by atypical endothelial cells.

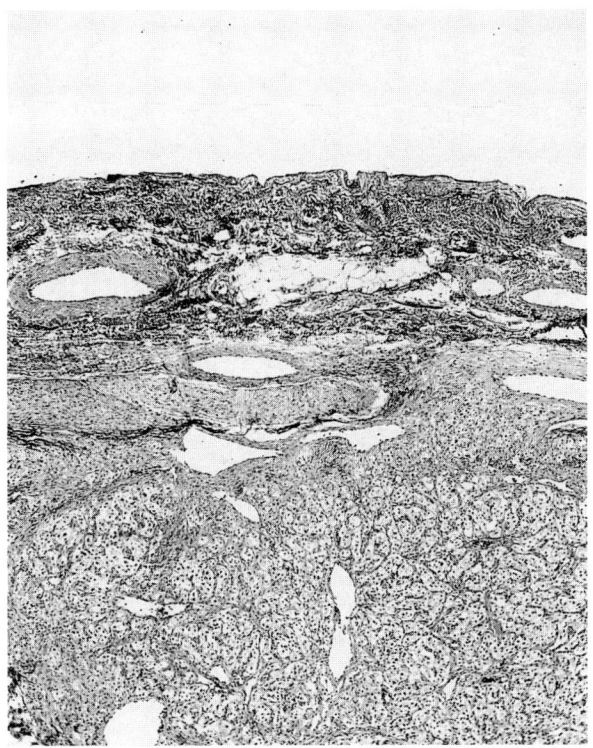

Figure 16-13
AORTIC PARAGANGLIOMA
Paraganglioma (bottom of figure) is embedded within the aortic adventitia. The adventitial border is at the top of the figure.

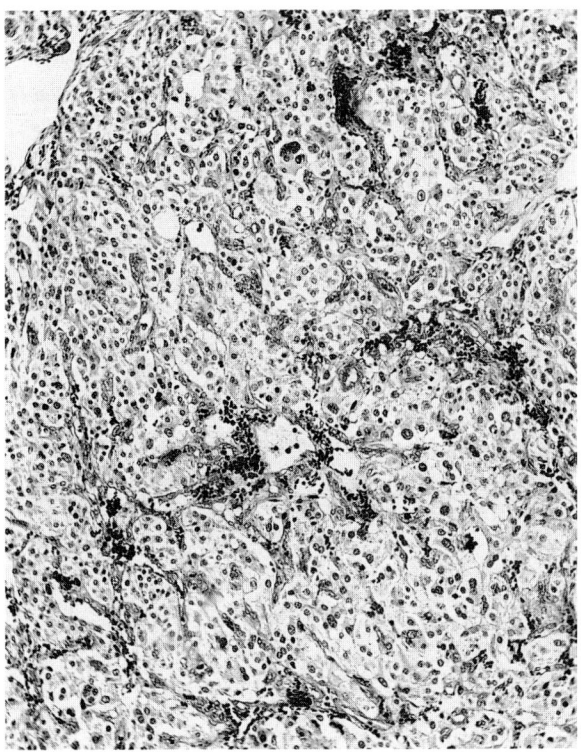

Figure 16-14
AORTIC PARAGANGLIOMA
A higher magnification of figure 16-13 demonstrates the typical features of paraganglioma, with neuroendocrine cells organized in small clusters separated by a delicate vascular stroma.

are located predominantly near the ligamentum arteriosum and at the inferior mesenteric artery (organ of Zuckerkandl). Occasionally, normal or hyperplastic paraganglia can confuse the surgical pathologist not familiar with the presence of paraganglial tissues near the aorta. Neoplasms of these paraganglia are even rarer than paragangliomas of the carotid body (19–21). Paragangliomas arising from paraganglia near the ligamentum arteriosum are usually termed *aortico-pulmonary* or *aortic paragangliomas* (21).

Both benign and malignant paragangliomas adjacent to the aorta have been described (19–21). Although not primary neoplasms of the aorta, paragangliomas should be considered in the differential diagnosis of tumors involving the aortic wall. The histologic (figs. 16-13, 16-14), immunohistochemical, and ultrastructural features of aortic paragangliomas are identical to those of other paragangliomas.

SARCOMAS OF THE PULMONARY ARTERY

Incidence. Approximately 120 primary sarcomas of the pulmonary artery have been reported in the world literature (22,34).

Classification and Histogenesis. Like those of the aorta, intraluminal pulmonary artery sarcomas are believed to originate from pluripotential mesenchymal cells of the intima. Because most sarcomas of the pulmonary arteries involve the pulmonary trunk, it has been hypothesized that they arise from primitive cells of the bulbus cordi (31).

Similar to aortic sarcomas, intimal pulmonary sarcomas are clinically distinct from mural sarcomas, and are, therefore, best classified independently. If there is evidence of specific differentiation, modifiers are added to the diagnosis. For example, a tumor may be designated "intimal sarcoma of the pulmonary artery, with focal osteosarcoma and chondrosarcoma," or "intimal angiosarcoma" of the pulmonary artery.

Similar to cardiac sarcomas, intimal sarcomas with two types of specific differentiation, in addition to fibroblastic cells, could be classified as malignant mesenchymoma of intimal origin (24,28,34). Sarcomas of the pulmonary artery frequently demonstrate osteosarcoma and chondrosarcoma and should not be classified as mesenchymoma unless there are areas of liposarcoma, myosarcoma, or angiosarcoma as well.

Rarely, pulmonary artery sarcomas arise from the wall of the pulmonary artery and are classified by their histologic subtype. These tumors are not considered to derive from intimal cells, and are very difficult to distinguish from sarcomas of lung parenchyma.

Clinical Features. A review of 110 sarcomas of the pulmonary artery showed a slight female predominance (1.3 to 1), with a mean age of 48 years at presentation (34). The age range in this review was 22 to 80 years, although subsequently, there have been reports of pulmonary artery sarcomas occurring in children (26). The mean age at presentation is younger than the mean age of patients with aortic sarcomas (62 years), and caval sarcomas (54 years).

Pulmonary artery sarcomas cause symptoms suggestive of recurrent pulmonary emboli (30). The most common symptom is dyspnea, followed by chest or back pain, cough, hemoptysis, malaise, weight loss, fever, and syncope (34); rarely, sudden death may occur in previously asymptomatic individuals (37). A systolic murmur is heard in slightly over 50 percent of patients (34). Chest radiographs may be normal or may show a hilar mass, prominent pulmonary artery shadow, hilar infiltrates, decreased pulmonary peripheral vascular markings, or pulmonary nodules consistent with metastasis. Perfusion scans demonstrate a lack of perfusion to the affected lung segment, which is best documented by angiography. Computed tomography may be helpful in identifying a tumor within the pulmonary artery, and is capable of distinguishing thrombus from tumor (32,34).

A diagnosis of pulmonary artery sarcoma is virtually never considered initially. The histologic diagnosis is usually made at autopsy, although it may be made at histologic examination of material removed from the pulmonary artery

at endarterectomy. Patients are often given anticoagulants for several months for presumed pulmonary emboli (25,31,35,37) before a tissue diagnosis is rendered.

Sarcomas of the pulmonary artery are less likely to metastasize to distant sites than are their counterparts in the aorta. However, metastases to lung, kidney, brain, lymph nodes, and skin have been reported (23), as well as bilateral adrenal metastases (33). Patients with intimal sarcomas of the pulmonary artery appear to survive longer on average than patients with aortic intimal sarcomas (23). A clinical course of over 2 years without metastases or treatment is common (23,27,29), but survival at 5 years is rare. In our series (23), the mean survival was 14 months, which is similar to the 18 months reported in a literature review (34). Patients in whom curative resection is attempted have a longer disease-free course than those without curative surgery. Currently, there is no evidence that chemotherapy or radiation therapy benefits patients with sarcomas of the pulmonary artery.

Gross Findings. The typical sarcoma of the pulmonary artery resembles a mucoid clot (figs. 16-15, 16-16). Bony or gritty areas may correspond to areas of osteosarcoma. The sites of attachment in the arteries are often multiple and difficult to define (34): the pulmonary trunk is involved in 80 percent of cases; the left pulmonary artery in 58 percent; the right pulmonary artery in 57 percent; both pulmonary arteries in 37 percent; the pulmonary valve in 29 percent; and the right ventricle in 8 percent. The tumor often extends distally along the lumen of the pulmonary arterial branches and occasionally infiltrates into pulmonary parenchyma.

Histologic Findings. Luminal sarcomas of the pulmonary artery are typically spindle cell proliferations that resemble myofibroblastic malignant tumors of the aortic intima, occasionally with malignant cells layered over dense collagen (fig. 16-17). A myxoid background is frequently seen (fig. 16-18), as well as osteosarcomatous (fig. 16-19) and pleomorphic areas (fig. 16-20). Approximately 50 percent are fibroblastic or myofibroblastic sarcomas that are not readily classified, and 20 percent have been reported as leiomyosarcoma (34). The remaining 30 percent have been classified as chondrosarcoma or osteosarcoma (7 percent) (fig. 16-19), angiosarcoma (7 percent),

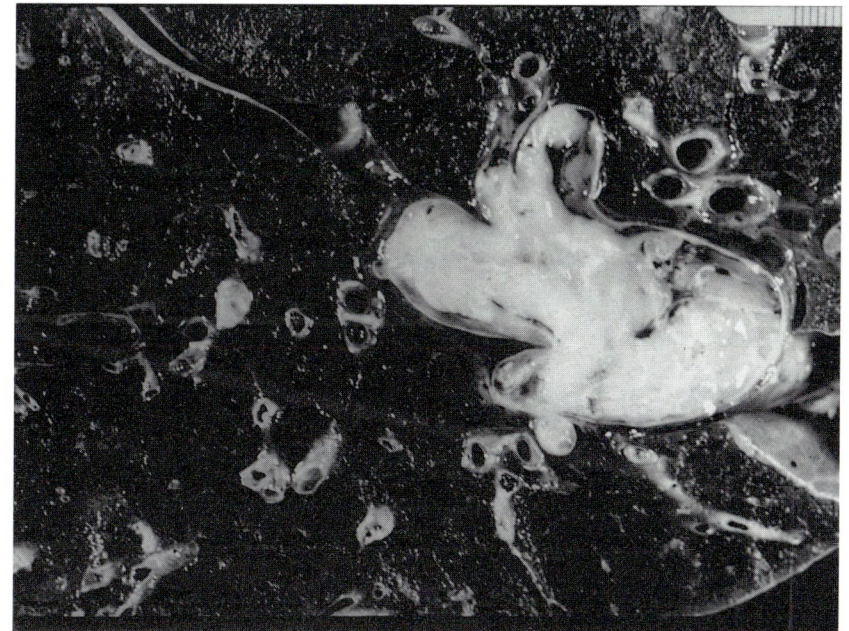

Figure 16- 15
SARCOMA OF THE
PULMONARY ARTERY
The tumor fills the pulmonary arteries with gelatinous masses.

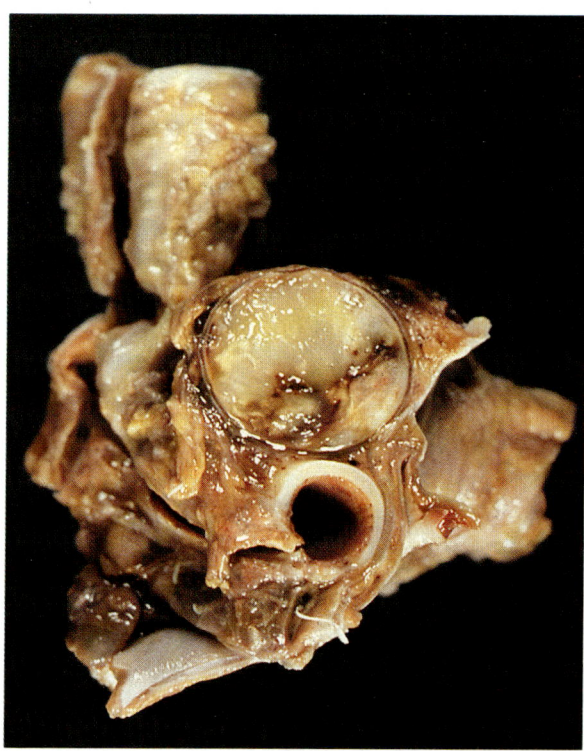

Figure 16-16
SARCOMA OF THE PULMONARY ARTERY

The pulmonary artery is markedly distended, and its diameter exceeds the accompanying bronchus.

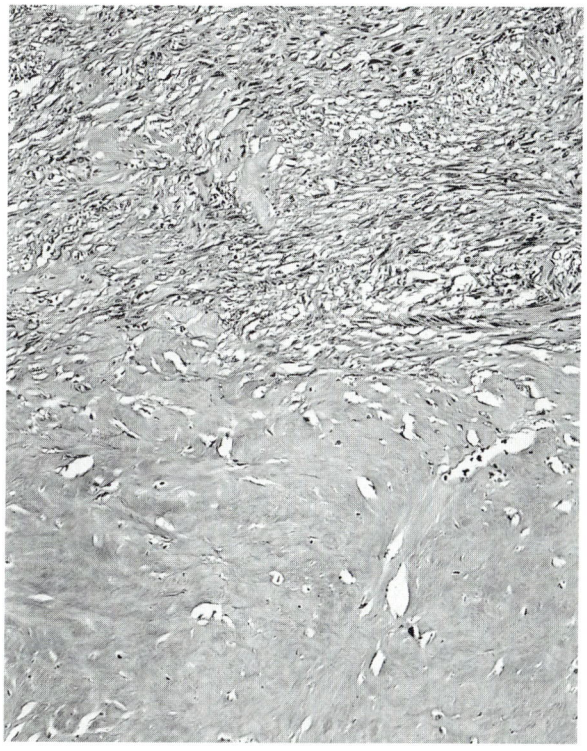

Figure 16-17
SARCOMA OF THE PULMONARY ARTERY

Like aortic intimal sarcomas, there can be densely collagenized areas. (Fig. 8 from Burke AP, Virmani R. Sarcomas of the great vessels. Cancer 1993;71:1761-73.)

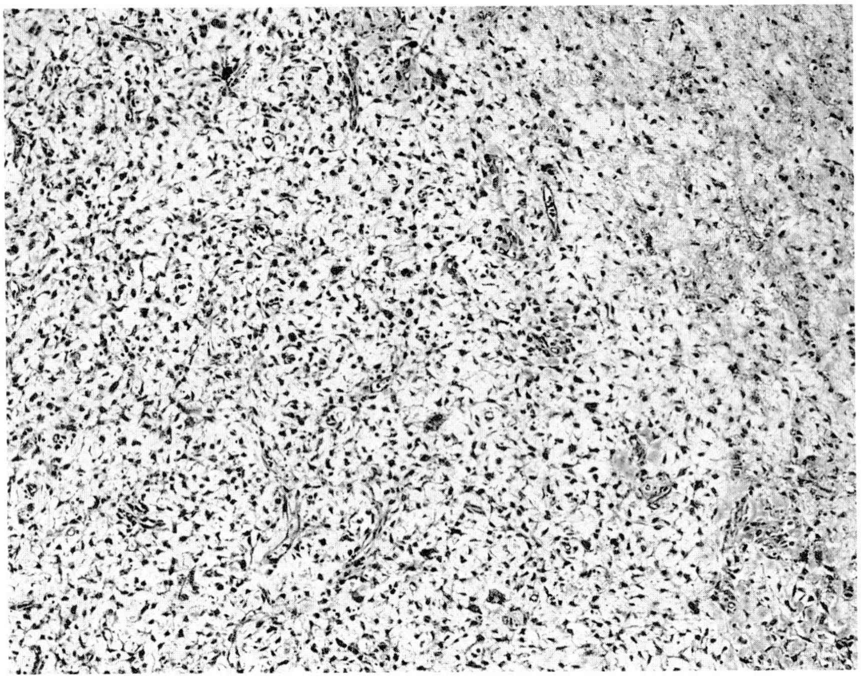

Figure 16-18
SARCOMA OF THE
PULMONARY ARTERY
Note the spindled cells with
hyperchromatic, pleomorphic nuclei
embedded in a myxoid background.

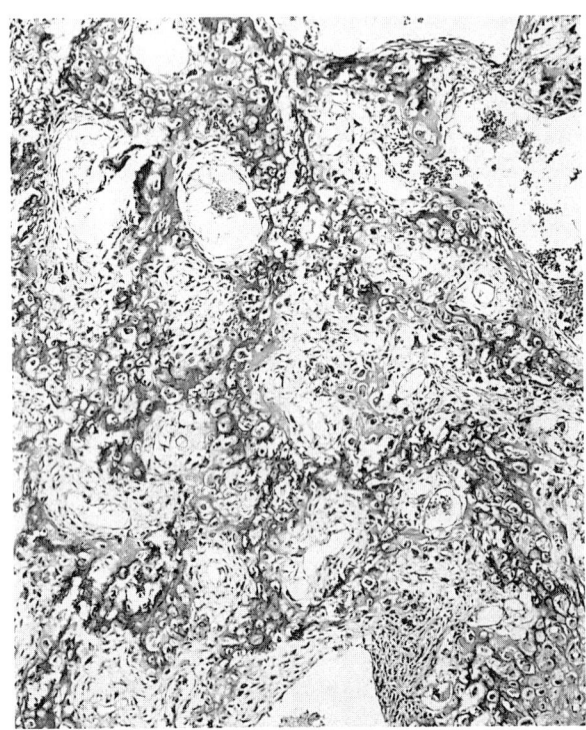

Figure 16-19
SARCOMA OF THE PULMONARY ARTERY
Osteosarcoma is more common in sarcomas of the pulmo-
nary artery than in sarcomas arising in other vessels.

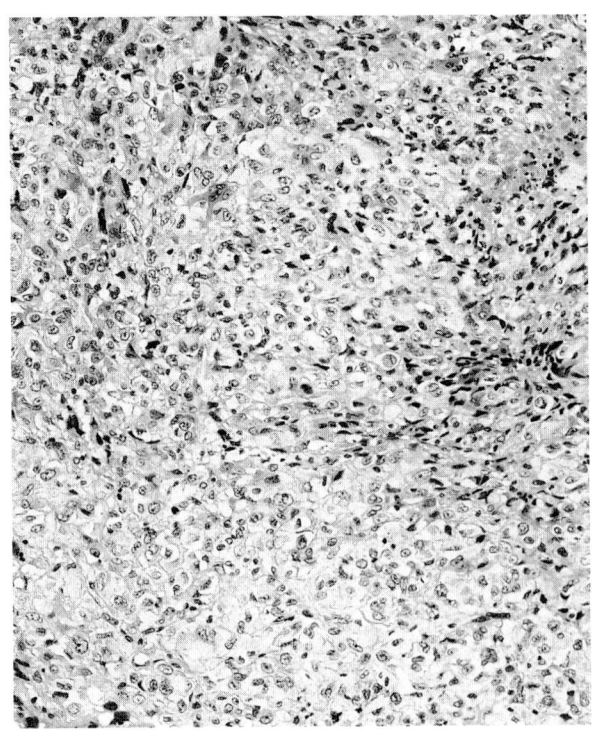

Figure 16-20
SARCOMA OF THE PULMONARY ARTERY
The tumor is composed of pleomorphic cells that do not
demonstrate differentiation of a recognizable cell type.

rhabdomyosarcoma (6 percent), malignant mesenchymoma (6 percent), malignant fibrous histiocytoma (3 percent), and liposarcoma (1 percent) (25,28,32,33,36).

Mural sarcomas of the pulmonary artery are far less common than luminal lesions. They have been described as angiosarcomas and leiomyosarcomas (23).

There are few immunohistochemical studies of pulmonary artery sarcomas (23,25,31,32,34). Generally, tumor cells express vimentin, smooth muscle actin, muscle-specific actin, and myosin, and lack desmin, cytokeratin, and neural markers. These staining patterns are not specific and are compatible with a myofibroblastic origin. Ultrastructurally, there may be microfilaments with dense bodies (32) within tumor cells, as well as a discontinuous basal lamina (34); these features are also compatible with a myofibroblastic derivation.

TUMORS OF OTHER ARTERIES

Primary tumors arising in arteries other than the aorta and pulmonary artery are exceptionally rare. Most are leiomyosarcomas (38); an aneurysmal bone cyst of the carotid artery has been reported (39).

SARCOMAS OF VEINS

Classification. Most sarcomas of the veins are leiomyosarcomas of the inferior vena cava that derive from medial smooth muscle cells (40–44,46–49). Rarely, sarcomas of the inferior vena cava are entirely confined to the lumen; presumably derive from pluripotent intimal cells, as seen in intimal sarcomas of the great arteries; and may not show muscular differentiation. Leiomyosarcomas of the superior vena cava, femoral vein, popliteal vein, and pulmonary veins are quite rare (42,44,45,47,50).

Incidence. The incidence of sarcomas of the venae cavae, based on reports in the literature, is somewhat greater than that of sarcomas of great arteries: 141 cases were collected from the world literature in 1991 (48). The true incidence is probably higher, because origin in the inferior vena cava may be difficult to prove. These lesions are typically larger than sarcomas of arteries, and often remain asymptomatic for a long period because luminal growth may be minimal. Many retroperitoneal leiomyosarcomas may have orig-

inated in the inferior vena cava, but their site of origin is obscured by their large size.

Clinical Features. Most leiomyosarcomas of the inferior vena cava occur in women: the female to male ratio is 4.5 to 1 (48). The average age at presentation is approximately 54 years (48), with a range of 15 to 83 years. The most common presenting symptoms and signs are abdominal pain, palpable abdominal mass, lower leg edema, weight loss, increased abdominal girth, and Budd-Chiari syndrome. The mean duration of symptoms is approximately 11 months prior to diagnosis. Thirty-four percent of tumors arise in the infrarenal, lower segment of the vena cava; 42 percent in the middle segment, extending from the renal veins to the hepatic portion of the vena cava; and 24 percent in the superior segment between the liver and heart (48). Although symptoms do not correlate precisely with tumor location, Budd-Chiari syndrome is most common in leiomyosarcoma of the upper portion of the inferior vena cava (41,46,48). Rare modes of presentation include recurring pulmonary emboli, metastatic disease, and jaundice; fewer than five reported cases were incidental findings during radiologic investigations or unrelated surgery (48).

Gross Findings. Leiomyosarcomas of the inferior vena cava are predominantly extraluminal in 73 percent of cases, and mostly luminal in the remainder (fig. 16-21) (48). Only rarely do they fill the lumen without significant spread into the vessel wall. Neoplastic thrombi occur within hepatic veins, right atrium, or iliac veins in almost 50 percent of cases (48). The tumors range in size from 2 to 30 cm, with a mean of 11 cm (48).

Microscopic Findings. Leiomyosarcomas of the inferior vena cava have been described as well, moderately, and poorly differentiated (48). Although a standardized grading system for these tumors does not exist, many leiomyosarcomas of the inferior vena cava are easily recognized as smooth muscle tumors (fig. 16-22). About 50 percent demonstrate intracytoplasmic desmin with the use of immunohistochemical techniques (42). Intimal sarcomas of the inferior vena cava that are confined to the vessel lumen histologically resemble intimal sarcomas of the great arteries (fig. 16-23).

Unusual venous sarcomas that have been reported include angiosarcomas of the superior

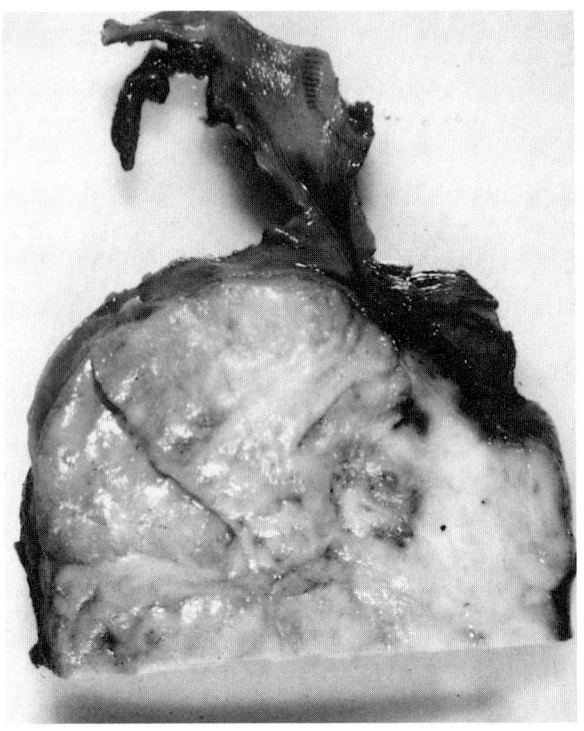

Figure 16-21
LEIOMYOSARCOMA: INFERIOR VENA CAVA
Site of origin in the inferior vena cava can be difficult to prove. This tumor was grossly attached to the inferior vena cava at excision.

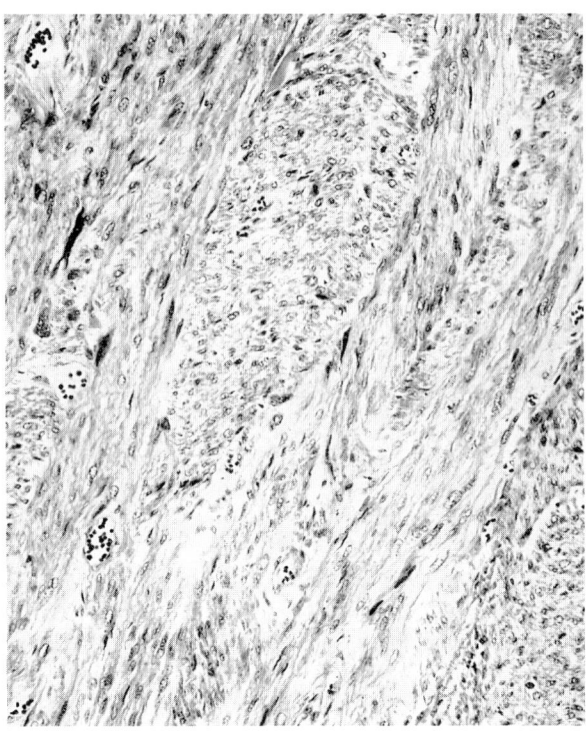

Figure 16-22
LEIOMYOSARCOMA: INFERIOR VENA CAVA
Generally, these tumors are well differentiated, forming fascicles of smooth muscle cells characteristic of soft tissue leiomyosarcoma.

Figure 16-23
LEIOMYOSARCOMA:
INFERIOR VENA CAVA
This particular tumor was predominantly luminal and demonstrated the layering effect typical of intimal sarcomas of the aorta and pulmonary artery.

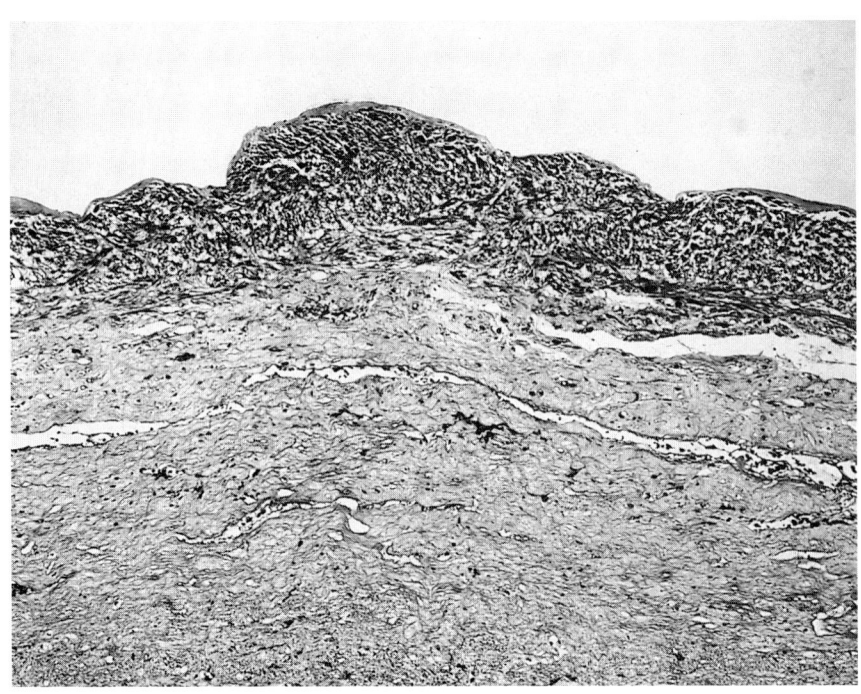

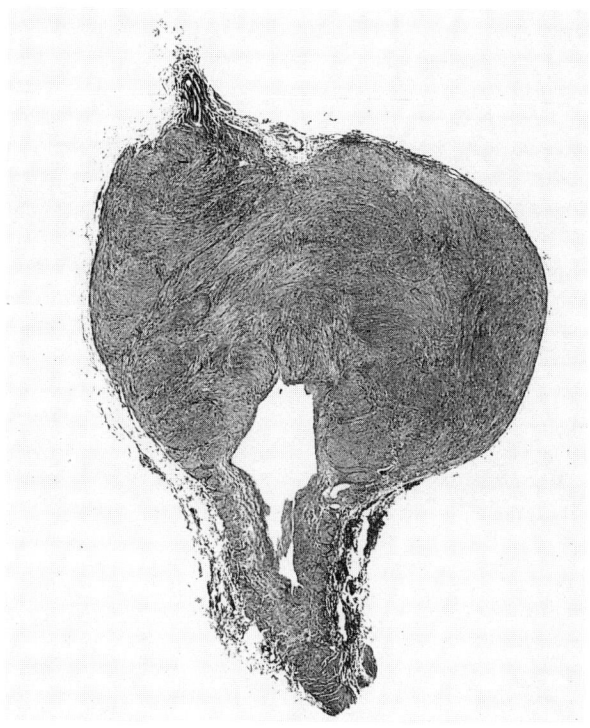

Figure 16-24
LEIOMYOMA: PERIPHERAL VEIN
The patient was a 21-year-old woman with a tender nodule on her right calf. The tumor consists of bundles of well-differentiated smooth muscle cells.

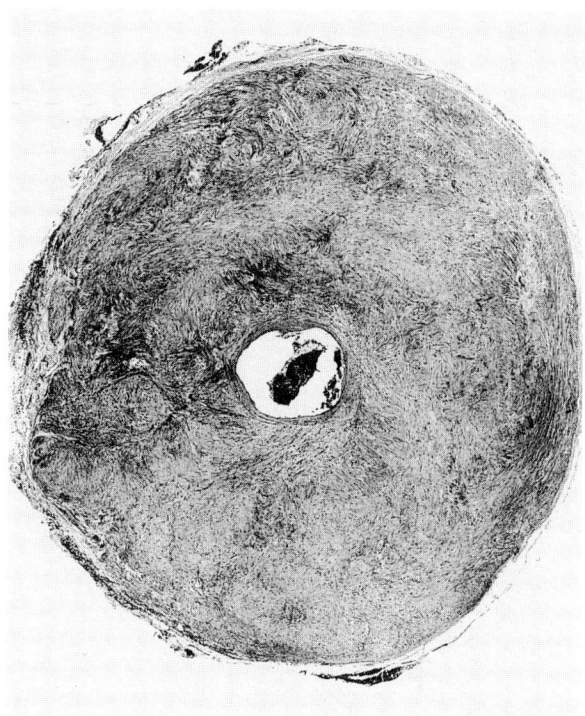

Figure 16-25
LEIOMYOMA: PERIPHERAL VEIN
This tumor was a painful subcutaneous mass similar to that shown in figure 16-24. This particular tumor is quite unusual because there is a circumferential smooth muscle proliferation around the lumen.

vena cava; synovial sarcomas of the superior vena cava; and leiomyosarcomas of the pulmonary, femoral, and iliac veins (42). A myxoid leiomyosarcoma of the pulmonary vein with cytoplasmic staining with antidesmin antibodies has also been reported (45).

Prognosis. Survival is longer in patients with sarcomas of the inferior vena cava than in patients with sarcomas of the aorta and pulmonary arteries, with an average of about 3 years. The 5- and 10-year survival rates for patients undergoing curative surgery are 28 and 14 percent, respectively (48). Variables associated with long survival are radical tumor resection, the presence of abdominal pain, the absence of a palpable abdominal mass, and patients with middle segment tumor (48). Metastases can occur in a variety of sites, including lung, kidney, pleura, chest wall, liver, and bone (42).

Treatment. Treatment consists primarily of surgery. Chemotherapy has been administered without any consistent protocol and is of questionable efficacy (48).

LEIOMYOMAS OF VEINS

Leiomyomas of peripheral veins are common (figs. 16-24, 16-25), and may present as painful masses. Leiomyomas of the inferior vena cava are rare (figs. 16-26, 16-27). They are generally luminal (53,54), in contrast to leiomyosarcomas of the venae cavae, most of which are attached to the vessel wall. The majority of leiomyomas that occur within the lumen of the inferior vena cava are extensions of uterine leiomyomas and represent so-called intravenous leiomyomatosis (52). Less often, they arise from the lining of the vena cava itself or are extensions of leiomyomas that originate in the hepatic, femoral, or more distal veins (51). With intracardiac extension, these tumors can cause obstructive symptoms and even sudden death (see chapter 10).

Table 16-1

**SARCOMAS OF THE GREAT VESSELS
CLINICAL AND PATHOLOGIC CHARACTERISTICS:
AFIP EXPERIENCE***

Location	Number	Males: Females	Mean Age (years)	Histologic Type (number)	Mean Survival (months)
Aorta					
Intimal (luminal)	17	10:7	67	Undifferentiated (9) Angiosarcoma (4)** Malignant fibrous histiocytoma (3) Myxoid chondrosarcoma (1)	7
Mural	3	0:3	37	Angiosarcoma (2) Leiomyosarcoma (1)	114
Pulmonary artery					
Intimal (luminal)	21	14:7	46	Undifferentiated (12) Osteosarcoma or chondrosarcoma (6) Malignant fibrous histiocytoma (2) Angiosarcoma (1)	14
Mural	2	2:0	22	Leiomyosarcoma (1) Undifferentiated (1)	109
Inferior vena cava					
Intimal	2	0:2	54	Undifferentiated (1) Leiomyosarcoma (1)	42
Mural	16	4:12	53	Leiomyosarcoma (16)	35

*Since publication of the previous Fascicle.
**Three with epithelioid features.

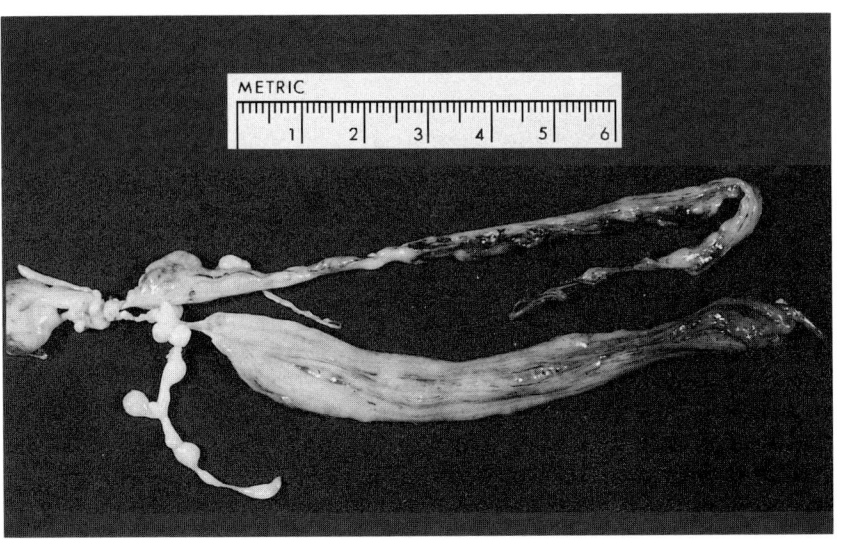

Figure 16-26
GIANT LEIOMYOMA:
INFERIOR VENA CAVA

This tumor, which grossly resembles a large clot, was removed from the inferior vena cava and its ramifications. The tumor is identical to intravascular leiomyomatosis, although in this particular case, no origin in the uterus or peripheral vein was noted. (Courtesy of Dr. John English, Vancouver General Hospital, British Columbia.)

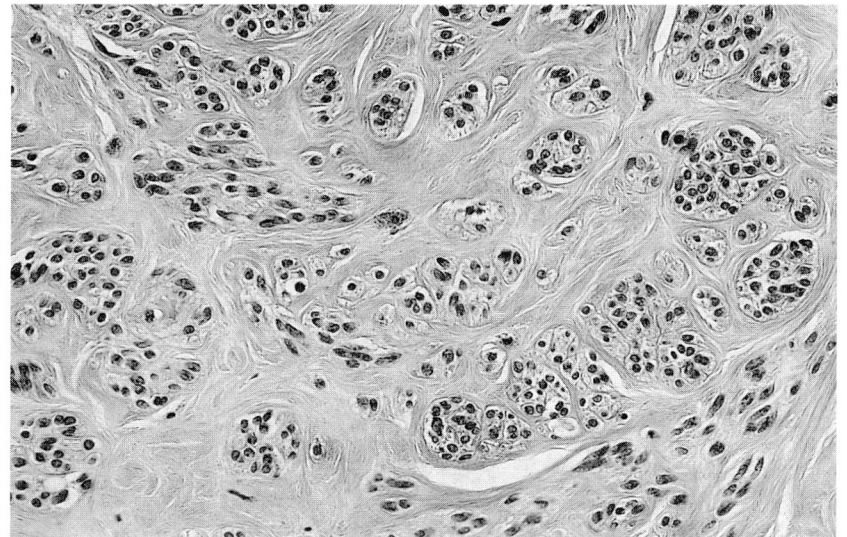

Figure 16-27
LEIOMYOMA:
INFERIOR VENA CAVA
Histologically, the tumor illustrated
in figure 16-26 demonstrates smooth
muscle bundles in a fibrous stroma.

REFERENCES

Introduction

1. Becquemin JP, Lebbe C, Saada F, Avril MF. Sarcoma of the aorta: report of a case and review of the literature. Ann Vasc Surg 1988;2:225–30.
2. Burke AP, Virmani R. Sarcomas of the great vessels. A clinicopathologic study. Cancer 1993;71:1761–73.
3. Fenoglio JJ Jr, Virmani R. Primary malignant tumors of the great vessels. In: Waller B, ed. Pathology of the heart and great vessels, Vol. 12. New York: Churchill Livingstone 1988:429–38.
4. Mingoli A, Feldhaus RJ, Cavallaro A, Stipa S. Leiomyosarcoma of the inferior vena cava: analysis and search of world literature on 141 patients and report of three new cases. J Vasc Surg 1991;14:688–99.
5. Nonomura A, Kurumaya H, Kono J, et al. Primary pulmonary artery sarcoma. Report of two autopsy cases studied by immunohistochemistry and electron microscopy, and review of 110 cases reported in the literature. Acta Pathol Jpn 1988;38:883–96.

Sarcomas of the Aorta

6. Becquemin JP, Lebbe C, Saada F, Avril MF. Sarcoma of the aorta: report of a case and review of the literature. Ann Vasc Surg 1988;2:225–30.
7. Burke AP, Virmani R. Sarcomas of the great vessels. A clinicopathologic study. Cancer 1993;71:1761–73.
8. Fenoglio JJ Jr, Virmani R. Primary malignant tumors of the great vessels. In: Waller B, ed. Pathology of the heart and great vessels, Vol. 12. New York: Churchill Livingstone 1988:429–38.
9. Fitzmaurice RJ, McClure J. Aortic intimal sarcoma; an unusual case with pulmonary vasculature involvement. Histopathol 1990;15:457–62.
10. Haber LM, Truong L. Immunohistochemical demonstration of the endothelial nature of aortic intimal sarcoma. Am J Surg Pathol 1988;12:798–802.
11. Herzberg AJ, Pizzo SV. Primary undifferentiated sarcoma of the thoracic aorta. Histopathol 1988;13:571–4.
12. Josen AS, Khine M. Primary malignant tumor of the aorta. J Vasc Surg 1989;9:493–8.
13. Nishikawa H, Miyakoshi S, Nishimura S, Seki A, Honda K. A case of aortic intimal sarcoma manifested with acutely occurring hypertension and aortic occlusion. Heart Vessels 1989;5:54–8.
14. Pruszczynski M, Coronel CM, Naudin ten Cate L, Roholl PJ, van der Kley AJ. Immunohistochemical and ultrastructural studies of a primary aortic intimal sarcoma. Pathology 1988;20:173–8.
15. Taegtmeyer H, Schroth G, Dickerson CA, Farhood AI. A middle-aged woman with dyspnea, cachexia, increased abdominal girth, pericardial effusion, and a continuous murmur. Circulation 1994;89:484–92.
16. Tejada E, Becker GJ, Waller BF. Malignant myxoid emboli as the presenting feature of primary sarcoma of the aorta (myxoid malignant fibrous histiocytoma): a case report and review of the literature. Clin Cardiol 1991;14:425–30.
17. Weinberg DS, Maini BS. Primary sarcoma of the aorta associated with a vascular prosthesis: a case report. Cancer 1980;15:398–402.
18. Wright EP, Glick AD, Virmani R, Page DL. Aortic intimal sarcoma with embolic metastases. Am J Surg Pathol 1985;9:890–7.

Nonsarcomatous Aortic Neoplasms

19. Duff C, van Segesser L, Schmid ER, Ziegler W, Turina M. Surgery of retroperitoneal pheochromocytoma. Helv Chir Acta 1989;56:151–3.
20. Faure G, Carpentier E, Berthet E, Chirpaz A, Revol M. Paraganglioma of the organs of Zuckerkandl. A case report. J Urol (Paris) 1980;86:671–4.

21. Lack EE, Stillinger RA, Colvin DB, Groves RM, Burnette DG. Aortic-pulmonary paraganglioma: report of a case with ultrastructural study and review of the literature. Cancer 1979;43:269–78.

Pulmonary Artery Sarcomas

22. Baker PB, Goodwin RA. Pulmonary artery sarcomas. Review and report of a case. Arch Pathol Lab Med 1985;109:35–9.
23. Burke AP, Virmani R. Sarcomas of the great vessels. A clinicopathologic study. Cancer 1993;71:1761–73.
24. Ceretto WJ, Miller ML, Shea PM, Gregory CW, Vieweg WV. Malignant mesenchymoma obstructing the right ventricular outflow tract. Am Heart J 1981;101:114–5.
25. Eng J, Murday AJ. Leiomyosarcoma of the pulmonary artery. Ann Thorac Surg 1992;53:905–6.
26. Farooki ZQ, Chang CH, Jackson WL, et al. Primary pulmonary artery sarcoma in two children. Pediatr Cardiol 1988;9:243–51.
27. Fer MF, Greco FA, Haile KL, et al. Unusual survival after pulmonary artery sarcoma. South Med J 1981;74:624–6.
28. Hagstrom L. Malignant mesenchymoma in pulmonary artery and right ventricle. Acta Pathol Microbiol Scand 1961;51:87–94.
29. Klinke WP, Gelfand ET, Baron L. Primary sarcoma of the pulmonary trunk: successful surgical intervention and prolonged survival. Clin Cardiol 1985;8:437–40.
30. Kruger I, Borowski A, Horst M, de Vivie ER, Theissen P, Gross- Fengels W. Symptoms, diagnosis, and therapy of primary sarcomas of the pulmonary artery. Thorac Cardiovasc Surg 1990;38:91–5.
31. McGlennen RC, Manivel JC, Stanley SJ, Slater DL, Wick MR, Dehner LP. Pulmonary artery trunk sarcoma: a clinicopathological, ultrastructural, and immunohistochemical study of four cases. Mod Pathol 1989;2:486–94.
32. Nakazawa K, Itoh N, Shigematsu H, Kanbayashi T. An autopsy case of pulmonary artery leiomyosarcoma. Acta Pathol Jpn 1993;43:76–81.
33. Nerlich A, Permanetter W, Ludwig B, Remberger K. Primary leiomyosarcoma of the truncus pulmonalis. Report of a case with typical features and unusual metastases. Pathol Res Pract 1990;186:296–9
34. Nonomura A, Kurumaya H, Kono J, et al. Primary pulmonary artery sarcoma. Report of two autopsy cases studied by immunohistochemistry and electron microscopy, and review of 110 cases reported in the literature. Acta Pathol Jpn 1988;38:883–96.
35. Promisloff RA, Segal SL, Lenchner GS, Cichelli AV, Wendell G, Aaronson G. Sarcoma of the pulmonary artery. Chest 1988;93:207–8.
36. Van Damme H, Vaneerdeweg W, Schoofs E. Malignant fibrous histiocytoma of the pulmonary artery. Ann Surg 1987;205:203–7.
37. Varriale P, Chryssos B. Pulmonary artery sarcoma: another cause of sudden death. Clin Cardiol 1991;14:160–4.

Tumors of Other Arteries

38. Leeson MC, Malaei M, Makley JT. Leiomyosarcoma of the popliteal artery. A report of two cases. Clin Orthop 1990;253:225–30.
39. Petrik PK, Findlay JM, Sherlock RA. Aneurysmal bone cyst, bone type, primary in an artery. Am J Surg Path 1993;17:1062–6.

Sarcomas of Veins

40. Basu SK, Scott TD, Wilmshurts CC, MacEachern AG, Clyne CA. Leiomyosarcomata of the popliteal vessels: rare primary tumours. Eur J Vasc Surg 1988;2:423–5.
41. Bruyninckx CM, Derksen OS. Leiomyosarcoma of the inferior vena cava. Case report and review of the literature. J Vasc Surg 1986;3:652–6.
42. Burke AP, Virmani R. Sarcomas of the great vessels. A clinicopathologic study. Cancer 1993;71:1761–73.
43. Fenoglio JJ Jr, Virmani R. Primary malignant tumors of the great vessels. In: Waller B, ed. Pathology of the heart and great vessels, Vol. 12 New York: Churchill Livingstone 1988:429–38.
44. Fischer MG, Gelb AM, Nussbaum M, Haveson S, Ghali V. Primary smooth muscle tumors of venous origin. Ann Surg 1982;196:720–4.
45. Gonzalez-Campora R, Rubi-Uria J, Mora-Marin J, et al. Pulmonary vein myxoid leiomyosarcoma. Pathol Res Pract 1989;185:900–4.
46. Griffin AS, Sterchi JM. Primary leiomyosarcoma of the inferior vena cava: a case report and review of the literature. J Surg Oncol 1987;34:53–60.
47. Leu HJ, Makek M. Intramural venous leiomyosarcomas. Cancer 1986;57:1395–400.
48. Mingoli A, Feldhaus RJ, Cavallaro A, Stipa S. Leiomyosarcoma of the inferior vena cava: analysis and search of world literature on 141 patients and report of three new cases. J Vasc Surg 1991;14:688–99.
49. Peh WC, Cheung DL, Ngan H. Smooth muscle tumors of the inferior vena cava and right heart. Clin Imaging 1993;17:117–23.
50. Taheri SA, Conner GW. Leiomyosarcoma of iliac veins. Surgery 1983;94:516–20.

Leiomyomas of Veins

51. Dunlap HJ, Udjus K. Atypical leiomyoma arising in an hepatic vein with extension into the inferior vena cava and right atrium. Report of a case in a child. Pediatr Radiol 1990;20:202–3.
52. Norris HJ, Parmley T. Mesenchymal tumors of the uterus. V. Intravenous leiomyomatosis. A clinical and pathologic study of 14 cases. Cancer 1975;36:2164–78.
53. Payan MJ, Xerri L, Choux R, et al. Giant leiomyoma of the inferior vena cava. Ann Pathol 1989;9:44–6.
54. Roman DA, Mirchandani H. Intravenous leiomyoma with intracardiac extension causing sudden death. Arch Pathol Lab Med 1987;111:1176–8.

INDEX

*Numbers in boldface indicate table and figure pages.

✧ ✧ ✧